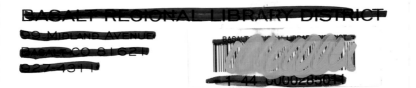

DATE DUE

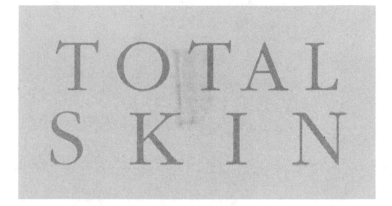

TOTAL SKIN

THE DEFINITIVE GUIDE TO WHOLE SKIN CARE FOR LIFE

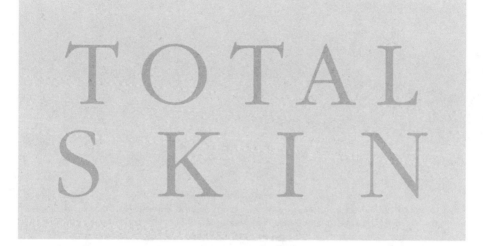

TOTAL SKIN

DAVID J. LEFFELL, M.D.

Professor of Dermatology and Surgery,
Yale University School of Medicine

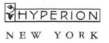

NEW YORK

The world of medicine changes rapidly as research provides new information about disease and
ways to treat it. Accurate indications, adverse reactions, and dosage schedules for drugs are provided in this book, but these may change. The reader should consult the package information data
from the drug manufacturers of the medications mentioned. In addition, consult your physician
for specific medical advice that applies to your personal situation.

Copyright © 2000 David J. Leffell, M.D.

Illustrations by Katie S. Atkinson

All rights reserved. No part of this book may be used or reproduced in any manner whatsoever
without the written permission of the Publisher. Printed in the United States of America. For information address: Hyperion, 77 West 66th Street, New York, New York 10023.

Library of Congress Cataloging-in-Publication Data

Leffell, David J.
    Total skin : the definitive guide to whole skin care for life / by David J. Leffell.
      p.   cm.
    Includes index.
    ISBN 0-7868-6504-0 (hc)
    1. Skin—Care and hygiene.
    RL87 .L366 2000
    616.5—dc21

                                                    99–047396

Designed by Lisa Stokes

FIRST EDITION

10 9 8 7 6 5 4 3 2 1

This book is dedicated to

the memory of my father, Bernard, and to my mother, Freda,
and to
C. Lane Fortinberry

Contents

Acknowledgments

The making of a doctor depends as much on the information gleaned from books and gained from teachers as it does on the experience obtained by caring for patients. To all my patients, I would like to extend a sincere thanks for their confidence in me and for what they have taught me, in all ways, about the practice of medicine. Similarly, no physician practices alone. When I developed the Dermatologic and Laser Surgery Unit at the Yale School of Medicine, I was joined by Diana Glassman, R.N., Anne McKeown, R.N., Kristina Heintz, R.N., and Jacqueline Artuncs—all highly trained, experienced, and compassionate professionals. Together we have cared for patients with conditions as diverse as melanoma, non-melanoma skin cancer, cosmetic issues, and concerns about aging. Throughout we have tried to do for our patients what we would want done for members of our own families.

The process of educating young physicians is quite unpredictable. Fresh-faced medical students and residents arrive one day, and it is sometimes hard to predict what kind of doctor each will turn out to be when the day is done. I am sure this is what my own teachers in dermatology must have felt when I arrived on their doorstep. Now that I stand in their shoes, I especially appreciate the responsibilities of teaching young doctors and recognize the commitment of my own teachers. I would like to acknowledge the former chairman of dermatology at Yale, Aaron Lerner, M.D.; my teacher Neil Swanson, M.D.; and the current chairman at Yale, Richard Edelson, M.D.; who gave me the opportunity to develop academically and professionally. I would also like to thank Jean Bolognia, M.D., a dear friend, colleague, and world-renowned expert in melanoma, for her ongoing contribution to this book and other projects.

Others who have contributed to this effort include Dr. Steven A. Kolenik III, a former resident and fellow and assistant clinical professor of dermatology at Yale, who provided superb advice and guidance, especially with respect to liposuction. Dr. Ivan Cohen, an associate clinical professor of dermatology at Yale and a nationally recognized expert in hair restoration, was extremely valuable in helping to develop the chapter on hair.

As a teacher and professor my greatest satisfaction derives from seeing a medical student or resident mature with knowledge and wisdom into a full-fledged physician. To my residents through the years, I extend a sincere thanks for challenging me to be clearer and more informative and to expand my own base of knowledge. Dr. Thomas McGovern was my dermatologic surgery fellow in 1998–1999 during the writing of this book; his contribution in research and his perspective have been extremely valuable, and for that I am much indebted. Similarly, Dr. Karynne Duncan, assistant professor of dermatology at the University of Colorado Health Sciences Center and former chief resident in dermatology at Yale, provided valuable input.

Dr. Glenn Goldman, professor of dermatology at the University of Vermont and former chief resident in dermatology at Yale, reviewed the manuscript in whole. Dr. Timothy Johnson, professor of dermatology at the University of Michigan, and Dr. Jeffrey Magnavita also reviewed material, for which I am grateful, as did Dr. John Carucci and Diane Ruben.

Total Skin was written during spare moments that I could cobble together between clinical practice, administrative responsibilities, and research. In writing the book, I have been privileged to have worked with several individuals with superb editorial credentials. Meg Blackstone was of great assistance, as was Trent Duffy. I am deeply indebted to Leigh Haber, my editor at Hyperion, for her patience, humor, understanding of my vision for this project, and willingness to help me publish the reader-friendly book that I hope has resulted. David Chalfant, my agent at IMG Literary, has been a steadfast source of support from the time that we first developed the book concept together.

Easy reading of complex information has been an important goal of *Total Skin*. To this end, I have relied on graphics more than is customary. Rather than commission technical illustrations, I sought the services of a highly skilled illustrator. I am deeply thankful to that wonderfully talented artist, Katie Atkinson, for her images.

I would like to thank Joy Deloge, my longtime transcriptionist, for her accurate transcription and special skill at deciphering my recorded mumblings. To Grace Camire, my superbly able assistant whose skills have enabled me to juggle practice, research, administration, and writing this book, I owe a special thanks.

Finally, I owe the greatest debt to my wife, Cindy. She has been a true partner in this effort from the beginning, a believer in its vision and a contributor of ideas. Cindy has also been a relentless researcher of material and a gentle editor as well. This book would not have been possible without her equal commitment to it. I would thank my two young children, Alexander and Dahlia, but they are still refusing to read.

To the best of my knowledge the information in this book is accurate, and any errors are exclusively my own. It should be noted that medicine changes rapidly and for any given condition there are likely to be areas of legitimate controversy among physicians about the proper treatment or approach. In cases where recommendations in this book differ from those of your physician, I advise that you follow the recommendations of your physician—he or she knows you the best.

Thank you for reading this book. I hope you enjoy discovering the world of skin as much as I have enjoyed writing about it!

This book is a guide to caring for your skin throughout life. It is based on the idea that you, the reader, will be best able to manage your own health if you have accurate, readable, and useful information. For over a decade I have been privileged to practice dermatology, a medical specialty that includes the art and science of skin disease and the realm of aesthetics and skin rejuvenation. I care for people with serious skin disease and work, as well, on ways to turn back the skin signs of aging we are all eager to reverse. Looking healthy is an important step to feeling younger, and this book seeks to provide useful advice about keeping your skin healthy.

We all should know our skin like we know the backs of our hands. By area, it is our largest organ. Our skin also reflects our internal health. If we are in good health, it will radiate from us. Helping you understand how best to live in your skin and keep it healthy is the purpose of this book. With the rapid advances in medicine and the unquenchable popular thirst for knowledge, it becomes increasingly important to convey breaking scientific information and approaches to health in ways that are understandable to everyone.

When it comes to your health, knowledge is power. As a teacher and physician, my goal is to provide you with what I consider the essential information for achieving and maintaining healthy, young-looking skin. The explosion of medical information in this area can indeed be daunting: the shelves of bookstores are filled with self-help books written by a wide range of authors; magazines are stuffed with articles about health and longevity; the amount of medical material on the Internet grows by the hour. The need to filter all this information and distinguish the correct from the dubious or the just plain wrong is now more important than ever. In this book, I will tell you what I tell my patients in practice.

Skin care can be confusing to today's consumer. A range of providers are involved with care of the skin: aestheticians, facialists, dermatologists, and plastic surgeons are the ones that come most quickly to mind. In general, it is best to get your information about skin health from physicians who are specially trained in the science of this, our largest organ. Facialists and aestheticians provide important care that supplements the program that your dermatologist can plan for you. Given the range of skin conditions that arise, it is fortunate that many different skilled people are available to focus on everything from grooming to wrinkle prevention, from rejuvenation of the aging face to management of skin disease.

In fact, the world of dermatology and skin is so vast that it is not possible in one volume to effectively communicate all that you are entitled to know and would want to understand. For this reason, this guide focuses on the most common conditions in dermatology and on ways that the science of skin can help you look your best. The website for *Total Skin*, www.totalskinmd.com, provides an opportunity to obtain information about many topics not covered here.

For me, skin is a fascinating field. Dermatology reflects the medicine of skin, but our skin is linked to far more than just the medical and cosmetic challenges that arise. There is history. There is sex. There is the rainbow of ethnicity. There is politics. In all, I have attempted to flavor the health content of this book with interesting side notes and tips that I think will distinguish it from the traditional home medical guide.

Total Skin can be read from beginning to end or used as a reference by accessing the index. My hope is that you will find the most enjoyable way for you to learn the information I've tried to convey.

Most important—read, learn, and be healthy!

THE BASICS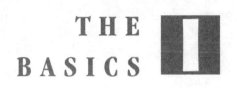

1 Why Skin?

Skin. The word conjures up many things—beauty, youth, grace, sex, illness, even art. Perhaps this is because our skin is the part of our body that we know best. We see it daily. We feel it. We feel through it. We groom it. We know right away when it's broken. We envy those whose skin is smooth as silk. We feel badly for those who are disfigured.

We think and speak daily about skin in ways we never pause to consider: Smooth as a baby's bottom. By the skin of our teeth. No skin off my nose. Shirts and skins. Skin, it seems, is both a part of our body and a metaphor for so much that goes on in our lives.

Medically, skin is the resilient living fabric that envelops our entire self. It is defined as the "tough, membranous tissue that forms the external covering of the animal body." But skin is a lot more than just a membrane that covers. It is much, much more than plastic wrap that holds in our bones, organs, and blood like so many boxes on a pallet. In fact, the skin, our largest organ, is biologically *very* complex. Consider, for example, these amazing qualities:

- When we cut skin, it heals and makes new skin.
- Skin's complex layers of cells keep germs out 24 hours a day.

- Skin can tell if it has met an unwelcome plant, like poison ivy, and can remember the encounter years later.

Our skin, or integument, has molecules to shield us from the harmful rays of the sun, and it can change in specific ways to provide us with clues about how our insides are functioning.

In concert with our blood vessel system, skin helps retain moisture when necessary, just like a cactus, or diffuses excess body heat when we are exercising. In short, our skin is the house in which we live and our first interface with the world around us.

When we think of complex organs, the brain usually comes to mind first. Some might be impressed by the repetitive consistency of the heart or the amazing chemistry laboratory that is the liver. But in many ways, as you shall see, the skin itself is as complex as any of these other organs, steadfast in its service, and amazing in its chemistry.

The ultimate adaptability of the skin is due to its several layers. The *epidermis* is the top layer of skin cells. These cells divide and restore themselves at regular intervals, creating at the same time a protective layer called the *stratum corneum*. A second layer, called the *dermis*, depends heavily on a stretchy molecule called *elastin* and strong, cable-like bands called *collagen* to give skin its flexibility and strength. The dermis includes miles of tiny blood vessels that skirt to the surface of the skin, then plunge down into the deeper layers to transport nutrients and heat. Coursing through the dermis, as well, are lymph channels that escort away germs and other noxious elements. Throughout the skin one also finds unique cells that form an immunologic guard for the body, as well as a skein of specialized nerve endings, each with its own purpose. Some of these nerves can tell you you've been pricked by the pin of a dry cleaner's tag; others can warn that you are about to singe the side of your hand over a low gas flame; a third variety mediates the sensation of pressure and, unbeknownst to you, reminds you to turn while you are asleep so that you won't develop a pressure sore.

There is yet another dimension to skin: it is the medium through which we initially introduce ourselves to others. Our skin—close to four square meters of it—is the canvas upon which we craft our introduction to the world, often embellishing or altering it with makeup, dyes, tattoos, and other adornments. Skin can be the focus of religious rite, as in ritual circumcision, and the nexus of touch and thus an important means of conveying love and affection. Our skin has enormous social, sexual, and political implications.

It is, of course, through scientific discovery that our knowledge of skin advances. It was fascination with the science of this durable organ that led me eventually to choose to specialize in diseases of the skin. That choice in itself is a tale of discovery. When I was completing my residency in internal medicine at New York's Memorial Sloan-Kettering Cancer Center, I realized how much of the diagnostic knowledge in internal medicine is inferred from tests and scans. I decided that I was more comfortable examining and working with what I could see than what I *thought* I could see.

During my training at Memorial Sloan-Kettering Cancer Center in the early 1980s I was caring for young men dying from a condition then called Gay-Related Immune Deficiency, or GRID. Many had developed purplish skin lesions called Kaposi's sarcoma, which until that time had been seen almost exclusively in elderly men of Mediterranean extraction. The deep purple spots and lumps were popping up everywhere, and the pattern was different than the Old World type of Kaposi's sarcoma.

Something was up, but no one could figure it out. We thought there was a viral connection with the condition affecting these young men, but at that time no one had identified the human immunodeficiency virus (HIV) as a possible cause. Because of my awakening interest in skin and the opportunity to spend some extra time in the lab, I embarked on a project to transplant the tumor cells of Kaposi's sarcoma into immunologically neutered mice. The idea was that the tumors would grow in these mice because their immune system could not reject the tissue. We would then be better able to study the cancer and figure out its cause. I never got the tumors to grow, but my interest in the science of dermatology had been forged forever, as I learned to appreciate how the specialty combined the diagnostic skills of an internist, the technical skills of a surgeon, and the analytical skills of a pathologist.

I'm not sure when I first became aware of skin, but I have come to value the fact that on good days caring for the skin is an art, like the practice of medicine in general. The important difference for us dermatologists is that the results of our art are usually more readily apparent than those of the internist, radiologist, or pathologist.

During my dermatology training in the late 1980s enormous changes were taking place in the field. It might be said that dermatology had finally begun to emerge from being a minor character in the galaxy of medicine to becoming a shining star. New research technology made it possible to better explore some of the mysteries of the skin. For example, one special area of developing knowledge was of the skin as an organ of immunity.

As a dermatology resident at Yale–New Haven Medical Center, I did experiments on a factor isolated from blood that was responsible for fever and other mechanisms that help fight infection. I found that this compound, a type of immunologic chemical called *interleukin*, was elevated in patients with a severe form of psoriasis. Since then, it has become clear that our skin is not only an important component of our immune system, but that it manufactures a broad range of compounds in health and disease.

Another new development that began to focus attention on dermatology in the 1980s was a dramatic increase in the rate of new skin cancer cases. Deterioration of the ozone layer had become an important environmental and political concern and some epidemiologists suggested a link between skin cancer rates and this environmental change. More ultraviolet radiation was reaching the earth's surface, and thus potentially your skin's surface, whether you were lugging bags from the market to your car or golf clubs from the tee to the green.

A third factor affecting the increased importance of dermatology was a direct result of the famous baby boom. As this large group of Americans ages, our desire to continue to look young and turn back the clock of time becomes more pressing, and there are many, many more of us than ever before pursuing the goal of looking young while growing older. Dermatology is the medical field in which the scientific and medical bases for the vast majority of cosmetic procedures have been developed.

For all these reasons dermatology was a legitimate medical career choice for me. Nonetheless, I recall vividly a telephone conversation with my parents around the time I decided not to become a cardiologist or neurologist. When I advised them that I would be entering yet another residency, this time in dermatology, their reaction was dead silence—you could hear a toenail drop. You might have thought I had said I wanted to chuck medicine altogether, buy a motorcycle, and rip across the fruited plains with no meaningful goals. I knew what they were thinking: Dermatology was not really *medicine*. Dermatology was not practiced by "real" doctors. Dermatology was . . . well, it wasn't prestigious.

As my parents' initial reaction showed, dermatology is an area of medicine that in the past was not fully understood by the public. Interestingly, these stereotypes have nothing to do with the complexity of caring for skin.

Over more than a decade—sixteen years that have included collaboration on the discovery of the skin cancer gene, publication of numerous research articles, and involvement in clinical trials assessing new technologies and pharmaceuticals—I have been privileged to experience the breadth of dermatology and its strong foundation in medical science. The study of skin is, in its own right, the lens through which a wide range of human health and disease problems are continually being addressed.

My goal is that this book will be a handy and useful guide for the skin problems of greatest concern to you and that you will come away from even a brief glance at a specific topic knowing more than you expected. For example, when I discuss poison ivy, a form of contact dermatitis, you'll learn how in many ways it is similar to that rash around your wrist or on your earlobes that developed from your chronic exposure to nickel (and you thought those earrings were pure silver!). When I teach you how to take care of a wound, I will bring to bear all that is currently known about the science of healing. Please don't become skeptical of my credentials if some of the things I advise are at odds with what your grandmother taught you about taking care of wounds (at other times, I assure you, I will be able to corroborate Nana's wisdom).

I hope you enjoy this journey, that it will bring you in closer touch with your own body, and that you will begin to feel more in control of your health and appearance. At the same time, I hope you'll enjoy our brief forays into the world of science and discovery and realize how closely advances we take for granted are related to the research done in university laboratories throughout the world.

Dermatology is a medical specialty of deduction based on observation. What you see is not always what you get, but it is a good place to start. Describing what you see is the challenge for the physician and the patient, since so much of figuring out what is going on depends on an accurate description.

From earliest times, especially when the Roman Catholic Church or superstition forbade autopsy, all medical knowledge derived from what could be observed. That meant that the skin, and the diseases that afflicted it, were the primary source of direct medical information.

The essence of medicine, like all science, is classification. There are hundreds of types of roses, but they can all be grouped together best as roses, then as flowers, then even more broadly as plants. So it was with dermatology in the beginning. But classification in this field depended first on description. In dermatology, more than in any other field, words have a special burden because we need them to describe what is essentially a visual problem. Practicing in the second century, Galen was one of the first physicians to classify skin disease, doing so by color, smoothness, and thickness. That was a little bit like flying low over a parking lot and classifying the cars either as

Toyotas, GMs, or Fords—it told us virtually nothing about the individual vehicles, but it was a start.

More information was needed about the nature of skin disease. In the seventeenth century, Marcello Malpighi made good use of the microscope to describe oil glands and other structures in the skin. Eventually there was enough information for Robert Willan at London's Public Dispensary to classify all the diseases he saw. His classification of the different types of eczema, for example, is still in use today. At the beginning of the nineteenth century, a Frenchman by the name of J. L. B. Alibert published a twelve-volume system of dermatology based on his observations at the Hôpital St. Louis, a Paris hospital founded to nurse plague victims.

Because observation is so important in dermatology, a home guide such as this book can be especially valuable. In this chapter, you can learn the language dermatologists and others use to describe and explain different conditions or ailments. If you incorporate this language when you report what you see in your self-exams to your doctor, it will make your care that much simpler and more accurate.

I've included a glossary at the end of this book for easy reference, but this chapter attempts to go one step further. Here you will learn about some key terms that will be used throughout this book and will help you understand your skin. I don't aim to transform you into a skin expert, but by knowing what to call "things" on your skin you will be that much closer to understanding the problem and helping your doctor work with you to get it better.

There are three main layers to the skin—the epidermis, the dermis, and the fatty subcutaneous layer, which is also called the *subcutis*. In addition, we use specific terms to describe texture, color, size, and shape in dermatology, as in art—not that you would want to paint masterpieces of your skin problems. Having said that, there is a famous painting that hangs in the Louvre in Paris by Domenico Ghirlandaio (1449–1494) called *An Old Man and His Grandson*. It depicts an elderly man whose most notable feature is a bulbous fleshy nose. Ghirlandaio skillfully portrays the abnormal features with ruthless accuracy while at the same time conveying compassion and tenderness. No dermatologist can walk by that painting without instantaneously making a diagnosis of rhinophyma.

Based on the natural parallels between art and medicine, Dr. Irwin Braverman and his colleague, Linda Friedlaender, devised an exercise for Yale medical students that involved a visit to the Yale Center for British Art in New Haven. Students would spend an afternoon carefully viewing some of the paintings; afterward they would describe what they saw, using the tool of precise vocabulary. They soon found out that it was not so easy. Braverman, an internationally renowned expert in skin conditions and internal disease, thus taught his students how to improve their powers of observation, to truly see what they were looking at. This experience was valuable to the future doctors, whose professional success would depend on their ability to observe keenly and describe what they see.

Another episode conveys how important description is for doctors. When my son was three years old, he developed a high fever. I called our pediatrician. When he phoned back, he advised me on how to care for my son but quickly shifted to something dermatologists hear all the time:

"Now that I have you on the phone," the pediatrician began, "I wonder what you think of this. . . ." He described the condition of a boy he had in his office with him at the time. "He has multiple tiny spots on his whole left arm."

"What size?" I asked.

"About one millimeter," he said, using the metric system, which is the way we measure and weigh things in medicine. There are about 25 millimeters to the inch, so the spots he was describing were quite small.

"And the color?" I inquired.

"Red."

"You're sure it's not rust colored?" I asked.

"Well, maybe a bit," he said.

"Are they raised or flat?"

"I'm not sure. They feel just a bit raised when I run my hand over them."

I probed further: "Are there any new ones?"

The ability to distinguish new lesions from old is critical in determining how long a condition has been present. In this way, dermatology is often marshaled for forensic purposes. By knowing the stages through which a lesion or a normal skin element progresses, and how long it spends at each stage, it is sometimes possible to deduce facts that are of medical-legal importance. For example, it is possible to detect the presence of certain elements, such as lead or arsenic, in hair; then, by determining the length of the hair and where along the shaft the element is found, one can use the growth rate of the hair to determine the time of actual exposure to the compound.

"I think there might be a couple of new ones," the pediatrician responded.

I was trying, through my questioning, to determine whether we were dealing with a life-threatening condition or a more benign skin problem, one related perhaps to trauma or a bleeding disorder. Many times, as in this case, the child gets better and we never make a definite diagnosis. By using a common language of description, we can at least narrow the possibilities of what is wrong. In this case the child most likely had a temporary disorder of his blood platelets that was causing the particular rash.

In learning the language of dermatology, probably the most basic term to understand is the word *lesion*. Doctors use this term all the time with each other and with patients and their families. It is a general word and simply refers to a specific physical finding that is abnormal.

Keep in mind that in dermatology any abnormal skin growth is a lesion, but the term doesn't say anything about how serious the abnormality or the growth itself is.

For example, a lesion can be a tumor. A Latin word that simply means "growth" or "mass," tumor is probably one of the words the public least understands. It can be benign and noncancerous, like a cyst, or it can be malignant, in which case the lesion is referred to more precisely as a cancer. A melanoma, therefore, is a malignant tumor, while acne cysts are benign tumors (even though we rarely refer to them as tumors). Doctors may use the word *tumor* when they are referring to a specific cancerous growth, or when they are talking about a benign mass, such as a fatty tumor (also called a *lipoma*), or a normal mole, more properly called a *nevus*. To avoid confusion and, more important, unnecessary anxiety always ask your doctor what he or she means. Over the years I've learned that most people think of a tumor as something more often benign than cancerous; when I refer to a skin cancer as a tumor, patients often say, "Oh, so you mean it's benign." Unfortunately, of course, this isn't always the case. All of which serves to emphasize the point that so much of good medicine is good communication. It's essential for you to be sure you understand what your doctor is saying, and just as important that your doctor understands you.

The term *cancer* refers to any growth that expands in an uncontrolled fashion and overtakes normal tissue. Because skin cancer is the most common cancer in humans, it is a key part of the practice of dermatology. Fortunately, the majority of skin cancers do not travel in the body, in a process known as *metastasis*. Death from most skin cancers is rare, but any melanoma is quite serious and can pose a real risk of metastasis.

A good way to learn the language of skin is to look at and think about a patch of normal skin on your own body—say the back of your hand. There are hairs growing out of hair follicles. If you look closely under a magnifying glass, you can even see the markings of the skin that look like interconnecting patio blocks. You might also notice some different colored spots. Any flat lesion that is noticeable because its color is different from its surroundings is a *macule*. A freckle is a good example of a *macule* because it is small, flat, and colored. A "liver spot" is another example of a macule.

If you can see something that is raised above the surface, like a small mound, and it is less than a quarter of an inch high, it is a *papule*. Many

[Macule]

benign moles fit this description, one of the most famous perhaps being the nevus on Cindy Crawford's face (if you're older, think of Khrushchev). A *nodule* is a larger version of a papule, where some of the substance of the lesion is felt to be in the second layer of the skin, or dermis, or even the subcutaneous layer.

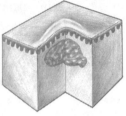

[Nodule]

An *erosion* is a moist, red shiny area in which the top layer of skin has come off. Abrasion or scrape is a common term for erosion. Your kitchen cabinet door can cause an erosion on your forehead if it's left open and you don't watch out. When an erosion gets deeper, it's called an *ulcer*.

A *crust* is what most people know better as a *scab*, a dried covering over a wound that is adherent and rough. It is made up of old white blood cells that were at the wound to help it heal, some skin that is no longer alive, and fluid that was produced by the wound in the process of healing.

Purpura are red or purple marks that develop in the top layer of the skin when hemorrhage or bleeding has occurred. Small pinpoint lesions of purpura are called *petechiae* and larger areas of the same process are called *ecchymoses*. Mike Tyson has been responsible for causing many cases of ecchymoses in his day, mainly around the eyes of his opponents. Many older people are familiar with ecchymoses on their arms, where the skin, thinned by age, is susceptible to simple trauma. The black-and-blue marks that result can take weeks to resolve

[Erosion]

and will pass through stages, turning green then yellow

before fading completely. This is because the color of
hemoglobin, the iron-carrying molecule in blood,
breaks down as it changes.

In dermatology, *scales* are not something you
practice but white to brown flakes that can result from
the normal shedding of skin. They are best known
when they occur on the scalp as dandruff. If you look at
your skin after you've been sitting in a dry heated house in
the middle of winter, you will see skin flaking—a perfect
example of scale and a sign that the skin is regenerating itself
on an ongoing basis.

[Ulcer   ]

Language and precision are nowhere more important than when talking about skin cancer. Indeed, how often do you hear someone say, "Aunt
Millie had breast cancer ten years ago and now she has brain cancer."
That's probably not what has happened. Rather, through a complex process
we don't yet fully understand, but which will be important to explore when
we talk about melanoma, cancer can not only divide and grow where it sits
but can travel elsewhere in the body as well. This process is one of the
lethal behaviors of cancer.

To this end, it is helpful to know the term *in situ*,
which refers to cancer cells which exist in the top
layer of the skin or epidermis and thus *do not* have
access to the blood vessels or lymph channels of the
dermis. No access, no entry—and therefore no risk of
metastasis or spread. Similarly, *invasion* is a term that
we use when we talk about skin cancer; it refers to the
fact that the cancerous cells have divided sufficiently so

[Scab   ]

that they now extend into the dermis and can gain entry to
blood vessels and lymph channels. At this point, sadly, the
rapidly dividing abnormal cells can be whisked away to other organs, where
they can set up house, divide, and cause misfortune.

Other words dermatologists employ are simpler to grasp: *erythema*
means redness. A reddened patch of skin is helpful because it tells us much
about what is going on. Skin turns red if it is inflamed, and inflammation is
the process by which the body tries to repair itself after an injury. Think
about what happens after you accidentally cut yourself while preparing for
that special dinner party. The incision hurts; you run it under cold water
and put a Band-Aid on it. When you replace the bandage the next morning,
you notice that there is redness on either side of the wound. This results

from a whole cascade of chemicals that are released by cells that have marched to the site in response to a signal that something has gone awry. One of the first things these chemicals do is increase blood flow in order to remove debris and bacteria while providing a channel for internal healing compounds to get to the scene of the accident. Erythema also occurs after sunburn, where the blood vessels dilate to help dissipate heat, and it's certainly a classic sign of infection, when the skin is working overtime to get rid of bacteria and reestablish a normal state of affairs. (It is interesting to consider that the language we use today to describe medical problems has changed little since the time of Hippocrates. The cardinal signs of infection continue to be *rubor* or redness, *calor* or warmth, *tumor* or mass, and *dolor*, pain.)

Other colors are important in dermatology: *pigmented* usually means brown, though it can refer to other colors caused by pigment-producing cells in the skin. *Hypopigmented* means lighter than the skin around it. *Hyperpigmented* means darker than the surrounding normal skin. *Depigmented* means there is no color whatsoever. Individuals who lack pigmentation completely are called *albino*; they may be at special risk for skin cancer.

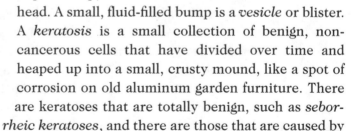

[Pustule]

[Vesicle]

There are also a host of terms to describe lesions in more detail. These single words convey a lot to the dermatologist. A *pustule* is a pus bump, a *comedone* is a blackhead. A small, fluid-filled bump is a *vesicle* or blister. A *keratosis* is a small collection of benign, noncancerous cells that have divided over time and heaped up into a small, crusty mound, like a spot of corrosion on old aluminum garden furniture. There are keratoses that are totally benign, such as *seborrheic keratoses*, and there are those that are caused by the sun and are precancerous, actinic keratoses. The former occur with age (or, as I say to my age-sensitive patients, "the passage of time"). I liken them to barnacles on the hull of a ship—in fact, they can be easily scraped off in a simple office procedure.

These words, along with a good eye for color, will help you describe virtually any skin problem. They will also help you get the most out of this book.

3 "You Know, Doc, I Have This Thing"

You know, doc, I have this thing . . ."

No matter where I go—a party, a social function, a business meeting—I am invariably offered the opportunity, once my profession becomes known, to examine and comment on a range of skin "things" that friends, colleagues, and acquaintances have become concerned about. Typically, interest in particular skin lesions follows on the heels of a news story about a famous individual who has been diagnosed with melanoma or the knowledge that a family member has had "something" removed. Alternatively, concern about skin things relates more than ever to a preoccupation with the signs of aging. In a social setting, it has been my personal policy not to be offended by individuals seeking reassurance that their "things" are not serious. At least twice, people I met outside of my office showed me lesions that proved to require prompt attention. That they felt comfortable enough to raise the question may have been lifesaving. Nonetheless, it is true that the vast majority of lumps, bumps, and spots that we all have (and continue to accrue as time passes) are not malignant and bear no risk of cancer. However, they serve an important medical purpose: they often bring people in to see the dermatologist, who then has an opportunity, through a full-body skin exam, to identify whether more serious conditions exist.

In this chapter, I will describe the most common spots, the lesions that individuals bare in the host's kitchen, the restaurant's bathroom, or even in a corner of the hotel's meeting hall. Full-color examples of many of these are provided in the "Color Atlas of Your Skin" (see insert).

The best way to think about any spots you may have is to identify the color. Does the color disappear when you put pressure on it? Is it a single spot, or are there many others just like it in the same area or elsewhere? Do the spots occur only where the skin is exposed to the sun? How long has the lesion been there? Did it occur within the past 24 hours or has it been present for the past several weeks or months?

▪ BROWN SPOTS

Spots that are brown have pigment in them. The brown coloration is caused by the pigment-producing melanocyte cell, or it can be the result of pigmentation from previous injury or even a side effect of certain medications. Blue spots may also result from the presence of pigmentation in the skin, but the pigmentation is deposited deeper, in the dermis, so as light reflects off it in a process called the Tyndall effect the growth appears blue rather than brown.

Brown spots on sun-exposed areas can be one of several things: so-called liver spots, which are due to chronic sun exposure; freckles; melasma, which appears as patches of pigmentation as seen in the mask of pregnancy; or lentigo maligna, a condition that requires serious attention because of the risk that it could turn into invasive melanoma.

Solar lentigo, also called liver spot or sun spot, generally occurs on the face and the backs of the hands. It can occur in men and women and begin in middle age, occurring mostly in fair-skinned individuals of northern European descent.

Freckles are often present throughout life and are manifested by numerous small brown non-scaly spots that become darker with sun exposure. They begin in childhood and are most common in fair-skinned children with blond or red hair and blue or green eyes. The tendency to get freckles is probably inherited.

Of all the brown spots that can develop on the face with age, the one that is most alarming is *lentigo maligna*. This type of flat, dark patch is often present for many years; it may have variation in pigmentation including brown, blue, black, and sometimes red. The edges of the patch are frequently irregular and maplike.

Lentigo maligna occurs in sun-exposed areas, most often on the face and neck. Although it is usually seen in older, fair-skinned individuals, recently it has become clear that there has been an increase in this condition in younger individuals, even in their forties. Over many years lentigo maligna can transform into invasive melanoma, and for this reason it should be approached aggressively.

Melasma is a blotchy tan discoloration that affects the cheeks, primarily under the eyes and cheekbones. It can affect the chin and upper lip as well, but is usually not seen on the backs of the hands or the chest. Melasma is very common in women who have been pregnant. In fact, it usually appears first during pregnancy, when it is known as *chloasma* or the *mask of pregnancy*. Melasma can be exacerbated by taking oral contraceptives. All this tells us that the pigmentation in some way is related to estrogen, but we are not certain about what that mechanism is since melasma is occasionally seen in men too. The treatment options for this condition are relatively limited, which makes melasma a frustrating condition to dermatologists. We have tried using laser, chemical peel, and bleaching creams, and the best thing that can be said is that treatment must be customized to the individual. This condition is not in any way dangerous.

Another common pigmented patch is the café-au-lait spot. These smooth, benign, uniformly pigmented, tan patches are usually larger than half an inch. Although they occur most frequently on the trunk, they can be seen anywhere on the body. About 10 percent of all people have one to three spots like this. Rarely, café-au-lait spots are a sign of an inherited condition. Albright's syndrome, which includes premature puberty and bone abnormalities, can have a café-au-lait spot as a skin sign. Neurofibromatosis, a condition incorrectly thought to be "elephant man disease" may also be associated with multiple café-au-lait spots. In this condition, spots are only a small part of a syndrome that includes multiple fleshy nodules or fibromas over the whole body.

Sometimes pigmentation changes arise after an inflammatory event has taken place. Inflammation is simply the process by which the body tries to fix a problem. For example, if you scratch yourself, your body immediately senses that something has gone wrong and sends cells into the area that release chemicals, which set about fixing the problem and restoring the skin to its normal state. In doing so, there is redness, the result of the ingrowth of new blood vessels and release of compounds that assist in warding off any infection, which might now take advantage of the break in the skin. Under normal circumstances the body goes about its business and corrects the problem. What is often left is something called postinflammatory hyperpigmentation, in which the pigment melanin has been deposited in the dermis. This will take time to resolve, but is otherwise not a problem.

When pigmented spots occur in areas that are not sun-exposed, we usually think of less serious conditions, such as a fungal infection, benign moles, or congenital nevi (the moles with which we are born). Any new or changing brown spot on the palms or soles should be investigated immediately because of the possibility of melanoma. Your dermatologist will be able to determine if there is any reason for concern.

Another common complaint is a black nail. People often think that this represents a melanoma, and indeed it can. More often, however, it is so-called *talon noir*, which is the result of a stubbed toe or other trauma. The bruise or hemorrhage under the nail can look just like melanoma.

Pigmentation can color the skin more broadly than just in particular spots. When *hyperpigmentation* occurs over the whole body, it can be an indication of an internal problem. For instance, Addison's disease, the condition that afflicted President John F. Kennedy, can cause generalized darkening of the skin. This is due to failure of the adrenal glands, which sit on the top of the kidneys, to function properly. Another internal condition with brown skin discoloration is arsenic poisoning. The accidental ingestion of arsenic was far more common when the chemical was used as an insecticide on farms and elsewhere. While internal cancer could develop as a result of this poisoning, it was the outward manifestation—rough pits on the palms and the development of skin cancers—that often signaled that something was wrong.

A few more conditions merit a brief mention. Cushing's syndrome, in which the adrenal gland produces excessive amounts of cortisol, can manifest itself with facial hair, new outbreak of acne, black-and-blue marks, and stretch marks. A rare blood condition called hemochromatosis can result in bronzing of the skin, hair loss, and spoonlike changes in the nails.

▪ LIGHT SPOTS AND WHITE SPOTS

On the other end of the color spectrum are spots that lack pigmentation completely or are lighter than the surrounding skin. So-called depigmented areas can be indicative of a condition called vitiligo, which has been made most famous by Michael Jackson. Hypopigmented macules are spots that have decreased pigmentation and could represent a superficial fungus infection called tinea versicolor or some other disease.

Conditions that represent the absence of pigmentation include albinism. In this inherited condition there is a total body loss of pigmentation. People with albinism are especially at risk for developing skin cancer because they lack the natural pigmentation that protects their DNA from the damaging effects of the sun.

▪ RED SPOTS AND PATCHES

Red spots generally reflect the presence of new or active blood vessels. In children, small spider angiomas may develop, which eventually clear up on their own. These are about 1 millimeter in size with a central "body" from which vessels extend just like the legs of a spider. With the advent of safe lasers many parents often opt to have these patches treated. Lesions like this can also develop during pregnancy and are believed to be related to increased blood levels of estrogen.

Probably the best known example of a red patch is hives. Hives are red, often raised patches that sometimes have a surrounding white halo. They can be as small as the point of a pencil or as wide as an egg. Hives, which can occur anywhere on the body including the lips and tongue, are frequently itchy. Medications, especially aspirin and penicillin, and preservatives in foods, fish, nuts, and berries can cause hives. Other culprits include viral infections, intestinal infections, bug bites, and even environmental factors such as sunlight, cold, and pressure. Hives normally go away on their own without any special treatment, but occasionally an oral antihistamine is helpful.

Raynaud's phenomenon is a condition in which the fingertips and toes are very sensitive to cold. As a result these areas turn white, then become purple and red within several minutes. Other terminal ends of the body, such as the ears and nose, can also be affected. Although more common in females, it can occur in males. If an actual ulcer develops on the fingers, Raynaud's may signal an underlying medical problem.

Flushing syndromes are quite common, and the most notable of them is rosacea. In this condition, the central facial redness is hard to control. Many individuals, especially those of northern European descent, develop telangiectasias, often referred to as broken blood vessels. These can be due to heredity, rosacea, or chronic sun exposure. Telangiectasias develop quite often on the face as small broken capillaries. The term comes from Greek words meaning "dilated ends of the blood vessel."

A rare condition called HHT (standing for Hereditary Hemorrhagic

Telangiectasia) is being investigated at Yale and elsewhere. People with this condition have multiple telangiectasias on the lips, face, fingers, and the rest of the skin. The special problem is that the same lesions may exist inside the body, in the brain, lung, and elsewhere, where they can cause serious problems—they can lead to hemorrhage and stroke. Individuals with multiple telangiectasias that fit this pattern should be evaluated for Rendu-Osler-Weber syndrome, which is the traditional name of HHT.

▪ FLESH-COLORED BUMPS

The most common flesh-colored growths are skin tags, which appear with age around the neck and in the armpits.

On the face, a common dome-shaped, flesh-colored bump is the fibrous papule. It's important for your doctor to recognize these, because they can be confused with basal cell cancer.

Seborrheic keratoses and warts are two common, benign growths that are often flesh-colored.

[Seborrheic Keratosis]

Note: For more on each of these dermatologic growths or to locate additional information see the index.

4 Skin, Very Close Up

*I'm interested in how the skin works because it's
the part of my body I'm most familiar with, and I
think the better I understand it, the better I can
take care of it.*

—Camille, 48, book publisher

Until you suffer a bad sunburn, have a close encounter
with a patch of poison ivy, or notice you don't quite
look the way you'd like to look, you probably don't think
much about your skin. If you're a runner, your joints are
on your mind daily. If you lift weights, you visualize
your muscle mass growing with each repetition. If your
vision is changing, you probably fuss with decisions
about your eyewear or laser eye surgery. But skin is an
organ that, in the words of a retired surgeon I know, "we
take for granted."

Among the many reasons that we are able to take our
skin for granted is the amazing reliability and durability of
this important organ. Our skin weighs only about nine
pounds but buttresses us against all manner of slings and
arrows: sun, cold, a razor's edge, viruses, germs, and little
burns. It varies in thickness with such remarkable precision that it can be flexible where needed (around the eyes,

for example) and stiff and rigid where flexibility would be a handicap (the palms and soles). The skin on our eyelids is about half a millimeter thick (1 millimeter is about the thickness of the lead in a standard No. 2 pencil). The skin on the soles is about 5 millimeters, ten times the thickness of the eyelid skin. In general, where the skin is sensitive, it is also very thin. In areas where it is subject to friction and calluses might form, it is likely to be thicker. Where the skin is always moving and subject to stress like the back of the neck, it is also thicker. Most people are thick-necked, at least dermatologically speaking.

The protection the skin provides us as our first defense against the outside world is due as much to its complex physiology as to its physical strength and flexibility. The skin has a remarkable array of nerves that sense pressure, pain, heat, and cold; cells that wander from the bone marrow to the skin and back; cells that produce pheromones to attract the opposite sex; cells that make sweat to cool us off; blood vessels that can constrict to keep us warm on a wintry night. The skin, in short, is a vast, dynamic organ. To take good care of it, it helps to understand how it functions. Learning about the skin, very close up, is certain to heighten your appreciation of this most obvious of organs.

▪ INSIDE OUR HOUSE

Most of us have a good basic knowledge of the body's important organs. Our heart has four chambers and serves as a pump. Our brain has two halves and functions like an enormous computer. Our kidneys are bean shaped, nestle just below our ribs in the back, and function as efficient filters, much like a sewage treatment plant. Our eyes work just like a camera.

But what about our skin? The wonder of skin resides in its clever design. Imagine how you would construct a covering for a house that was to be built in an area with a climate of extremes. The winters are very, very cold and during that time the interior of the house is heated artificially. In summer, the exterior temperature rises high as the sun beats down upon the outside, while the inside of the structure must maintain a constant temperature. The heat and cold cause expansion and contraction on the outside of the structure, putting more stresses on the covering. (This is similar to what happens to bridges in northern climates, which crack and deteriorate sooner than the roadways leading to them. Because they hang out in open air, they freeze first in cold weather and are more subject to expanding and contracting, which causes cracking in the surface material.) Add to the challenge of temperature the fact that this house you are building is in the middle of a war zone. At any moment sharp objects or exploding missiles could land on and even penetrate the surface. Sometimes the missiles are so tiny they are unnoticeable. At other times the threat to the outside of the house even comes from within. Surely, the sheathing on

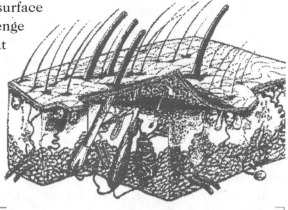

Cross-section of skin showing its complexity with hair follicles in different stages of growth, sweat glands and ducts, blood vessels, and nerves.

this building would have to be dynamic, combining the strength of Tyvek with the reflecting features of aluminum and the mass and strength of bricks.

Skin sets the standard for how a complex, multilayered structure, embedded with specialized parts, can serve a host of functions. While the heart pumps, the kidneys filter, the brain thinks, and the eyes see, the skin must do many different things at once. Here are four examples of specialized parts of the skin, each performing its own task.

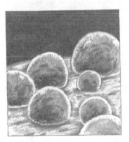

Beads of sweat under the electron microscope

1. Our *sweat glands* allow heat to evaporate, so that we don't get overheated. (More amazingly, in winter we don't have to fill up with antifreeze and we never rust.)

2. Our *lymph channels*, integral to the design of the skin, perforate every inch of skin and whisk away bacteria, other germs, and even the residue such microorganisms leave behind.

3. Our *hair follicles*, proud reminders of our fine-feathered evolutionary cousins, not only serve to make us attractive to the opposite sex but are important for the sensation of touch, yet another job of skin.

4. Our *nails* allow us to pick up a dime (or the tab) and let us scratch, a paradoxically pleasurable experience.

The skin, then, is not just a complex covering. In this brief journey down through the layers of skin, think about your own special skin nuisance and where the problem might reside. Later chapters will tell you how to fix it.

▪ MILLE-FEUILLE OR NAPOLEON

Regardless of the word you use to order this rich pastry, the mille-feuille (or napoleon) has a structure that can illustrate the layers of the human skin. The hard white frosting is analogous to the stratum corneum, the compact but scaly surface produced by the epidermis. The top layers of thin, undulating pastry leaves are similar to the epidermis. The thicker, denser layer of custard is like the dermis. Once your fork strikes the hard ceramic surface of the plate, you've reached the bone under the skin.

To get a complete sense of the complexity of the skin, let's continue with more food imagery. Imagine a cutaway side view of a summer garden. Imagine that after being planted with potatoes, carrots, and radishes, the garden isn't very well tended. Eventually it becomes overgrown with a variety of plants whose roots extend under the surface and intertwine extensively. In our cutaway view the top layer of fertilized soil represents the epidermis. The various tubers represent the appendages of the skin, such as the sweat glands, the oil glands, the hair follicles, and even the nerves; these *adnexal* (pronounced add-NECK-sull) structures form during the third month of fetal development, growing down like roots from the brand-new epidermis. Sweat glands develop in certain parts of the body while apocrine sweat glands—the kind that produce body scent and pheromones—develop in specialized areas. This web of structures adds purpose and dimension to the skin as a whole.

▪ THE HORNY LAYER AND THE EPIDERMIS

Although we speak about the epidermis as the top layer of skin, it also comes with a covering. Take a look at the ball of your foot. Do you see how thick the skin is? Much of the thickness is due to this very top layer, called the stratum corneum or horny layer, which forms a protective covering. In certain parts of the body, this covering can be dense, while it may be barely noticeable elsewhere. Under the microscope it looks like a basket weave. If you want to see the stratum corneum, take a look at your hairbrush. The many flakes you see (in fact, they're dandruff) is the keratin that has survived after production by the keratinocytes (also called the epidermal cells) and includes some dead keratinocytes as well. In some skin conditions, the body makes too much keratin and little rough bumps or patches can develop. In general, though, we best know it on a daily basis when it develops in excess in the form of callus.

How many layers does the skin have? That depends on whether you are talking about the big layers or the layers within layers. Broadly speaking, the skin consists of three layers: the epidermis, the dermis, and the subcutis, or fatty layer. But the epidermis itself, thin as the book page you are holding in your hand, has itself many layers of cells.

Cells are the basic building block of the body. In any local pond you could find small, single-celled organisms; any one of these amoebas contains all the machine parts for daily activity. In humans and in other vertebrates, billions of different cells, each with its own function, join together in a tight confederation to make organs, all of which add up to a full-blown, complex body. In humans, cells are what doctors and scientists study to understand in part how the body works. They can be seen only under the microscope, where it becomes quite obvious just how busy each cell is. To give you an idea of how small cells are, it would take about 750 million to fill an area the size of a pencil eraser.

The outermost layer of the skin, the epidermis and its horny covering, is in constant contact with the environment. Snow melts on it, water rolls off it, sunlight darkens it, sharp edges scrape it, and aging etches lines in it. The epidermis is formed by multiple layers of single cells called *keratinocytes* (pronounced KER-a-tin-o-sites) whose job it is to make keratin, a family of tough proteins. The job of keratin, in turn, is to protect the epidermis.

The keratinocyte is also important to understand because it is the origin of most skin cancers. Keratinocytes also make hair and nails, which are composed of keratin. Keratinocytes make up roughly 95 percent of the cells of the epidermis and originate as basal cells just where the epidermis fuses with the dermis.

The epidermis is not impermeable. It is not supposed to be. Were it like latex, we would all walk around overheated and uncomfortable. Although it does share the property of flexibility with latex, there are other features to its fine design that make it especially adaptable to the ever-changing, always threatening circumstances of our environment.

It is the epidermis that we assault with abrasive pads, astringents, facials, crushed apricot pits, chemicals, the new miracle creams, the old miracle creams, natural miracle creams, makeups of all kinds, and oils. That the epidermis can tolerate these attacks, and in some cases even respond positively to them, is remarkable. Such resilience is made possible because the epidermis is designed to regenerate itself regularly.

Within the epidermis are four specific layers: the basal layer, the prickle layer, the granular layer, and the horny layer. Basal cells, so called because they are at the lowest level, produce two new cells each time they divide. One remains in the basal layer to make more new keratinocytes, while the other slowly moves in step fashion through the full thickness of the epidermis, changing its shape as it does so. Originally a small round cell, a basal cell flattens out as it passes up through the skin to the surface of the epidermis. Normally, epidermal cells take about fourteen days to travel from the basal layer to the surface. By the time this keratinocyte makes it to the top layer of the skin it has lost its nucleus or DNA material and is very, very flat.

How these keratinocytes hold together is extremely important. Were they not able to adhere to one another you would not be able to hold this book, much less read it. We know that the cell membranes, or outer envelope of keratinocytes, make specialized plates, which look almost like door hinges. In this fashion, cells link up one to the other, creating a continuous covering over the body but one that is permeable to a variety of compounds. When there are problems with this networking of keratinocytes, certain rare but serious skin diseases result.

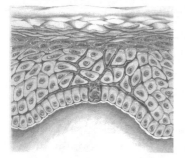

A single melanocyte or pigment cell among many keratinocytes

The epidermis itself includes two other cell types besides the keratinocytes; these are melanocytes and Langerhans cells. *Melanocytes* (pronounced MEL-a-no-sites) are the cells of the epidermis that produce pigment. These small, octopus-shaped cells dot the basal layer of the epidermis, populating it at a frequency of one melanocyte for every ten basal keratinocytes.

Melanocytes are responsible for the color of our skin; without melanocytes, there would be no races, no people of color, and the absence of these cells can make sun a serious hazard for people not of color. The number of melanocytes in the epidermis is the same, regardless of race or color. It is the number and size of the pigment granules manufactured by these melanocytes, called *melanosomes,* that determine racial difference in skin color. Pigment cells of dark-skinned individuals synthesize larger melanosomes than those produced in light-skinned individuals.

The social, political, and historical issues raised by melanocytes go beyond race. The function of these cells can have an astounding impact on the quality of human life. The absence of pigmentation, or *vitiligo* (pronounced vit-i-LIE-go), is especially important worldwide because of the association of depigmented patches or even large areas of pigment loss with leprosy, and the fact that lepers have been shunned throughout history. Albinism is another condition in which the number of melanocytes is normal but individuals are unable to fully manufacture melanosomes—a total absence of color occurs. Just as lepers have been shunned, albinos have also suffered social and cultural prejudice.

One purpose of skin pigment seems to be to protect against the sun. For example, chronic sun exposure can fool the pigment-producing cell into making larger melanosomes, thereby causing a tan. A tan is the body's response to injury from ultraviolet radiation. When one looks at epidermal cells under the microscope after they have been exposed to the sun, it is amazing to note how the granules of pigment sit over the nucleus of the keratinocyte like a skullcap. It appears that the pigment is attempting to shield the DNA of the nucleus from the harmful mutating effects of the sun.

Despite the admirable purpose of melanocytes, they, like everything else in the body, can at some point go awry. When melanocytes behave badly, they turn into melanoma, a high-risk skin cancer that is increasing in incidence.

The *Langerhans cell,* named after the scientist who discovered it, is a member of another class of cells that populate the skin as well. The Langerhans cell is found scattered among keratinocytes in the middle region of the epidermis, as well as in the dermis. It is believed that Langerhans cells monitor immune reactions of the skin, functioning not unlike an alert police officer. Prominent among these reactions are rashes, such as poison ivy.

The immunology of the skin is an area where remarkable scientific advances have been made over the past two decades. For some time we have known that there had to be some connection between our skin and our immunity. For example, certain diseases of the immune system, such as lupus erythematosus, often are accompanied by skin changes. Many other diseases in this category also cause changes that are sometimes first detected in the skin. A sort of information superhighway runs from the

THE HOLY GRAIL OF ARTIFICAL SKIN

The complexity of our skin is demonstrated by the difficulty in developing artificial skin, which is considered the Holy Grail of skin biotechnology. Several products have been developed, but so far we have failed to create anything more than a sandwich of epidermis and dermis. In one such material epidermis is formed from skin cells cultured from the foreskins of circumcised infant boys and the dermis or collagen is made in the test tube from collagen derived from cows. So far, clinical trials indicate this serves as a good biological dressing that can help heal leg ulcers. Nevertheless, it is not yet possible to make skin with all the bells and whistles—hair follicles, sweat glands, lymph channels, and blood vessels—that would make it function as the "real thing."

skin through to the bone marrow and the spleen, and on even into the brain; this system ties in our skin with the daily immunologic surveillance that protects us from external invasion. Langerhans cells play an important role in reactions as common as poison ivy and allergy to nickel or other compounds that come in contact with our skin.

▪ THE DERMIS

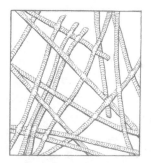

Collagen fibers as seen magnified thousands of times under the microscope

The dermis is the second layer of the skin. It is the resilient, durable, and flexible infrastructure upon which the epidermis sits. Epidermis alone is rather flimsy. If you have ever fallen off a bicycle, palm outstretched to break the fall, and emerged with a huge scrape, you know how thin the epidermis is. Strength is provided by the dermis, which essentially holds everything together. The dermis is also home to all the specialized parts that make skin what it is and that have proven so hard to imitate in our search for artificial skin.

The main component of the dermis is *collagen*. Collagen is not just an ingredient in the latest anti-aging cream. It is first and fore-

most a protein that is found in skin, tendons, ligaments, and lining covering bones throughout the body. In fact, 70 percent of the dry weight of skin
is made of collagen, a very versatile protein.

It is collagen that degenerates with age, leading to wrinkles and sagging
skin. It is collagen that heals skin wounds. It is collagen and its partner,
elastin, that are so damaged by excessive sunlight that lines, wrinkles, and
even small yellowish bumps can develop on the skin. It is collagen that
overproduces in people who make bad scars. And it is because collagen is
so important to the health and appearance of skin that the cosmetics
industry has spent millions attempting to re-create it, control it, inject it,
stimulate it, capture it in cobalt blue designer bottles, and apply it to the
surface of your skin—all in an effort to make it right once again.

Collagen is made by *fibroblasts*, small cigar-shaped cells that populate
the dermis throughout the body. Each fibroblast cell produces a spiral
chain of collagen molecules that join together like thick braids. Once the
braids of collagen are woven into bundles and the bundles are in turn
woven into netlike arrays, the final collagen has been synthesized.

Collagen is rich in amino acids, such as hydroxyproline, hydroxy-
glycine, and glycine. I mention these specific names because it is not
uncommon to see these amino acids on sale in health food stores, with
the promise that they will improve skin quality and enhance appearance.
But current science does not support the claim that these amino acids,
when taken by mouth or applied as a cream, can actually improve collagen in the skin. To date, the only FDA-approved agent that has been
shown to stimulate collagen production in skin is Retin-A, known chemically as tretinoin. This is a vitamin A–type compound; it is not the same

MEASURING AGING SKIN

Over a decade ago, while still a research fellow, I teamed up with a cardiologist who was studying the use of lasers to diagnose arteriosclerosis, or
hardening of the arteries. Elastin is important in our blood vessels, but we
knew it was important in skin as well. We developed a laser device that
could detect changes in elastin and collagen in the skin just by shining a
light on the skin. From the pattern of light that was reflected back and measured we could tell if damage to the skin was due to aging alone or the
effects of ultraviolet radiation from the sun as well.

as retinol or other vitamin A chemicals that are sold in over-the-counter anti-aging creams.

Another vital element of the dermis is *elastin*. The stretchy fibers of elastin are different from collagen. They consist of fine filaments of protein that do what the name implies: act like an elastic band. When stretched, healthy elastin allows the skin to snap back into place. With time and sun, elastin in the skin deteriorates; this is a primary cause of the loss of "snap" in your skin.

In certain disorders, there are congenital abnormalities of collagen and elastin. In these situations, healing can be impaired. Other abnormalities of elastinlike molecules can lead to loose joints. President Abraham Lincoln is thought to have suffered from Marfan's syndrome, which is due to an abnormality of this sort.

As far as I know, elastin cannot be replaced or fixed with creams applied to the surface of the skin. What remains unalterably true is that the effects of sun can be devastating. Under the microscope, skin exposed to the sun shows broken fragments of elastin where there should be long, wavy bands.

▪ WAIT, THERE'S MORE!

The dermis consists of more than just collagen and elastin. It is also home base for an extensive network of blood vessels and lymph channels. The dermis is rich in nerves. Special bulbs of nerve tissue, each serving a particular sensation, are distributed throughout the skin.

Pacini corpuscles are among the most amazing nerve endings. Located deep in weight-bearing areas, they detect pressure. Other nerve endings provide for the exquisite sense of touch. To see just how, put this book down for a moment. Can you tell precisely where on your fingertips you were holding the pages? Of course you can. What's even more amazing is that you can probably distinguish the exact spot within a millimeter. That is how precise these nerve endings are.

Other sensations transmitted by nerves in the skin include temperature, pain, and itching. These sensations pass to the brain by way of nerves that track back to the spinal column. When this system works well, it works very well. When it is shaken up by illness, it can be troublesome—for instance, in the case of shingles and the pain that comes with it.

SWEAT OR PERSPIRATION:
IT ALL DEPENDS ON WHO'S MAKING IT

The old rule of thumb is that men sweat, women perspire. Don't sweat it. It's really all the same. Perhaps sweat is what causes social problems, while perspiration is what makes up, according to Thomas Edison, 99 percent of the creative process.

That sweating is viewed as undesirable is proven by the huge variety of antiperspirant deodorants that are on the market. Certainly, individuals who sweat excessively have a major social problem. Happily, new work with botulinum toxin, known commercially as Botox and already used for treating wrinkles, may benefit people with excessive sweating. Another abnormal situation occurs in people who are born without sweat glands. Such individuals have major problems with regulating heat; their body temperatures rise very high, with all the attendant discomfort.

The truth is, we must sweat it. Sweating is our air coolant system, keeping us from overheating. By regulating body heat, our sweat gland system is our ticket to normal body temperature. The millions of sweat glands and ducts that are studded throughout our skin are there for a very important reason: to keep us comfortable and, by perspiring, keep us from expiring.

The sweat gland itself is complex and found at virtually all skin sites. We all know from personal experience that sweat glands are most common on the palms, soles, forehead, and armpits. But why do some of us seem to sweat buckets while others look dewy fresh on the hottest of days? How much you sweat is dependent on the nerve fibers that supply the sweat glands. These fibers, called *cholinergic fibers*, respond primarily to heat. Emotional stress can be an important factor as well, highlighting the close connection between your mind and your skin.

SCENT, AROMA, OR SMELL? AGAIN, IT ALL DEPENDS

Ironically, the gland in the skin that is probably the least understood may have the greatest impact on our social interactions. The *apocrine* (pronounced AP-o-krin) glands secrete a fluid that contains protein, carbohydrate, ammonia, fats, and iron. This secretion is milky and odorless until it reaches the skin surface. There, bacteria interact with it to create a unique scent, one that varies from individual to individual.

In most cases, this scent is either unnoticeable or mild. In some people, because of the nature of their secretion and the bacteria that live on their skin, a foul smell can develop. This condition, called bromhidrosis, can be controlled to some degree with antibiotics.

Apocrine secretion is affected by the nervous system, particularly chemicals like adrenaline that circulate throughout the body. In animals, apocrine glands have a protective and sexual function. The most common sites of these glands in people are the armpits, the nipples, and the anal area.

Pheromones are the scent molecules produced by animals that serve a role in sexual attraction. Since skin is our largest erogenous organ, it makes sense that it should bear fibers for touch and glands to attract those who touch, though we are not yet certain of the role of pheromones in humans.

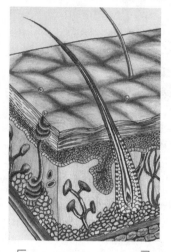

Hair follicle and
spiral sweat gland
growing in skin

▪ HAIR TODAY, HOPEFULLY NOT GONE TOMORROW

Hair—and I don't mean the Broadway musical—reminds us from where we came and who our relatives are. Whether we are fair-skinned with light hair or darkly pigmented with thick curly hair, each of us is covered with hair follicles.

Fur is one of the distinguishing features of mammals. Through evolution human beings have lost the thick pelage that characterize other mammals and even birds, but the follicles remain. All you have to do is study a chicken's skin more closely the next time you're preparing dinner to see how similar our feathered friends are to us. Next time you have occasion to see a fish up close notice the difference.

In human life, hair is an extremely important social and sexual attractant. The desire to have—and retain—hair has been with us always, as proven by the number of ancient remedies for baldness. Ironically, even as we scramble to retain the hair on our head, some people are bothered by unwanted hair in other places (for instance, on the upper lip in women and on the back in men). And it's in hair removal, with the popularity of laser devices, that dermatologic science and technology have made large strides. Laser hair removal isn't yet perfect, but it is an important step in the right direction.

Wanted or unwanted, hair remains a fascinating part of the structure of skin. Each hair grows from a follicle, which generally develops at an angle to the skin surface (think fur). At its base is the hair bulb, from which the hair itself actually grows. On one side of the hair follicle is a sebaceous gland, which produces oils (think duck) that lubricate the hair and the skin as well. Attached to the other side of each follicle is something called the erector pili muscle (think shivering).

The actual hair shaft develops from the very active cells that are in the center portion of the hair bulb. The sheaths and contained hair are derived from different parts of the hair bulb and form concentric cylindrical layers. Think of a telescoping radio antenna and you'll have a sense of what it's like when the hair sheath grows and moves outward toward the surface of the skin. The epidermis that surrounds the hair follicle is a potential source of new keratinocytes. For this reason, patients with third-degree burns, in whom the hair follicles are destroyed, cannot regenerate epidermis. In burns that are not as deep epidermis can regrow.

The speed of hair growth depends on how fast the cells of the hair bulb divide. Interestingly, the shape of hair varies racially. The scalp hair of Caucasians is round while their pubic hair, beard hair, and eyelashes tend to be oval in cross section. The scalp hair of blacks is also oval but its curliness is due to the curvature of the follicle just above the bulb.

Hair color is due to the distribution of pigment granules within hair bulb cells, which become the cells of the hair shaft. The intensity of color is probably due to the number of fully developed granules produced by the melanocytes of the hair. Hair turns gray when a decreasing number of melanocytes produce fewer melanosomes.

While it is true that human hair growth is cyclical (when your dog sheds isn't it fall?), each follicle functions independently. Hair follicles operate in a fashion best described as hurry up and wait. There are stages of activity and stages of peace and quiet. During the growing phase, or *anagen*, the cells of the hair bulbs are dividing rapidly to produce the growing hair. As the division of these cells slows down the follicle goes into *catagen*, a transitional phase, where the cells stop dividing and the hair shaft develops a clublike appearance. During the final resting phase of the cycle, called *telogen,* the follicle gets ready for new hair to grow. The newly formed hair dislodges the club hair that was present during the previous phase.

The average scalp hair grows for three or four years and the resting phase lasts for about three months. On average, 85 to 90 percent of all scalp hairs are in the anagen phase, but of course this figure gets much lower with age and decreases even faster in individuals who have male-pattern baldness. (For more information, see chapter 14, "Hair.")

▪ THE BASEMENT MEMBRANE ZONE

What keeps the epidermis attached to the dermis? Why doesn't our epidermis just slide off? Why do you get a scar when you cut yourself, but not when you scrape yourself superficially? The answers lie in the fascinating structure where the epidermis meets the dermis, an area that is visible only under the electron microscope. Special attachment plates are identified in the so-called basement membrane zone where the epidermis comes in contact with the dermis.

The basement membrane zone is considered a porous filter; it permits exchange of cells and fluids between the epidermis and dermis. The most important thing to note, however, is that scarring will only occur if the dermal-epidermal junction has been damaged. A simple injury in which just the epidermis is scraped off but in which the basement membrane zone is not harmed will not result in a scar; on the other hand, any incision that traverses or violates this junction will most certainly result in some sort of scar. The extent of the scar depends on the wound care and the nature and location of the injury. Cosmetic claims notwithstanding, it is impossible to cut through the skin at this level without getting a scar. The question for the person having cosmetic or reconstructive surgery is not whether there will be a scar but whether that scar will be noticeable. Hiding the scar and helping it fade as much as possible are all in the province of wound healing and the techniques of dermatologic and plastic surgery.

▪ FINALLY, FAT

The subcutis is the third layer of the skin. Also known as the panniculus, it consists of fat cells, or lipocytes, separated by bands of collagen or fibrous strands. It is these fat cells that have made liposuction so popular since it is in this layer of skin that unwanted fat accumulates so easily (see chapter 16, "Liposuction").

Subcutis is a reservoir of energy for the body. It is both the tissue that shapes us into who we are (but might not want to be!) and an important source of insulation.

No aspect of the subcutis has received more attention than that called *cellulite*. Cellulite is not a formally accepted medical term, nor is it a distinct anatomic structure or abnormality. Cellulite refers to the puckered appearance of the skin, usually on the thighs in women. This puckered appearance is thought to result from the fibrous bands that divide the lobules of fat and extend from the base of the subcutis to the top of the skin, pulling down like an upholsterer's button does on the back of your sofa or favorite chair.

I know of no cream, pill or procedure, wild claims notwithstanding, that will eliminate cellulite. Enough said. That doesn't mean that progress will not be made in understanding the anatomy of this tissue, allowing us to do so in the future.

Suffice it to say that beneath the subcutis is usually muscle, bone or cartilage. For all practical purposes this book will not go further than where the subcutis ends.

H ere are some questions asked most often of dermatologists.

Q. I heard that there are different types of skin and that I should know what kind I have to best take care of it. What are the different skin types?

A. There are six traditional skin types that dermatologists use to classify people. They are based on the way your skin responds to the sun. Each of the skin

KNOW YOUR SKIN TYPE LIKE THE BACK OF YOUR HAND

Thomas Fitzpatrick, professor emeritus of dermatology at Harvard University and a pioneer in the field of pigment biology, defined six types of skin.

Skin Type	Natural Skin Color	Response to Sun Exposure
I	White	Always burns, never tans
II	White	Always burns, tans minimally
III	White	Burns minimally, tans gradually and uniformly
IV	Light Brown	Burns minimally, always tans well
V	Brown	Rarely burns, tans darkly
VI	Dark Brown	Never burns, tans darkly

types has a different risk for skin cancer and premature aging from the sun. The table on page 36 shows the six types.

Q. I have a lot of different spots and bumps. How can I tell if I have skin cancer?

A. A common sign of skin cancer is a spot that bleeds. Another red flag is a spot that heals up only to come back in a few weeks (that is a favorite trick of basal cell cancer and squamous cell cancer). Although most of the growths on your skin are not skin cancer, you should learn the warning signs of early melanoma, another form of skin cancer (see chapter 22, "Melanoma"). Ask your dermatologist to teach you what to look for. Most will be glad to oblige. Also see the "Color Atlas of Your Skin," in the insert.

Q. I've been told that I have a skin cancer on my nose. I'm confused about the treatment because my doctor told me there are different ways to remove it. How can I know what is best?

A. The two most common types of skin cancer are basal cell cancer and squamous cell cancer. The majority of these occur on sun-exposed areas such as the face. Treatment options include scraping and burning it off, excision, or excision with the Mohs micrographic surgery technique. In the Mohs method the cancer is removed layer by layer and the tissue checked under the microscope until complete elimination of the cancer cells is confirmed.

Q. My doctor told me I could go to a Mohs surgeon or plastic surgeon for treatment of my skin cancer. What should I do?

A. Treatment of your skin cancer really involves two stages. The first, removal of the skin cancer in its entirety, is often best accomplished with the Mohs micrographic technique, if indicated (see page 262). After the skin cancer is removed, repair of the wound must be addressed. Most Mohs surgeons in the United States are trained in plastic reconstruction of skin cancer wounds. An advantage of Mohs micrographic surgery is that the reconstruction can be done at the same time as the cancer removal. In the case of very large or complex cases it makes sense to involve reconstructive plastic surgeons who have experience working with Mohs surgeons. In these circumstances, you will benefit the most from the team approach. One main advantage of the Mohs method is the high cure rate and optimal cosmetic result. In fact, sometimes the limited wound that results may heal well naturally, without any plastic surgery.

Q. My doctor says he does a treatment "just like Mohs surgery." What does he mean?

A. *Although the Mohs method is used only for certain skin cancer situations, it is very specific. Individuals are specially trained in this technique in the course of a full fellowship that lasts a year or more. Doctors must be board certified before being eligible for the fellowship. It is best to determine if the person doing the Mohs surgery has done a fellowship in it.*

Q. If I have plastic surgery, will that mean there will be no scar?

A. *No. All plastic surgery results in a scar. What most patients mean by this question is whether the scar will be disfiguring or noticeable. Many different specialists use the same plastic surgery techniques that are designed to hide the scar and make it as unnoticeable as possible. Remember that after any surgery the healing process continues for up to twelve months, so no conclusions can be made about the final cosmetic results until the surgery site has had a chance to mature.*

Q. I am concerned that if the basal cell cancer on my nose is treated it will be disfiguring. Right now I can cover it with makeup and it is growing very slowly if at all. It has been present for two years, I think. Why not leave it alone? I am sixty years old now and if it continues at this pace I should be OK.

A. *It is important to remember that basal cell cancer is a cancer, even though it doesn't spread in the bloodstream. If neglected it will continue to grow. It is already likely larger under the surface than it appears to you. If you delay treatment it will only be more of a problem later.*

Q. Can you recommend a good cleanser and moisturizer?

A. *The market is now filled with good products—indeed, there may be too many to choose from. To help you select a product that does the job without damaging your skin, follow these simple guidelines:*
   1. *Use a nonsoap cleanser that is hypoallergenic. This should be marked on the label.*
   2. *Use a moisturizer that is unscented and hypoallergenic.*
   3. *Wash your face with cleanser no more than once a day.*
   4. *Apply moisturizer sparingly. If your sheets are stained in the morning, you're using too much.*

Q. What are these brown spots on my skin?

A. *Many people are concerned about different brown spots they notice on their skin. This is in part because people are now educated about how to look for melanoma, and because such spots, often signs of aging, are disconcerting. There are many different types of "brown spots": freckles, moles, liver spots, even skin cancers. So it is important to bring any dark spot of concern to you to your dermatologist's attention.*

Q. Is there anything I can do to prevent wrinkles?

A. *There are four basic things you can do to help:*
   1. *Practice good sun protection.*
   2. *Don't smoke.*
   3. *Get lots of rest.*
   4. *Keep your skin well moisturized; it will lessen the appearance of fine lines.*

Q. My skin is so dry—what can I do?

A.   *1. Avoid forced-hot-air environments.*
2. Keep your shower brief—less than three minutes.
3. Avoid hot water.
4. Pat yourself dry.
5. Use a good moisturizer, applying it right after you shower or bathe. Moisturizing at this stage, when your skin has already been hydrated, helps lock in the moisture. Be careful when you use bath oils, as oily skin combined with a wet tub or bathroom floor is a hazardous situation. Slipping is easy.

Q. How can I make my pores smaller?

A. *You can't, at least not permanently. However, facials, astringents, and Retin-A may help decrease the amount of debris from your follicle that builds up in your pores, making them more noticeable.*

Q. Are fruit acid peels helpful?

A. *Fruit acid peels are widely used now and the active ingredients, alpha-hydroxy acids, have found their way into many over-the-counter moisturizers. They are effective to some degree as peeling agents. To eliminate many fine facial lines, consult with your dermatologist about laser resurfacing, chemical peel, or newer techniques such as coblation.*

Q. What should I do for sun protection, and will it help?

A. *Avoiding the sun will help you minimize aging of your skin and decrease your chances of skin cancer. It is not a magic program, however. Since most sun exposure is acquired in childhood, make sure you protect your children from the sun. Even if you are over sixty-five, it still pays to protect yourself from the sun.*
Here are some tips:

1. *Use a sunscreen with an SPF (sun protection factor) of 15 or higher and make sure that it filters out both ultraviolet A and B radiation.*
2. *Stay out of the sun when it is strongest—read in the shade. New guidelines suggest avoiding the sun between 10 A.M. and 4 P.M.*
3. *Wear a broad-brimmed hat.*
4. *Wear sun-protective clothing if you are outside frequently.*

Q. Is there such a thing as a safe tan?

A. *No. A tan is a sign that your skin has been damaged by the sun. To avoid premature lines and wrinkles, practice good sun protection.*

Q. Are tanning booths OK?

A. *No. Tanning booths make use of artificial ultraviolet radiation that can be as damaging to the skin as natural sunlight.*

Q. Are self-tanning products helpful and safe?

A. *These compounds used to make you look like a walking carrot. They have improved a great deal over the years and are easier to apply. The active chemical, dihydroxyacetone, interacts with proteins in the epidermis to darken the color of the skin.*

It's important to realize that these compounds provide no sun protection. When you go out in the sun, you must wear sunscreen as well. Self-tanning products are helpful if they give you the color you want and help you avoid the sun.

Choosing Your Dermatologist

Finding a physician is a bit like figuring out who to call when the IRS comes knocking. Except for one thing—all you've got to lose to the IRS is your money and your property. When issues of health knock at your door, you've got your life and well-being to think about. Choosing your doctor carefully is especially important in an era of managed care, overburdened schedules, and contradictory health information in the media.

In stressful moments of illness (or worry about illness), our minds focus on only one thing: getting the best help fast. Particularly when under pressure, it is difficult for the average consumer to know how to judge the quality of a dermatologist, let alone whether he or she has the appropriate expertise for the problem at hand. Because we so often leave such choices until the last minute, we may panic. Most people spend more time selecting a vacation destination or buying a car than they do choosing a family physician or specialist.

Meanwhile, a small industry has arisen around the desire to rank, rate, and reveal the "best" doctors. Magazine articles and books attempt to tell you who is the best doctor in America, the best doctor in your city, the best doctor in a given specialty, the best doctor anywhere for anything. Such reports can provide some guidance as long as you know that the information is not collated scientifically but represents the results of casual polls.

While you may use these publications as an aid in identifying doctors, it's important to gather all the information you can from all the sources at your disposal. It's also important to understand what goes into the making of a good physician. To begin with, you want to make sure your doctor knows what he or she is doing.

All physicians licensed in the Unites States today have completed college, medical school (which usually includes four years of training), plus postgraduate training in their chosen specialty. It used to be sufficient to perform one year of internship in general medicine and then become a general physician, but as medicine has grown more and more complex and a whole world of medical specialization has developed, such training is now inadequate. Advances in technology, massive proliferation in new medications and procedures, and an explosion in our understanding of disease have made it virtually impossible for any physician to have a complete grasp of the whole "nut" of medical knowledge. Specialization has become critical to providing the public with focused expertise.

In order to become a dermatologist, a medical student must complete a year of internship as well as three years of residency. If he or she chooses to specialize in surgical dermatology or in the pathology of the skin (dermatopathology), tack on an additional one- to two-year fellowship in that subspecialty. When all the training is done and the physician is considered qualified to take care of patients, he or she will have completed a total of eight or nine years of schooling after college.

Such a rigorous program notwithstanding, there's more to making a good physician. Beyond the knowledge and wisdom rooted in the science and art of medicine, a good doctor makes the patient feel comfortable and at ease. Having the right bedside manner can be every bit as important as being an expert in the field. Some people say, "Hey, I'm looking for a doctor that can fix my problem, not someone to marry," but in the case of serious or chronic illness, your confidence and belief in the doctor as healer is extremely important.

Although the patient-doctor relationship and its impact on healing has been studied, it is hard to quantify. A woman I saw recently perhaps best described the importance of good chemistry between doctor and patient. She had just been to another doctor but she was unhappy with him. "He didn't seem to care about me as a person," she said. I think that says it all. All things considered, find a doctor who seems to care about you as a person.

Your dermatologist should have the ability to understand you, your body, and what you can or cannot tolerate. For example, certain therapies for skin conditions are complex and require a great deal of attention, while others permit—even require—you to participate. The benefit in the latter case is that you may feel a greater sense of control. It is the wisdom and judgment of the physician that will help in selecting which therapy is best for you.

Physicians may become defensive about patients who seem to be putting them through a job interview, but the important point for you to remember is that any good physician believes that your health and comfort come first. Don't be intimidated by a new doctor; at the same time, use common sense and treat the doctor with the respect you'd like to receive. You don't want to alienate someone who could actually help improve your life.

When considering cosmetic surgery, don't necessarily choose the physician-to-the-stars you've seen featured in a magazine article. He or she probably won't have the time to give you the attention you deserve (unless you are a star yourself!). Quality does not necessarily go hand in hand with notoriety.

Follow-up is a hallmark of quality care. Medical care does not end when the prescription is written or the last suture is placed. In my view, those physicians who practice good follow-up care are good physicians.

Practicing medicine, in many ways, is very simple: do what is right, know what you're doing, and care about the patient. Find a dermatologist who works by these rules, and you'll probably be in pretty good shape.

▪ BOARD CERTIFICATION

The public is often confused by the issue of board certification. In the United States a formalized system of board certification developed in the 1930s. Extending to most major specialties, board certification ensures that a doctor has completed the formal specialized education and training required beyond medical school and has passed examinations to attest to a minimum body of knowledge and judgment to practice in the specialty. Many people who have been involved in training the new specialist have input into the final approval of a doctor to practice in the specialty as a board-certified physician.

I think that this system of close observation ensures that those who do become board-certified are truly "quality controlled." *Choose a physician who is board-certified.*

Many medical specialties provide medical services that overlap. Care of the skin is something that is performed by a wide range of physicians—for example, doctors in family practice and general internists may see more routine skin problems than dermatologists do. Nonetheless, for skin problems other than poison ivy, mild acne, or the like you'll want to consult a board-certified dermatologist.

In the realm of skin surgery, no one specialty holds a monopoly. General surgeons, dermatologists, plastic surgeons, ophthalmologists, ear, nose, and throat surgeons, and properly trained primary care doctors are all qualified to remove skin lesions. The techniques each kind of physician uses, however, may vary. The formal surgical training that every dermatologist receives is rooted in knowledge about the biology of the skin. As you will see in this book, we have many techniques that have been developed to minimize scarring and ensure the best results with the least risk. And sometimes, just by knowing what a lesion is, dermatologists will be able to tell you that surgery isn't required.

Which kind of specialist to see becomes a trickier issue when the subject is cosmetic surgery. Historically, plastic surgeons have been responsible for developing areas of cosmetic surgery (face-lift, breast augmentation, etc.), but office liposuction, hair transplant, and laser surgery all developed within dermatology. So many cosmetic procedures are performed by different specialists that it is hard for patients to know which doctor to choose.

When it comes to cosmetic surgery it is the quality of the results that matter. The volume of experience that a particular physician has with a procedure can also be a guide. Some of the busiest liposuction experts I know are dermatologists, and there are even obstetricians who practice this procedure. If he or she has performed the procedures many times, you are likely to have found an expert. Similarly, in a non-cosmetic area such as skin cancer, you'll want to identify a specialist with extensive experience treating skin cancer, such as a determatologist.

In addition, patients undergoing complicated procedures benefit the most when specialists with different expertise combine their efforts in the care of patients when needed. One good example is Mohs micrographic skin cancer surgery. Although I perform an extensive number of such cases including plastic reconstruction, in many instances the extent of the cancer is such that I collaborate with highly qualified plastic surgeons, ophthalmologists, head and neck surgeons, and radiation cancer experts. The patient always benefits from this team approach.

▪ A NOTE ON REFERRALS AND CASE PHOTOGRAPHS

In the cosmetic arena, many physicians are unwilling to give the names of patients that they have worked on because of confidentiality issues. Similarly, for two reasons, many physicians do not want to show before and after pictures of other patients who had a similar procedure. First, by showing photographs there is, our lawyers say, the implicit suggestion that a guarantee is being made about the final result in your case (needless to say, no guarantee is possible; there are great variations from person to person with respect to healing and final outcome). Second, no two cases are the same, so photographs of other patients may not be very meaningful.

In the end, the best way to find the appropriate physician for you is:

1. Ask your primary care physician for a referral.

2. Ask friends for names of doctors they have been happy with. Be careful here, because quality and congeniality are not equivalent. In general, however, patient referral is a good bit of information to add to the process.

3. Call the office of the physician candidate and determine whether he or she is board certified. Ask what the physician considers his or her area of expertise.

What matters ultimately is whether you are confident in the physician's skills and whether you click on some level. For this reason the consultation visit is very important.

I am always amazed at the number of highly educated, wealthy, or sophisticated patients who end up choosing a physician out of the Yellow Pages. The Yellow Pages are good for identifying some things, but it is not a source of information on medical expertise. There is a range of organizations that you can contact to get information about physicians. (See Appendix 6: Further Information on the Web.)

Finally, do not be unduly swayed by the increasing tendency of state licensing agencies to post disciplinary actions against physicians on the Web or publicize them in other ways. As an individual who has reviewed many cases of this sort, I can tell you that the threshold for bringing action on the part of patients can be very low. Often action can be initiated just because of dissatisfaction with an outcome.

Most physicians strive to provide excellent care and are deeply concerned about their patients. Yet the human body is an inexact organism, and no one can guarantee what results will occur—all the more reason to spend time and effort in finding the doctor who can meet your needs.

RADIANCE

7 Radiance, Youthfulness, and Beauty

I don't want to look like a Vogue *model. I just want to look less tired.*

—Anne Marie, 47, attorney

I'm in a business where youth matters. It's cutthroat. If I don't look young, clients will think I can't act young. I need to get rid of these lines and bags.

—Louis, 60, real estate agent

I can't think of the word *radiant* without thinking about *Charlotte's Web*. In that classic children's tale about aging and friendship, this powerful word is used again and again. In fact, I think radiance is the best way to capture what we all strive for in our lives: youthfulness, health, and, as important, inner vitality. It is impossible to separate our quest for vitality from appearing radiant and youthful. While we all recognize that we are on a continual march toward aging and becoming older, increasingly medicine offers us effective detours. Although feeling good on the inside often results in radiance there are still some areas where our "outside" can use extra help.

▪ IT'S YOUR CHOICE

Whatever your personal reason for wanting to look younger, be assured of one thing: it is *your* choice. Don't be embarrassed about wanting to improve yourself in some way. Don't let others tell you you don't need a face peel, a face-lift, or a hair transplant if your gut tells you it would make you feel better about yourself. On the other hand, be certain to learn as much as you can about the procedures available and the doctor who will be performing them. It is essential that you do everything you can to develop realistic expectations of what can be achieved.

There are dozens of books and countless magazine articles covering such topics as anti-aging therapies and keeping your skin looking young and fresh. Some books, articles, and television newsmagazine shows are accurate; others are not. Some are promoted by commercial interests (be careful!); others reflect the views of experts. Whatever your source of information, it helps to keep both eyes open. In addition, as you consider ways in which you would like to improve your appearance, it is important to reflect for a moment on self-image: How do you actually see yourself? How do you think others see you? (This is often very different from what you might think.) What is your own threshold for risk? (Any procedure or treatment you decide to pursue has some level of risk, but in most cases the benefits outweigh the risks, or the procedure would not be commonly done.)

▪ DO YOU CARE ABOUT LOOKING YOUNGER?

On a typical day how much time do you spend in front of the mirror washing your face, applying makeup or shaving, styling your hair, worrying about a new blemish, line, or wrinkle? No time at all? Half a minute? Five minutes? Half an hour? The time we take caring for our skin is a measure of how important it is to us that our appearance be as good as it can be. Our desire to look good to others is natural and has strong biological roots. The desire to be attractive continues throughout life, long after we've married, had children, and worry no more about dating or finding a mate. Why is this?

How we *view* ourselves affects the way we *feel* about ourselves. And that is especially important because it reflects on how others see us. For this reason we place a special emphasis on appearance. A healthy, attractive appearance tells others we are lively and spirited.

In truth the quest for beauty and youthful appearance is more than skin-deep. There is an internal side of wanting to look good and feel young that is driven by our desire for immortality. While we spend time in front of the mirror every day to improve how we look that particular day, we receive other messages back from that silver-plated sheet of glass, messages about how we are coming along in life and how, in fact, life is moving along.

From the day we are born, we begin to die, biologically speaking at any rate. The processes of growth and dying stand in counterpoint to each other. Aging is what we as organisms experience with the passage of time. While there is a net growth in the number and size of the cells that make up our body, cells die on an ongoing basis and are replaced. As we age and begin to feel the effects of aging, each cell divides a bit less well, like an aching back first thing in the morning. The DNA may not get it quite right and the cell may even make a mistake while it is dividing, leading either to a cell that just dies or, short of that, becomes cancerous. (Cancer is really a disease of aging.)

▪ HOW WE AGE

In the early 1960s it was first shown that the cells that make up our bodies actually go through a predictable, controlled process of aging. If cells are grown on a petri dish, they will divide about fifty times—with each division taking a little longer—until division ceases and the cell actually dies. In general, this process in a single cell affects the whole body, since we are those cells.

In the 1970s scientists demonstrated that a small piece of the chromosome called a *telomere* (pronounced TEEL-uh-mir) seemed to change as the cell aged. There is evidence that if one alters the length of the telomere, one can actually modify the aging process of the cell. As you can imagine, this has amazing implications. Although there are many factors involved in physical aging, being able to identify such a critical piece of the puzzle at the DNA level holds much promise for treatments that can affect aging.

In coming years, you will probably read a lot about *telomerase* (pronounced TEEL-ah-mer-ayz). This is an enzyme our cells make to control the length of the telomere. If we can find a way to control the enzyme we can possibly keep cells dividing indefinitely, finally achieving the goal of slowing the aging process. Longevity seems to run in certain families, sug-

AGING OR MATURITY

I often refer to wrinkles as "lines of maturity." It always inspires at least a polite chuckle. I use this phrase to emphasize that the lines and furrows we develop over time have not come unearned. Even though we would all prefer to wear such medals and stripes on our epaulets and coats and not our foreheads, there are things we can do about the range of changes that indicate aging.

gesting that aging is genetically controlled. In one experiment, altering just two genes increased the life of the flatworm six to eight times. When you think of the normal life span of a worm (which I am sure you do daily) compared with our own life span, you realize the magnitude of this life extension. (OK, I'll tell you: it's equivalent to extending human life to 600 to 700 years.)

Research into the telomere is still in the early stages. Since it seems to time how the cell divides, it will likely prove important in cancer therapy as well as aging. The actual role of telomerase in aging is not yet clear, and further research may yet identify other enzymes or genes that are critical. Nevertheless, the exciting message here is that since the dawn of time we were conceived, born, matured, and died all within a well-defined time period or life span. In the past, we never had a clue about how aging was controlled or predestined. Now we are honing in on ways that the aging of cells is regulated by our chromosomes. When we find a sufficient number of pieces to finish the puzzle, our problem will likely be finding enough food on the planet to feed all the 200–year-old men and women who are golfing, tending gardens, or working the slot machines.

▪ COSMETIC SURGERY OR ANTI-AGING THERAPY?

Dermatology is a medical specialty concerned with the health of the skin, the canvas upon which we paint the picture we would like to present to others. In my practice I deal with those skin problems that reflect concerns of aging. These can be called "cosmetics," "cosmetic surgery," or "aesthetic surgery"—but this aspect of the practice really is *aging therapy.*

While aging is hardly a disease, in some people it causes *dis*-ease, and much of medicine addresses the *dis*-ease that we feel as a result of certain physical or psychological circumstances. A good term for this aspect of dermatology, taking a cue from the use of ancient languages to describe terms in medicine, would be kronotherapy (from *kronos*, the Greek word for "time"). I go to the trouble of newly defining this area because I believe that the traditional term of "cosmetic surgery" has gained a cheapened, narcissistic meaning. For example, there are those who contend that only the vain pursue cosmetic surgery and that people with a strong sense of values don't worry about how they look. I disagree.

It is true that there are many people who don't put their appearance as a number one priority, but I think we all care about how we look. Taken to the extreme, I think the popular musical *The Phantom of the Opera* would not have been so successful had it not appealed both to our fear of ugliness and our rootedness in deeper values of acceptance.

We all age, but some of us show the signs of aging more than others do. Often this is due to environmental and lifestyle causes (sun exposure, stress, smoking, etc.), but sometimes the tendency to wrinkle is simply in our genes. Aside from treating skin cancer and other "medical" problems, one of the satisfactions of being a dermatologist these days is having so many options for improving human appearance. There are many productive ways that dermatologists, plastic surgeons, and others in the field can contribute to your quality of life and, yes, happiness.

▪ LISTENING FOR THE REAL AGENDA

QUESTIONS TO ASK YOURSELF

1. What feature of my appearance is it that really bothers me?
2. Why don't I like the way it looks?
3. How would I feel if it disappeared or got better completely?
4. Does it bother me enough to undergo a surgical procedure and take the risk of possible temporary discomfort and scarring?
5. If I don't change it, how many times a day will I notice it?

Because aging is so complex and how we feel about how we look is a crucible for so many personal issues, I try to listen carefully to patients who come for cosmetic consultations. There are several reasons for this:

1. Any procedure we might do would be purely elective and, by definition, not medically necessary. Therefore the risks we are willing to take are much less than if we were attempting to cure a medical problem on a non-elective basis.

2. Because no procedure is without risk, it is critical to be sure that you really *want* the procedure. There is so much misinformation about anti-aging treatments that some people arrive in my office with hugely incorrect ideas of what procedures involve, including the recuperation period and what can actually be achieved.

3. I have found that just talking about people's cosmetic concerns gives them a new outlook. Occasionally, talking allows the person to be happier without a significant procedure. For instance, a sudden need to look younger can often follow on the heels of a major life change, such as the death of a spouse or divorce. If that is the case in your situation, it is critical that no decisions about surgery be made until you have reached a new level of equanimity or balance in your life. Don't use surgery to fix a problem or concern it can't really improve. Such "proxy surgery" should be avoided.

▪ CHANGES IN AGING SKIN

It might not seem so each birthday when you say to yourself, "I can't be *that* old . . ." but one of the great pleasures of life is to age well. Certainly aging well is far superior than growing old and looking old before your time. But before you hop on the operating room table, there are some obvious things you can do to help stay in shape: eat well; don't smoke; if you drink alcohol, drink modestly; keep your weight trim; and get enough rest.

Some of the skin changes associated with aging you can do little, if anything, about. It is important to make the distinction between those intrinsic changes that you can't fight and others over which you have some control. One of the latter is photo-aging, or the effects of exposure to sunlight on your skin. For now, protecting yourself from the sun is still the best policy.

Your oil glands, which keep your skin moist, slow down their activity with age. Thankfully, the increasing dryness of your skin is also something you can have some control over. You can replace the decreased amount of

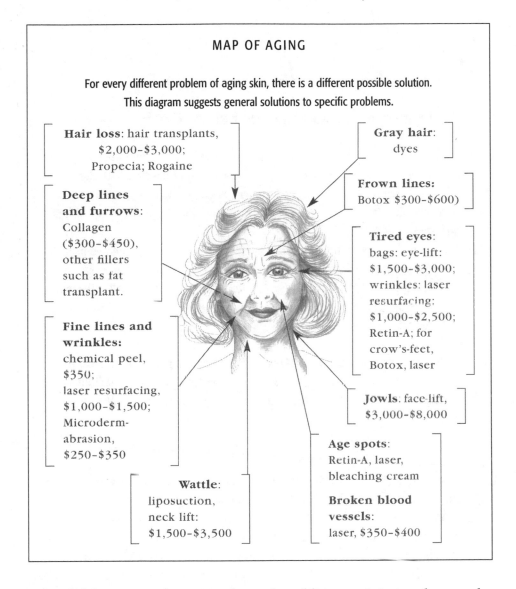

MAP OF AGING

For every different problem of aging skin, there is a different possible solution.
This diagram suggests general solutions to specific problems.

Hair loss: hair transplants,
$2,000–$3,000;
Propecia; Rogaine

Gray hair:
dyes

**Deep lines
and furrows**:
Collagen
($300–$450),
other fillers
such as fat
transplant.

Frown lines:
Botox $300–$600)

Tired eyes:
bags: eye-lift:
$1,500–$3,000;
wrinkles: laser
resurfacing:
$1,000–$2,500;
Retin-A; for
crow's-feet,
Botox, laser

**Fine lines and
wrinkles:**
chemical peel,
$350;
laser resurfacing,
$1,000–$1,500;
Microderm-
abrasion,
$250–$350

Jowls: face-lift,
$3,000–$8,000

Age spots:
Retin-A, laser,
bleaching cream

Wattle:
liposuction,
neck lift:
$1,500–$3,500

**Broken blood
vessels**:
laser, $350–$400

natural lubricant with moisturizers. In addition, minimize dryness by avoiding environments that are very dry.

PROFILE OF A WRINKLE AND WHAT YOU CAN DO ABOUT IT

What keeps our skin taut and smooth is its elastic properties. Elasticity of skin comes from elastin tissue and collagen that make up the dermis (see chapter 4, "Skin, Very Close Up"). As a result of natural

---

A MIRROR EXERCISE

To get an idea of the way in which you have aged, try this exercise:

- Get photographs of yourself at three or four stages including high school graduation and now.
- Lay out the photos in front of you and look at them in order, from the youngest to most recent. Study how you've changed. Make a note of how you feel after doing this—e.g., happy, disgusted, saddened, content.
- Next, scramble the pictures and look at them again. How do you feel? To which picture are you most drawn?
- Finally, line the pictures up so you can see them in a mirror. Whom do you see? To which picture are you drawn the most? (Seeing the picture in the mirror reverses your facial features, which are naturally asymmetric. When you view yourself in the mirror you are seeing yourself not as others see you—only as you see yourself.) How do you feel seeing these images?

The odds are that you will be ultimately drawn to the current picture of yourself. That is good. Who we were twenty years ago is a part of us we can relive in our minds but never re-create. This is a key point to remember when it comes to cosmetic surgery and kronotherapy.

---

aging and because of the damaging effects of ultraviolet radiation, both elastin and collagen deteriorate. When they do, skin becomes less stretchy—more like an old sock that has lost its elasticity and can no longer hug your calves. Your skin begins to develop fine lines, then wrinkles. Jowls are due as much to this change in the skin as they are to the effects of gravity. (Jowls are relatively uncommon among two-toed sloths that sleep upside down.)

Given what we know about the causes of wrinkles, it makes sense that the best way to improve them is to reconstitute the collagen and elastin tissue

TWO KINDS OF AGING SKIN

- **Intrinsic:** Natural, or chronological, due to biological changes in the skin cell's DNA.
- **Extrinsic:** External, due to outside causes. The sun is the main culprit here, stimulating a process called photo-aging.

that we grew up with and took for granted. Several approaches have been developed to accomplish this. Some are topical creams, others are surgical. It should also be noted that in addition to the changes in the dermis that result in "weaker" skin, many changes occur in the epidermis—chief among them dryness—that contribute to the appearance of fine lines and wrinkles.

LINES

Lines are wrinkles' first cousins. They can first appear as incipient, creaselike indentations around the mouth, which are politely called *laugh lines*. Many people notice delicate creases across the forehead, which are reasonably called *worry lines*. If you are a frowner, you may also find that as you grow older the corners of your mouth may turn down and a crease or two may appear across the chin.

Needless to say, it is far better for your mental health and thus for your skin to collect laugh lines rather than worry lines. We already know that smiling uses approximately half the muscles of the face compared with frowning—certainly a boon for the skin.

> **TOP FIVE SIGNS OF AGING SKIN**
>
> 1. Fine lines and wrinkles
> 2. Mottled brown discoloration
> 3. Broken blood vessels or capillaries
> 4. Roughness
> 5. Deep wrinkling

Fine, early lines may be softened with a good moisturizer and eliminated for a time with collagen treatments. If shallow enough, they may also be removed by laser or other surgical procedures (see chapter 13, "Medical Lasers").

WRINKLES

Wrinkles are a natural part of life's aging process. In Western culture they are often seen as a cardinal, unavoidable sign of aging. In other cultures, wrinkles are a sign of wisdom. This is well and good, but try convincing someone who is unhappy with their changing skin that it is better to be wise than to have tight skin. A truly wise patient might say: Why can't I have both?

Be that as it may, not enough of us accept our wrinkles as a sign of having lived long enough to know what we're doing and to enjoy life. Until that time comes, we dermatologists will continue to be asked, "Doc, how can I get rid of my wrinkles?"

The simple answer is there is still no magic wand that will re-create the lost skin of your youth. The only way to prevent big-time wrinkling is to avoid sun exposure, and most of us adults have already exposed our skin to far too much sun. What began as your yearly tan has turned into the most common sign of extrinsic aging, photo-aging. Thus, the damage has been done.

What you can do now to reduce further fine lines and wrinkles is to avoid the sun and use a waterproof broad spectrum sunscreen with an SPF of 15 or higher that protects against ultraviolet A radiation (UVA) and ultraviolet B radiation (UVB).

A clinical psychologist recently published an instructive study on attitudes about sun exposure. He found that beach-goers who would not otherwise apply sunscreen were far more likely to do so if they were told it would help them look younger, than if they were told to use it to prevent aging skin or cancer. The lesson, not surprisingly, is that people respond better to positive messages than to threats.

SMOKER'S FACE

Evidence now exists that links smoking to an increase in lines and wrinkles. Most dermatologists would agree that people who smoke appear to have more wrinkles, and that those wrinkles are coarser than the wrin-

---

HAVE REALISTIC EXPECTATIONS

To gauge how much of a concern a particular aesthetic problem is, I ask my patients how often they think about it. Some might become aware of the concern only when they catch their reflection in a store window, suffer a moment of disgust, and move on. Others might struggle in front of the mirror every morning with lines that become like lines in the sand: borders of confrontation between their appearance and their psyche. In general, if you have realistic expectations of the outcome of any kronotherapy you will be happy. If you have unrealistic expectations about what surgery can do, you will be unhappy. The trick is for the doctor to talk with the patient and listen carefully to be sure that expectations are realistic.

kles on the skin of a nonsmoker's face. In fact, it's very easy to spot what dermatologists call *smoker's face*. The skin of a chronic smoker's face is crosshatched with crevicelike wrinkles and lines, often giving the cheek a tic-tac-toe look. The skin may also be sallow because of decreased blood flow since chemicals in smoke constrict the blood vessels in the skin (they do the same to the blood vessels in the heart and brain). Another identifying mark of smoker's face is the fine lines that radiate from the upper and lower lip due to perpetual puffing. Clearly, it isn't easy to give up smoking, or more smokers would be successful at quitting. However, if there is one habit worth eliminating from your life, it's smoking. To get help, consult your primary care physician. There are also many groups you can go to for additional support. To find out more, contact the American Cancer Society, American Heart Association, or the American Lung Association.

▪ SIGNS OF AGING: FIRST, KNOW THE ENEMY

In order to fix your aging skin problems, it's helpful to first know all the different changes that take place that add up to looking older.

ENLARGED PORES

The medical term for a pore is a *follicular orifice*, but calling a pore a pore is equally acceptable in dermatological circles. Contrary to what many cosmetic companies and beauticians try to make you believe, it is impossible to change the size of your pores, self-stick patches or not. Although a toner, astringent, or mask may tighten pores for a few hours, they will then revert to their normal size.

In some people, large pores are present from youth; in others, they seem to become more prominent with time. Pore size is determined by genetics and age. Genetics determines the size of the sebaceous gland at the side of the pore and the size of the opening. As you age, pores become more noticeable because oils and skin cells accumulate that can plug up the pore and dilate it temporarily.

A common misconception is that the pore fills with dirt because you have not done a good job keeping your face clean. This is not true, so do yourself a favor—put the power washer away and keep the abrasive pads to clean your car.

Large or small, your best choice when it comes to your pores is to wash your face gently and avoid clogging them additionally with excess creams and potions. Do not pick, squeeze, dig, excavate, or otherwise molest your follicles yourself. A professional facial can go a long way to removing the pore contents temporarily, thus minimizing the appearance of pores.

BROKEN CAPILLARIES

A common change associated with aging is the appearance of tiny capillaries, or broken blood vessels, usually on the face. These fine red lines, which especially plague those with fair skin, appear most frequently on the cheeks and nose. The spidery networks are harmless, except to the self-esteem of those who find them unsightly. In addition, many people with red noses find that friends and acquaintances mistakenly believe that they drink alcohol excessively. Fortunately, it's quite easy to remove them with laser treatments.

SKIN TAGS

"What's that on my neck?" you may ask yourself with some alarm one morning. The "thing" is a skin tag. These are tiny growths of benign skin that protrude from the body, usually in the neck area and armpit. While unsightly to some, they are not dangerous and can easily be removed during an office visit.

If the tag is black, which can be due to the tag getting strangulated on its little pedicle, have it evaluated by a dermatologist.

RED DOTS AND DARK SPOTS

With age, we develop an abundance of spots and dots, most of which are easily removed for cosmetic reason.

Cherry hemangiomas are about 1–2 millimeters in diameter. They are small, red hemangiomas that appear on the trunk, arms, and legs as we get older, first becoming noticeable in our thirties. These spots are not precancerous and can be easily removed with laser or other methods in your dermatologist's office.

Seborrheic keratoses are rough growths that appear on the surface of the skin with the passage of time. I call them "barnacles of life" because they typically have the same stuck-on appearance. These harmless growths are usually scaly, brown, and raised; they may seem warty in appearance and texture. People sometimes become concerned about them because they can be quite dark, change in some way, or even fall off. When this happens, fear about melanoma can arise. These concerns can quickly be quashed when your dermatologist examines the keratoses. They don't have to be removed, but your dermatologist can easily scrape them off when they become unsightly. They *should not* be excised, or you will get a permanent scar in place of a very superficial "barnacle."

If these growths become irritated, turning red and itchy, your doctor can remove them simply by scraping them off.

LIVER SPOTS

Also called age spots, liver spots are flat and brown or tan in color. Harmless signs of aging, they usually appear on the hands, face, or other areas that have been continuously exposed to sunlight. Most dermatologists say, "Leave well enough alone," when it comes to liver spots. However, if you are truly bothered by their appearance, such spots can be treated by your doctor with acids, liquid nitrogen, laser, or you may have some success with fade creams.

Occasionally, a "liver spot" may become darker in one area or change in some way. Your dermatologist should evaluate this and a small biopsy might be performed to be sure that it is not an early form of melanoma called *lentigo maligna* (see chapter 22, "Melanoma").

WATTLES

A wattle is usually defined as a fleshy, vividly colored flap of skin that sags from the neck or head of some birds and lizards. Unfortunately, this indelicate word also serves as a somewhat humorous nickname for similar-looking sagging flaps of skin on the aging human face. The good news is that through advances in cosmetic surgery no one need suffer with a wattle. In most cases, a procedure to tighten up the muscle of the neck or liposuction can improve the appearance of these folds, which are due to gravity and loss of skin elasticity.

SAGGING JOWLS

Sagging jowls result from a combination of the effects of gravity and the natural breakdown in the elastin tissue of the skin that occurs over time.

A face-lift performed by a competent cosmetic surgeon—one who performs the procedure frequently—is still the only way to fight these signs of gravity and failing elasticity in the skin.

HAIR LOSS

Hair loss is a cardinal sign of aging. See chapter 14, "Hair," to learn more about what you can do.

VARICOSE VEINS

As we travel the journey of life, gravity and the fact that we walk upright conspire to give us road maps on our legs in the form of varicose veins. For details on how these can be treated, see chapter 17, "Veins or Vanity."

FEET

Corns and *calluses* are the painful results of not paying enough attention to the feet. These irritating culprits are caused by prolonged and persistent pressure and friction on the skin of the toes or bottom of the feet.

Corns and calluses are both hyperkeratoses, or thickened areas of skin. A corn is usually round or cone-shaped, with a tip that points into

---

CARING FOR DRIER SKIN

Once you hit forty, a major challenge is protecting your skin from dryness. Dry skin accentuates wrinkled skin, and no person I've ever treated has wanted to speed up that process. Here are some tips:

- **Avoid the sun.**
- If you must be in the sun, use a broad-spectrum sunscreen of SPF 15 or more.
- Quit smoking, if you haven't already.
- Do not use soap. Find a nonsoap cleanser.
- Remember to pay attention to all parts of your body, not just your face, when it comes to dry skin. Use your moisturizer on your arms (particularly drying elbows), legs (the calves of aging legs often grow scaly in winter), feet, and anywhere else on the body where dry patches of skin have developed.
- Take baths in a natural bath oil to moisturize the entire body.

the skin. This point digs into your skin like a pebble, making the corn extremely painful. Corns are found on the outside of your toes most frequently, but soft corns may be found between your toes, and seed corns may appear in clusters on the bottoms of your feet. Calluses are skin thickenings that form over bone protrusions, such as the ball of your big toe.

Both of these conditions can be caused by abnormalities in your gait or abnormalities of bones. For example, people with a hammertoe—one that is permanently bent upward in a flexed position—are especially prone to corns in the affected area. By and large, most corns and calluses are caused by wearing shoes that don't fit well.

Ill-fitting shoes are most likely to pinch the last two toes. While women often develop corns or calluses on these last two toes due to wearing high heels, men can develop the same condition, though in their case it's often because they tend not to change their shoes as often as women do. To avoid pressure and friction on your toes, you should wear a shoe that gives your toes room and has a low or flat heel, so that your toes are not constantly being pinched and pressed forward. You should also have more than one comfortable pair of shoes in your closet, so you won't have to wear the same pair every day.

For temporary relief, soak your feet in warm water until the corn or callus has softened. Then use a pumice stone to gently wear away the dead skin and shrink the corn or callus. Avoid razors, scissors, or "callus parers," and don't try a medically treated pad, unless your doctor advises you to. If your corns or calluses are extremely bothersome, consult your dermatologist or podiatrist. You may benefit from orthotics, which are custom-made insoles designed especially to accommodate the shape of your feet. In some cases, surgery may also be necessary. In general, pedicures are an effective way of keeping the skin and nails of your feet in good shape.

▪ TURNING BACK THE LINES

A wide range of exciting techniques is available to remove lines and wrinkles. Each works in a slightly different way with a different risk profile. Chemical peels, soft tissue filler substances, laser, and topical Retin-A are the most reliable ways of improving fine lines and wrinkles. Some of these procedures, such as peels, are simpler than conventional wisdom would have it. Others, like laser, can be more complicated, with more post-operative care and higher

risk than the media portray. Let's take a look at the more common procedures used to decrease or remove fine lines and wrinkles.

CHEMICAL PEELS

Carpenters and people who know fine furniture appreciate how the
gentle removal of the surface of a piece of rough wood can transform it into
a smooth, attractive piece of material. The same can be said of raw gem-
stones and marble. In fact, any material with imperfections can benefit
from gentle smoothing or buffing. In a sense this is what a chemical peel,
also called *chemexfoliation,* does for the skin.

The top layer of skin, the epidermis, is continually renewing itself; it
sheds dead skin daily. This sloughing of dead skin cells has absolutely no
effect on the development of fine lines and wrinkles or on the development
of actinic keratoses, which are sun-induced precancers. However, the
buildup of dead skin can leave a "less healthy" appearance to the skin in
the opinion of some. A chemical peel can be used to remove this top dead
layer of skin to rejuvenate the appearance of the skin. Depending on the
depth of the peel, new collagen production can be stimulated.

There are several types of chemical peels, categorized by how deeply
the chemical used penetrates the skin. You can think of a chemical peel
as causing controlled levels of destruction in the skin. With the deeper
chemical peels, you are in fact causing a mild and controlled chemical
burn. The three main varieties of chemical peel are superficial, medium-
depth, and deep.

A superficial chemical peel simply removes the very top layer of the
epidermis. It causes no permanent changes, although as I've mentioned, it
will improve the appearance of the skin. A medium-depth chemical peel
removes epidermis and affects the dermis, the middle layer of the skin.
Deep chemical peels extend deeper into the dermis. The risk of scarring
relates directly to how deep the peel is. In general, the risk of scarring is
low with superficial and medium-depth peels.

SUPERFICIAL CHEMICAL PEEL

Superficial chemical peels are also called "freshening peels" by some.
A variety of different acids are used. The goal here is to remove the top,
dead layer of the epidermis leaving the skin with a fresher appearance.

Superficial peels generally result in the feeling and appearance of a few hours in the sun. In fact, when undergoing a superficial chemical peel, no type of sedation or local anesthetic are required. Some facialists perform peels that may be considered superficial, but your dermatologist will use acids that are stronger and may be of more benefit if you want to be more aggressive in your treatment.

After the acid is applied to the skin, a light white frost briefly develops. A mild amount of stinging resolves quickly on its own.

> ### QUEEN OF THE NILE: TALK ABOUT SUN DAMAGE!
>
> Cleopatra is said to have had chemical peels done with milk that contained various amounts of lactic acid, a form of the popular class of "anti-aging" creams called alpha-hydroxy acids.

MEDIUM-DEPTH PEEL

The medium-depth chemical peel is performed much like the superficial peel. The main difference is that after preparation of the skin with a degreaser such as acetone and application of a solution to remove the horny cells on the surface of the skin (Jessner's solution), trichloroacetic acid 35% (or a similar

> ### LASER OR PEELS: WHAT DO I NEED?
>
> The choice of treatment that is best for you depends on several factors: the depth of the lines or wrinkles, your skin type, your tendency to scar, your doctor's expertise, and your risk threshold.
>
> In general, chemical peels will eliminate superficial changes in the epidermis but *will do nothing to deeper lines.* To eliminate these, actual destruction of dermis is necessary, so that new collagen will form. Laser resurfacing is the best choice here. A new technique called *coblation* may also be helpful.
>
> Superficial and medium-depth peels cannot help scarring, such as that related to acne, because they do not penetrate deep enough to alter the dermis or scar tissue.

agent, depending on the choice of your doctor) is applied with a cotton tip applicator. After application of the trichloroacetic acid, the skin surface frosts lightly. Ice packs are applied during the procedure to cool down the heat and stinging associated with the action of the peeling chemical. The white frost usually fades within two hours. The irritation and scaling that develops in the skin peaks between five and seven days after treatment, but residual redness may remain for up to two weeks. Approximately one week after the treatment, the peeling skin resembles the peeling that occurs after a sunburn.

The medium peel is the type that I perform most often. A series of four or five of them, spaced six to eight weeks apart, results in visible rejuvenation of the skin that can last for some time. It is an excellent way to smooth sun-damaged skin, making it less mottled and fresher looking, and it may even decrease the number of precancerous growths that might be present. My approach with chemical peels is "easy does it." I'd rather do five peels over time with relatively low risk than do one deep peel that could result in harmful effects.

DEEP PEEL

Deep chemical peels are usually performed using a chemical called *phenol*. While this type of peel can remove some of the deepest wrinkles on the skin, phenol can be potentially toxic to the heart. Therefore small areas of the face are done sequentially while the patient is sedated and monitored with a heart monitor.

Although a deep peel reduces the deep wrinkles there is an accompanying risk of scarring. This peel is not suitable for dark-skinned individuals, because when the epidermis regenerates, it is often lighter than the skin it replaces. These peels are less commonly performed these days because of the advent of laser resurfacing although there are skilled dermatologists who still prefer this approach.

PEEL RISKS

A chemical peel is no different than any other surgical procedure in that there can be side effects and no guarantee can be made about the final outcome. There is always the risk of scarring, increased or decreased pigmentation, and the possibility that you will not be satisfied with the result. Redness can persist for months. A chemical peel can induce an outbreak of cold sores, so if you are susceptible tell your doctor; he or she will typically put you on an antiviral medication just before the peel to help prevent an outbreak of cold sores. Some people get an impetigo-like infection after a peel, which can be treated with antibiotics.

THE LUNCHTIME PEEL

Recently, a new technique to smooth the top surface of the skin has become popular, promoted under names such as Powerpeel, Parisian Peel, DermaPeel, and UltraPeel; it is generally known as the micropeel or micro-dermabrasion. In this technique, minute crystals of aluminum oxide, like tiny beads of sand, are sprayed over the skin at regulated pressure—in a sense, the top surface of the skin is sanded off. No anesthesia is required and these peels have a low incidence of side effects. Unlike laser or chemical peels, the after-effects are such that one could actually have the procedure done at lunchtime and go back to work. The only immediate effect that is noticeable for several hours is slight reddening of the skin. The procedure, which is very gentle, may be repeated as often as necessary to maintain the benefit.

There is no doubt that people who undergo the procedure feel that their skin is smoother after the session. Without changes in the collagen, however, it is unlikely that any lasting benefit will accrue. The micropeel is more aggressive than home treatment with alpha-hydroxy acids and less aggressive than a traditional chemical peel.

Different techniques to rejuvenate the surface of the skin vary in effectiveness and risk. In general, the more effective a technique, the more risk.

▪ HOW TO TREAT DEEP LINES AND WRINKLES

Chemical peels and micro-dermabrasion are helpful to control or remove very fine lines. Deeper lines and wrinkles are more of a challenge.

The idea that we can fill out a depression or puff up a crease has captivated dermatologists for generations. If you can put back what's been lost, you should be able to smooth out the skin and restore it to its youthful luster. Because the skin is accessible, either by needle injection or minor incisional surgery, we have long sought the ideal material to make up for the shriveled elastin tissue and collagen that wanes with age.

The first attempt at using an injectable material for cosmetic purposes was performed in 1899 with paraffin. Soon after its initial use, it was discovered that paraffin caused a number of problems, including the forma-

---

FIVE EASY THINGS YOU CAN DO TO LOOK RADIANT

1. Practice aggressive sun protection.
2. Use Retin-A for fine lines and irregular skin surface.
3. Wash gently only once a day with a nonsoap cleanser.
4. Use makeup in moderation.
5. Regarding product claims, remember: If it sounds too good to be true, it probably is.

---

tion of lumps known as granulomas. The problems were significant enough that paraffin was no longer used after the 1960s. These days many other agents and techniques are used for filling in the depressions or contouring the defects that are a result of the aging of the skin.

MICRO-LIPOINJECTION

Micro-lipoinjection is the transfer of fat from one area of your body to another. The fat can be harvested during liposuction, or it can be extracted with a syringe from any site in order to reinject into another area.

Micro-lipoinjection is frequently used to fill in the groove that runs from the nose to the corners of the mouth. Filling in this *nasolabial* fold, which over time tends to sag, can have an impressive effect on making you look fresher and less tired.

Other popular sites for this procedure are the lines at the corner of the mouth, depressions on the cheeks, and the backs of the hands which gradually lose fat over time. The transplanted fat seems to last longest in areas with the least movement—for instance, hollows that some people have on their cheeks will retain the fat longer than will the lines around the mouth.

Complications are rare but include infection (hematoma or black-and-blue mark) and swelling. Keep in mind that multiple treatments may be required to obtain any type of long-term result.

DERMAL GRAFTING

The middle layer of the skin, the thick and tough dermis, provides such strength that certain contour defects can be treated with dermal grafting. This procedure may be used for furrows or certain acne scars.

Dermal tissue to be used in grafts is typically harvested from behind the ear. The tissue is then used where needed, much like a skin graft would be; the key difference is that it is placed *under* the surface of the skin for purposes of filling out a defect. For example, a scar such as an acne crater would be anesthetized and prepared to receive the graft by creating a small pocket. The dermal graft is inserted in the pocket, pushing the tissue above its previous level.

After dermal grafting, people should expect to have some bruising, crusting, and swelling. Some mild to moderate pain can also be expected, but this should be easily controlled with various pain medications. More than one session is typically required. The first procedure corrects from 40 percent to 70 percent of the defect on average, but after two sessions, the majority of patients are usually fully corrected. If any settling of the grafts is to occur, it typically happens between one and six months following the procedure. Acne scars and smaller folds or wrinkles seem to respond with the best results. Grafts last up to five years. Newer alternatives have made this procedure less common.

INJECTABLE BOVINE COLLAGEN

Collagen collected from cows is probably the most widely used injectable form of the substance. (Yes, that's *bovine* as in cow.) One of the common uses of injectable bovine collagen now is augmentation of the lips to give them a fuller, more sensuous appearance. Perhaps you never realized that leather is made almost completely of collagen. An anti-aging product containing bovine collagen was first used in the United States in 1977 and approved by the FDA in 1981 as the first soft tissue filler device. The collagen is derived from the hides of a specially raised American herd of cattle that does not intermingle with other cattle and cannot acquire veterinary infections. The cowhide undergoes many steps to purify and sterilize it. Bovine collagen is marketed under the trade name Zyderm and Zyplast.

Approximately 3 percent of individuals are allergic to this product. If you and your doctor are considering using bovine collagen to fix wrinkles or other skin defects, it is best to do two skin tests on the forearm, spaced four to six weeks apart. If you don't react to the collagen, then it means you can proceed safely.

The treatment itself involves no anesthetic. You usually sit in an upright position, so that the natural folds of the face may be seen. In general, 30 percent of people report an eighteen-month period of correction, while the other 70 percent require touch-up treatments at intervals of every three to twelve months.

Adverse reactions to bovine collagen can include redness for several hours and bruising that can last up to seven days. Rarer complications are very small needle marks, infection, superficial white marks, and swelling. Only 1 in 10,000 patients develops problems away from the site of injection. These may include joint or muscle aches. Less than 1 in 1,000 patients will have local reactions at the site resulting in a small scar.

If you are not comfortable using materials derived from cows, there are currently at least two forms of human collagen available for injection. In addition, other connective tissue, called *fascia*, is available commercially.

USING YOUR OWN COLLAGEN

In a new technique, your own collagen is harvested, grown, and then reintroduced into areas that need to be filled. The dermatologist removes a small specimen of skin 3 millimeters across from behind your ear. This piece of tissue is sent to a commercial laboratory where your cells are multiplied in a culture or test tube. Once the specimen has expanded, it contains a concentrated dose of your own collagen. The company returns it to your physician to inject into the area to be treated. Because the collagen is from your own tissue there have been no reported allergic reactions to it. No infections or scarring have been reported either. Another product uses collagen fibers obtained from skin bank tissue.

GORE-TEX: NOT JUST FOR YOUR PARKA

Expanded polytetrafluorethylene (ePTFE), commonly known by the trade name Gore-Tex, is an inert substance that is tolerated by human tissue. It has been used for grafting blood vessels together and repairing hernias.

In the cosmetic realm, the most common use for these ePTFE grafts is in blunting the nasolabial fold and augmenting the lip lines. In a simple procedure small slit incisions are made at both ends of the area to be augmented. A strip of ePTFE is threaded through from one end to the other and then clipped at both ends. Both small openings are closed with one stitch.

Mild redness can be seen at the entry and exit points for several weeks, but this will fade, and infection and extrusion of the implants are rare. Because ePTFE is permanent, it is expected that the cosmetic results will also be permanent.

BOTULISM: THE FRIENDLY POISON

Despite the fact that botulism is a much feared toxin, it has important medical uses. Botulinum toxin, the product of an especially dangerous form of bacteria, acts by blocking the action of a certain chemical and its receptor in a muscle, so that a muscle is paralyzed. This effect has been exploited for beneficial results in kronotherapy.

The motion of facial muscles creates unflattering lines on our faces. The frown lines on our lower foreheads and between the eyebrows, as well as the crow's-feet alongside both eyes, are caused—and then made worse— by overaction of muscles. Injection of *very small amounts* of botulinum toxin will paralyze muscles within two to three days. The maximum amount of paralysis is reached about one to two weeks after injection, when the injected muscle fibers have shrunk in size as a result of not being used. Reduction in wrinkles lasting up to twelve months has been noted in several studies. However, retreatment is usually required in three to six months to maintain the effect.

Complications of injecting around the eyes may include a temporary droop of the eyelid. With injection into horizontal forehead lines, several patients have commented that their eyebrows have drooped slightly or that their forehead felt heavy. When treating the frown line between the eyebrows, complications are uncommon but have included a little droop of the upper eyelid. The droop will happen one to two weeks after injection if some of the botulinum toxin migrates into that area. The droop lasts anywhere from two to four weeks and occurs in approximately 2 to 3 percent of people.

Botox, the brand name for commonly used botulinum toxin, has also proven helpful in controlling excessive sweating of the armpits and palms. The toxin paralyzes the sweat gland unit in the skin. Botox treatment is safe and can be easily administered by your physician. Just keep in mind that repeat treatments will be needed.

THE HOME FACIAL REJUVENATION PROGRAM

To smooth the surface of the skin and get a refreshed look follow these easy steps:

1. Wear sunscreen daily and practice good sun-safe habits.
2. Moisturize daily with moisturizer than will not cause pimples (non-comedogenic).
3. Wash your face with tap water and nonsoap cleanser once a day.
4. At night, apply Retin-A in one of its forms (I prefer the form Retin-A Micro) as follows:
   a. Rinse your face with tap water and pat dry.
   b. Apply a small pea-sized amount of Retin-A to each of the regions of your face:
      - right and left forehead
      - right and left cheek
      - right and left area around the eyes (avoid contact with the eye itself)
      - chin
      - upper lip and lower lip
      - jaw region
   c. Massage in well.
   d. When starting Retin-A treatment, begin with this application schedule:
      - two nights per week for two weeks
      - three nights per week for one week
      - five nights per week for one week
      - nightly thereafter

   If redness, peeling, or irritation develops, discontinue use. Be sure to apply moisturizer. After skin has settled down, consider starting again more gradually if your dermatologist advises.

8 Dreams in a Bottle: Caring for Your Skin

When my sister has a new boyfriend, she sleeps with her makeup on. I'm an actress and when I get off the set, I can't wait to take my makeup off, so I can't understand this. I nag her all the time to take better care of her skin. Besides, I say, what happens if you marry the guy? You can't wear makeup twenty-four hours a day for the rest of your life.

—*Claire, 32*

In general, what you put on your skin must come off. Yet with all the attention and money paid to make up the face to be beautiful, many of us forget that makeup removal and the cleansing of the skin need to be approached carefully, so that your skin will remain in good shape for years to come. Using the right cleanser is so important that we'll begin this chapter with a thorough discussion of the various kinds of soaps and other cleansers—a topic that should be of equal concern to men and women—before going on to look at cosmetics.

▪ KEEPING THE SKIN CLEAN

Every day the skin is bombarded with dirt and dust particles, and if you wear makeup, then you have to add grease to the list. Most makeups are very greasy and cannot be removed with water alone.

You can take your pick from soaps of all kinds (including deodorant soaps, medicated soaps, or soapless soaps), washing creams or lotions, and cleansers that come in cream or lotion form. And that's just the beginning. Toners, astringents, and what are called clarifying lotions are also available, depending on how much time and money you wish to invest in skin care.

Soaps work to remove dirt because of chemicals called surfactants and emulsifiers. These chemicals are composed of molecules that can attach to both water and grease and thereby dissolve grease and oils from the skin.

If you are in a pinch, any soap will do. Whenever you have a choice, however, you'll want to use soaps sparingly and ideally select a nonsoap cleanser. The same qualities in regular soap that help lift off external oils and grease will also dissolve away the skin's natural fats or lipids, which keep the skin's own moisture locked in. The key principles to remember are:

- Too much washing leads to dry skin.
- Too much soap leads to dry skin.

OF AIRPLANES, AIRPORTS, AND SITTING ON THE TARMAC

As any seasoned traveler knows, the air in airplanes is brutal on the skin. It is very dry and all the sloughed skin cells contribute greatly to the dust in the closed environment.

Mode of travel aside, travel in general can wreak havoc on your body. Here are some skin tips for travel:

1. Drink plenty of water.
2. Do not spray water on your face—it will only evaporate in the dry environment of the airplane leading to drier skin.
3. Use a very light moisturizing cream.
4. Don't use hotel soaps—pack your favorite nonsoap cleanser.
5. Travel with your own shampoo.
6. Try to get some rest.

Probably the best approach to cleaning your face is to wash once a day and rinse once a day:

1. Wash your face with tap water and a nonsoap cleanser, such as Neutrogena Extra Gentle Cleanser, Aquanil, or Cetaphil once a day.

2. Rinse gently with tap water (no cleanser), once a day.

3. Always pat dry with a soft towel—do not rub.

SQUEAKY CLEAR ABOUT SOAPS

Regular soaps, also known as toilet soaps, are made from animal fats, vegetable oils, or olive oils. Other oils, such as coconut or palm kernel oil, may be added to promote lathering. Toilet soaps are inexpensive and can clean off dirt, dust, grease, and most cosmetics. Because they are alkaline by nature, however, they often irritate the skin. Also, when combined with "hard" water, soaps can leave behind a filmy residue on the skin.

Superfatted soaps are toilet soaps to which a moisturizer has been added. These contain 5 to 15 percent fat, compared with 2 percent in most soaps. Some people find these soaps less irritating than ordinary toilet soaps, while others complain they leave a greasy residue behind.

Soapless soaps are less paradoxical than they may sound. Simply put, they substitute fatty acids, petroleum products, or other substances for the ingredients found in regular soaps. They tend to irritate the skin less frequently than ordinary soaps.

WASHING CREAMS AND LOTIONS

Washing or washable creams or lotions are not much different from plain old bar soap except in price and packaging. The major difference is that a moisturizer is usually added to a soap or detergent base. The lotions are just like the creams, with more water added. These products are very popular now, especially for shower use. I have not seen many problems from the use of these cleansers.

CLEANSERS

Cleansers come in creams and lotions. Many of them are soap-free and therefore appropriate for those people who have allergic reactions to most soaps. Cleansers contain water and a cleansing agent, such as cetyl alcohol. The cleanser is applied to the skin and usually rubbed in until it begins to foam; it's then wiped away with a soft cloth rather than washed off with water, and a thin layer of moisturizer is left on the skin.

If you use heavy makeup, it is a good idea to use a second, lighter cleanser to make sure the skin is clean before leaving a layer of moisturizer behind. If makeup is left on the skin, it can clog pores and cause pimples.

Abrasive or exfoliating cleansers are also available. These contain granules intended literally to abrade your skin, sloughing off the dead cells. These cleansers may contain up to 25 percent pumice, a nice word for ground volcanic rock. Needless to say, such aggressive cleansing is not ideal. If you need a jackhammer to remove makeup residue, you should change makeup products.

Most people with normal skin find that exfoliating cleansers dry and irritate the skin, rather than leaving it smooth and glowing. Do not use these products if you have active acne since the pumice will only aggravate the condition.

WHAT KIND OF SKIN DO YOU HAVE?

The most common comments I hear from patients about their skin are: "My skin is too oily" or "My skin is too dry." Here's how to figure out where you are on the spectrum:

Normal skin has small pores, is smooth to the touch, and is neither dry nor oily.

Dry and/or sensitive skin possesses little natural oil and small pores. It becomes dehydrated, dulls easily, and is prone to lines and wrinkles.

Oily skin is prone to excessive oil secretion and is generally shiny. Pores are large and open. The skin is coarse and subject to blackheads.

Combination skin has both oily patches, usually on the central forehead, nose, and chin (the so-called T zone) and dry patches, usually occuring on the cheeks, jawline, and outer portion of the forehead.

If you really feel better using these products, be stingy. No matter how good you feel about the results of a single usage, you should refrain from frequent use. You'll find that the more you use one, the drier your skin will become. It may even start to flake and, in some cases, you may begin to notice broken blood vessels. So, proceed with caution.

TONERS, ASTRINGENTS, AND CLARIFYING LOTIONS

This group of skin-care products are often alcohol-based. Toners and astringents remove excess oil from the skin because alcohol dissolves fatty chemicals. They are usually scented to cover the medicinal smell of the alcohol. While the coolness they impart may give the impression of tighter pores and better skin tone, this tends to be a passing fancy.

An astringent or toner may also include other ingredients. Menthol or camphor adds to the cooling sensation. Salicylic acid or witch hazel are strong astringents that may even have a light peeling effect on the skin. In general, keep alcohol-containing products away from your skin as much as possible.

CLEANSING MASKS

If you wash your face regularly with a good cleansing agent, most cleansing masks will add little to your cleansing regime. However, if you do have oily skin, you may want to use an antibacterial cleansing mask now and then to help minimize the oil on your skin.

Some facial masks claim to reduce the redness in the skin and tighten pores. Although there is no solid evidence that this is so, many people report that using a light facial mask helps them feel better about their skin. If you can afford it and find the feeling of a facial mask pleasant, that is a good enough reason to indulge yourself when you have a spare ten or fifteen minutes. Facial masks will not remove large facial pores but may temporarily remove accumulated cells and oils that enlarge the pores and make them look big.

BATHING AND WASHING

Contrary to what you might think after riding on a crowded bus or subway or squeezing through a large crowd at the football stadium, we probably wash ourselves too often, sometimes bathing twice daily. Such frequent bathing dries skin, and the problem can be compounded by the use of harsh soaps. Remember, dry skin looks older and may even "age" more rapidly.

A mild soap should be used to wash areas that perspire a lot, such as the neck area and under the arms, and to wash the genital area. The dirt and grime accumulated during the day on the rest of the body can be removed, *without soap*, by cleaning the skin gently with a soft wash cloth or skin massage gloves and then rinsing with water. Avoiding the frequent use of soap will help maintain the proper natural oils on the surface of the skin which provides protection in the skin's daily battle with the world. Soapless soaps or cleansers may also be substituted for traditional bath soaps.

▪ MOIST IS GOOD, DRY IS BAD

Our skin is cleverly designed to prevent evaporation of moisture from within its topmost layer. Yet when the skin dries out, this protective ability is lost and the integrity of our skin and our comfort suffer. For this reason, proper moisturizing is critical.

Moisturizers can't make you younger, but they can keep your skin hydrated. Dry skin is the result of water loss in the stratum corneum—the surface layer of the epidermis. As the stratum corneum loses moisture, your skin starts to become drier and drier, until it eventually begins to flake. A good moisturizer serves two important functions: it retards moisture loss and helps to draw water back into the stratum corneum.

There are two kinds of moisturizers, oil-based and water-based. Moisturizers contain different kinds of oil, and the ratio of water to oil varies from product to product. Obviously, which type you choose will depend on your skin type. If your skin is oily and adulthood has brought you little relief from the acne blues, you'll want to use a water-based moisturizer in order to avoid burdening your pores with more oil. If your skin is dry to normal, you can go ahead and choose an oil-based moisturizer.

People with so-called combination skin (areas of dry skin and patches of oily skin) should stick with a water-based product. However, in wintertime, I advise my patients with combination skin to spend a little extra time on skin care and use two moisturizers—a water-based one for general skin care, and an oil-based one for particularly dry patches of skin. Avoid moisturizers that contain alcohol. These can sting and dry the skin as well.

Once you get past the basics—oil-based vs. water-based—there are scores of moisturizers to choose from. There are moisturizing creams,

lotions, gels . . . you name it. There are moisturizers that contain a sunscreen. The best advice is to find a product you like—it doesn't have to
have an expensive label—and apply it after showering. Keep a small tube
of special hand cream such as Neutrogena Hand Cream at the ready
if you tend to have dry hands and chapped lips, especially during the
winter.

▪ COSMETIC OR "COSMACEUTICAL"?

No one would doubt that lipstick, blush, foundation and even hair col-
oring are cosmetics. They are removable or they wear off, and they don't
change the structure or function of your skin.

However, the issue gets a bit trickier when talking about those creams
that include vitamin C, enzyme CoQ 10, or any other agents that are
intended to function as antioxidants. This category of compounds—on
whose behalf claims are made about decreasing fine lines and wrinkles and
even, perhaps, preventing skin cancer—is increasingly being called "cosmaceutical." In time we will probably identify a class of compounds that
do live in the no-man's-land between true cosmetic and true drug. For now,
be suspect of claims that seem unreasonable.

▪ COSMETICS

Most women know what cosmetics they like, tolerate, and prefer to buy.
Every consumer has her own preferred product, but the search for new lipsticks, lip gloss, eye makeup, etc., nonetheless continues. Open any medicine cabinet and you will see proof of this. The cosmetics industry is
marketing-rich: just like the cereal industry it knows that people will likely
buy many different brands of the same product. What drives this is the
human desire to get the newest and latest, and there is nothing wrong with
that. Just be sure to follow some simple rules:

- When it comes to makeup, keep it simple. Don't overspend. Don't
  overapply.

- Use only non-comedogenic (non–acne causing) products that are
  also hypoallergenic. Usually, the label clearly states these features.
  Makeup that is very oily can clog pores and precipitate acne. Chemicals in non-hypoallergenic makeup can lead to rashes.

- Once you've found a product or product line you like, stick with it. If you bounce around from one to the other, you increase the risk that you will happen upon a product that your skin doesn't like.

- In searching for the ideal product, go with a major brand. These manufacturers have enough money to thoroughly research their products before bringing them to market. (Regarding buying animal-tested products, this is purely a matter between you and your conscience. There is nothing intrinsically better, from the scientific viewpoint, about products that have not been animal-tested.)

- If you are buying a product from your doctor's office, be sure he or she knows what is in it.

- If you are buying herbal or "natural" products, be sure that the ingredients are listed. If you develop a rash, it will be helpful to know what it might be due to.

There are usually three types of ingredients to be concerned with when choosing a cosmetic. Active ingredients actually do something for your skin, such as moisturize it or protect it from the sun. Inactive ingredients are there to thicken, stiffen, or preserve the product—in essence, they are necessary to make the cosmetic "work." Finally there are exotic ingredients that may be hyped but are not yet proven to be of value.

WHAT DOES HYPOALLERGENIC MEAN?

Strictly speaking, hypoallergenic means that the cream or lotion will not cause an allergic reaction of the skin, akin to poison ivy or some other reaction that your immune system causes. These days, however, this term is taken by the public to mean a broad range of things. The labels on cosmetic products contain many of the following words, which all intend to imply hypoallergenicity in the broad general sense:

Hypoallergenic	Preservative-free
Non-sensitizing	PABA-free
Irritant-free	Non-irritating
Allergy-tested	Allergy-free

WHAT ABOUT ALLERGIES?

When you have a true allergic reaction to ingredients in the cosmetics you use, some patches of scaling and redness may develop. Fragrances and preservatives within cosmetics are among the most common causes of allergic reaction in skin. In one study, two-thirds of people with facial rash had some form of allergic contact dermatitis—in other words, their rash was due to something they were putting on their face. If you do develop a rash and believe a cosmetic or fragrance is to blame, see your dermatologist. An elimination program may be followed by skin-patch testing with specific compounds; this will help you avoid purchasing products that contain the specific offending agent.

SKIN CARE OR SKIN HEALTH?

Cosmetics are used to make our skin feel better and look better. Pharmaceuticals and even certain cosmaceuticals are used in an attempt to actually change the biology of our skin. Cosmaceuticals don't require FDA approval; medicated creams do. The main things to watch for with any cosmetic are irritation, acne, and allergic reaction. Not all sensitivities are allergic, but a red, rough, stinging rash or a pimply outbreak should be enough to get you to switch products.

Here are suggestions to get the most bang for your makeup buck:

1. Use a moisturizer that has an SPF of 15 or higher. This way, when you apply your facial moisturizer daily you'll at least know you have that baseline sun protection. After all, sun protection is the most important thing you can do to keep your skin looking young.

2. Always use lip balms with an SPF of 15 or higher.

3. Clean makeup brushes regularly with a gentle shampoo, such as a baby shampoo.

4. To get a subtle but noticeable glow on your cheeks use about a peppercorn of Vaseline on your cheekbones.

5. Be alert to eyelid rashes. These can be due to an allergy to your nail polish, which comes in contact with your eyelids when you rub your

eyes. The thin skin of the eyelids is especially sensitive to allergic reaction.

6. As often as possible try to let your hair dry naturally. If you must use a blow-dryer, wait until your hair is just damp, virtually dry.

▪ MAKEUP

CONCEALERS

When it comes to face makeup foundations are the heavy hitters. They are applied to the entire face and, as the name suggests, provide a base coat of facial "paint" that helps to hide blemishes, scars, fine lines, and small irregularities. Think of foundation as a housepainter would think of primer.

If you don't use that much makeup, but do want to hide that telltale blemish or slight skin discoloration, concealers offer a choice. They also help hide dark circles and shadows. Because they are heavier and creamier than foundation makeups, concealers should be used sparingly and only on specific areas of the face. Concealers are usually oil-based moisturizers with added pigments. If you are prone to acne, it's possible to find oil-free, medicated concealers that will help clear your acne while covering it up.

COVER STICKS

Some cosmetic users find cover sticks an easier and more convenient form of concealer that can camouflage a multitude of minor sins. It should be noted, however, that cover sticks do contain a lot of wax. This gives the makeup body and thickness, but it can also irritate the skin and cause acne-prone skin to break out.

POWDERS

Powders are used to absorb oil and reduce shininess, but in the process they can also clog pores. The popularity of face powder is probably due to the widely held belief that a shiny nose or cheek is an uglier nose or cheek.

The active ingredients in powder cosmetics are pigments and powders. Iron oxides are a common pigment. Other ingredients include talc, clay, starch, and agents that hold the powder together.

For very oily, acne-prone skin, a powder alone should be used; it will cause less pore clogging than a base or pancake with a powder applied on top.

To wash off powders and cream-based makeup, you might want to use two cleansers to be sure that you have removed every trace of these pore-clogging cosmetics.

BLUSH

Blushes can be oil-based or oil-free. They are used to add contour and color to your skin. Find one brand you like and stick to it.

EYE SHADOW AND EYE PENCIL

These are composed of pigments mixed in oil-wax bases. Cream eye makeups should be applied with a soft brush or sponge and washed off thoroughly with a gentle cleanser.

The skin of the eyelid and surrounding eye region is perhaps the most sensitive of your body's skin. It is extremely thin and is thus easily irritated. Therefore, treat it with care and kindness. Watch for makeup that contains mica, which may irritate the eye. If your eye makeup causes even minor irritation, try another product.

LIQUID LINER AND MASCARA

Inorganic pigments are the basic ingredient in liquid liners; film-forming or plasticizing chemicals, acrylic copolymers and acrylates, are then added. Such chemicals help the liners adhere and provide sheen. Don't apply these products under the rim of the eyelid or too close to the corners of the eyes, or you may experience itching and irritation.

MASCARA

Applied to the eyelashes to add the illusion of thickness and luster to thin or short lashes, mascara is formed by adding pigment to a moisturizing base. Conditioning mascaras, which contain water-based moisturizers, are also available. Waterproof mascaras contain oil-based moisturizers to which shellacs and other hardeners may be added. Although many mascara manufacturers tout special mascara removal aids, you can easily remove mascaras with a gentle moisturizer.

LIPSTICK AND LIP GLOSS

Lipsticks can be the stuff of romance and seduction. They are basically wax, oil, and pigment mixed together.

Many of the new brands boast that they protect against chapped lips and the sun's rays. Select lipstick with sunscreen that does not contain PABA since some people are allergic to this ingredient. In the absence of PABA, the dye in lipstick should be suspected if you develop lip irritation.

Many natural lip glosses are available. These do not color the lips, but they do keep them moist and shiny. Plain cocoa butter is a fine lip balm. Eye sticks, used to moisturize the particularly sensitive skin under the eyes, also work well to keep lips moist and healthy.

If you have an active herpes lesion, don't share your lipstick or lip gloss with someone else. By the same token, don't borrow lip products from someone with a fever blister.

▪ COSMACEUTICALS

The many claims made for all sorts of over-the-counter products are hard to sort out. As an experiment, pick up a copy of your favorite women's magazine (or even men's magazine) and look at the ads that are designed to catch your attention. In general, those for skin creams convey the impression that in some way the product will stall or reverse the aging process in your skin or make you look younger. The wording is carefully phrased—close enough to keep the Feds (the Food and Drug Administration, actually) parked outside on lookout, but not so outrageous that they barge in with a battering ram. It's good that companies know their claims are being very carefully watched, since it helps keep them honest.

▪ CELLULITE

A wide range of products claim to reduce cellulite, or the puckered appearance of fat on the thighs. I know of no cream, however, that has an effective chemical that penetrates the skin and dissolves the fibrous tethers that cause cellulite.

Cellasene is an aggressively marketed herbal remedy for cellulite that the manufacturer claims increases circulation. It contains ginkgo, sweet clover, bladder wrack, grape seed extract, fish oil, and lecithin, among other ingredients. Keep in mind that each capsule contains 240 milligrams of iodine, so people with thyroid problems can be adversely affected by chronic use of Cellasene. Also, the sweet clover and ginkgo might increase the risk of bleeding for patients on aspirin or warfarin.

Cellasene costs about $300 for a full course of treatment. As far as I know no peer-reviewed study has been published confirming that use of this supplement reduces cellulite or thigh girth. Although the risks are low, pregnant or nursing women should of course not use it.

Endodermologie is not a pill or cream but a treatment that involves passing a probe over cellulite-ridden skin. SilkLight is another one of these massage therapies. Although the FDA permits manufacturers of these devices to say that they can help make the skin look better, this is certainly not the same as saying that in proper trials it is proven to eliminate cellulite.

CELLULITE CREAMS

Most cellulite creams, sold by reputable companies, include the words *firming* and *body* in the name of the product. These are pretty safe words to use, since they don't specifically say what they are firming (most moisturizers can be said to be firming the epidermis). People who use these products say that their skin feels smoother, if they notice any effect at all.

STRETCH MARKS

Stretch marks that develop after pregnancy can be very frustrating. If they are noticeable because of redness, laser treatment of the redness may help improve their appearance. Some dermatologists believe that even Retin-A can help build up the collagen in the area, just as it does in sun-damaged skin, and thereby improve the appearance. Others have tried resurfacing lasers, like the kind used to remove wrinkles. Most recently, a new cream is being marketed as a cosmaceutical to improve or remove stretch marks. It has not been proven to work in any clinical trials although the manufacturer is now conducting a survey to see if it works (kind of backwards, in my opinion).

Stretch marks result from thinning of the epidermis and loss of collagen. The only way to improve the problem is to actually replace what is missing.

▪ VITAMIN C

The rationale for including vitamin C, an antioxidant, in skin creams is that it may remove the free radicals that cells produce. These free radicals are associated with skin cancer and premature aging of the skin such as that due to sun exposure. Many cosmaceuticals advertise that they contain vitamin C, but most forms of vitamin C are unstable when exposed to the air. Cellex C is a product that claims greater stability and even penetration into the skin.

While topical vitamin C may help lighten solar lentigos and melasma, it has not been shown to help rebuild collagen in the skin. There has been some scientific evidence that the correct form of topical vitamin C provides additional protection against the harmful effects of the sun.

Until it can be reliably shown that vitamin C penetrates through the epidermis, there is no reason to believe that it will have an effect on collagen production, and thus on wrinkles.

▪ RETIN-A

The news regarding salvaging damaged skin is promising. Skin that has been regularly overexposed to the sun will never look as good as skin that has been consistently protected from the sun and other damaging environmental elements. I can safely say that some improvement of skin quality is possible through treatment with Retin-A.

The improvement Retin-A helps to make in sun-damaged skin begins reasonably quickly, within three months. Tretinoin, the active ingredient in Retin-A, and its cousins Renova and Retin-A Micro, is approved by the FDA as a safe and effective means to improve the appearance of sun-damaged skin. Many people have tried Retin-A but complain that it doesn't help improve the fine lines and wrinkles. Upon further investigation, it is clear that these people have usually discontinued use of the medication because of dryness or irritation. See recommendations for a home facial program on page 74 on how to step into the use of Retin-A slowly and carefully. When using Retin-A it is also important to keep your skin well moisturized (to minimize dryness) and use sunscreen regularly.

▪ WHAT ABOUT NATURAL INGREDIENTS?

Guess what? Retin-A is a form of vitamin A, which comes from carotene, which is present in carrots. Carrots come from the ground and are of course natural. So it goes with so many compounds in medicine. There are many "natural" agents that can be found in health care products.

Here are just a few of the natural ingredients you'll find in some of the most popular skin care products. Look for them when you read the labels before choosing a product.

- *Alpha-hydroxy acids (AHAs)*, an ingredient in a wide range of moisturizers and anti-aging creams, are as natural as they can be. Glycolic acid is derived from sugar cane. Lactic acid comes from milk, malic from apples, and tartaric from grapes. Citric is an AHA that has been around for a while. AHAs are thought to soften lines and wrinkles, improve skin tone, help erase age spots or sun spots, and even control acne.

- *Clay* is used as a base in many facial masks. It is rich in minerals and is known as nature's detoxifier. Clay masks may help improve circulation temporarily, cleanse the surface of the skin, and revitalize it. Clay is not considered a cause of allergic reactions in the skin.

- *Oat* is a natural grain that is rich in vitamins and minerals. This cereal protein, with an excellent balance of amino acids, is used in many cosmetic products. It is known to soothe sensitive skin and relieve itching and other irritations. It is also an effective moisturizer since it is a humectant, which means it promotes the retention of moisture—just what your skin needs.

- *Plant oils* were used to make the first cosmetics and are now back in vogue. You'll find them in many of today's most popular moisturizers. Some of the most popular plant oils used in cosmetics are almond, apricot, avocado, flaxseed, hazelnut, olive, sesame, and wheat germ oils. Some of these oils are comedogenic (see Appendix 4, Selective Guide to Skin Care Products).

- *Aloe vera* is a useful, versatile addition to the skin care world. The spearlike, fleshy leaves of this tropical plant contain a clear and viscous natural gel. When applied to the skin, this gel helps promote healing. The therapeutic properties of aloe vera gel in burn treatment have long been known, but now this rather remarkable plant is becoming recognized for other reasons as well. Aloe vera gel is also a humectant, helping the skin to retain moisture as it penetrates to the deeper layers. For this reason, it may help heal wounds other than burns, such as scrapes and abrasions.

9 Skin and the Environment Around Us

Q. When I was a teenager I relocated with my family to a tropical island for one year. During that time, I had a couple of blistering sunburns, which I still remember very well. I am fair-skinned, of Polish descent. Could this have led to the melanoma I recently developed on my shoulder?

A. *There is no question that a blistering sunburn can be associated with skin cancer. If you've had such experiences in childhood you should pay special attention to monitoring for the early signs of skin cancer.*

We often take our environment for granted. We believe that, like the weather, there is little we can do about it. It is only when we are confronted with changes we don't expect (such as the aging of our skin) or a medical problem we didn't anticipate that we suddenly become aware of the fact that we can run but we cannot hide. When it comes to the effects of the sun on the skin, this is especially true.

Sun is the source of all life on earth. Without it, we might as well be living on Mars: no flowers, no wheat, no bread, no life. Ancient Egyptians worshiped the sun,

IS FUN IN THE SUN DUMB?

It seems to be for one particular group: women between the ages of 16 and 24. These are the most frequent patrons of tanning salons. Guess what group has demonstrated the greatest increase in melanoma incidence? Women ages 24 to 35. While the link between sun exposure and melanoma is not as strong as that between ultraviolet radiation and non-melanoma skin cancer, this statistical observation probably represents a serious problem for women who seek youth and health in tanning salons, and in the end will age prematurely and may get cancer.

French monarchs adopted it as their icon (remember the Sun King?), and today we talk of a different kind of sun worshiper: the kind who "pray" on ocean beaches, mountain lakes, and even urban rooftops.

Even people who have had skin cancer cannot ignore the fact that we do *like* the sun. Lying out on the beach under an endless blue sky or feeling the warmth of the sun on our shoulders is a pleasant experience. The tingling warmth of the sun on our face somehow makes us feel alive. We enjoy the sun, I think, because it makes us feel good, and because deep down, rooted somewhere in our psyche, it makes us feel vital.

Research on seasonal affective disorder, or SAD, indicates that sunlight plays an important role in our moods and daily biorhythms. Through a complex process sunlight acts on a small gland between and behind our eyes, called the pineal gland, to make sure that our hormone system cycles properly throughout the day and night. When changes in the cycles of light and dark occur, our mood changes. Think about why we welcome Santa Claus and his reindeer to brighten the northern skies in winter. The short days and long nights of the North Atlantic nations make winter a dreary time. Something was needed to compensate for the lack of sunlight. Feasts of Saturnalia, decorations, special foods, gifts—what better way to fight off the blues of a dark and dreary winter?

Our love of the sun permeates our lives, our language: "My, that child has a sunny disposition," we might be heard saying. For this reason it is very hard to convince people that the sun has a dark side. Were this not the case, Club Med would have resorts in caves and architects who design buildings without windows would be the most sought after in the world.

The attraction of the sun goes beyond how it feels. It has to do with its

WHAT IS SPF?

This is what "SPF" means: a product with a Sun Protection Factor (SPF) of 15 allows you to stay in the sun 15 times longer than you normally would be able to before getting red. An SPF 30 allows you to stay out 30 times as long. If you normally get red after 10 minutes, an SPF 30 should allow you to stay in the sun 300 minutes (30×10 minutes) before turning red. The problem with these ratings is that they are inexact.

SOLUTION: Find a product you like and determine how much protection one application provides. Then, apply regularly at proper intervals being certain to apply the sunscreen about 30 minutes before first going outdoors.

tanning effect as well. Isn't it a little strange that so many of us, whether we are light or dark-skinned, seem to have this overwhelming desire to literally change our color? Those who are pale want to grow dark, and in many cultures, those who are dark want to grow pale so intensely that they will use strong bleaching creams and ointments to try to do so. This desire to change color is also reflected in the attraction of opposites. When Fletcher Christian arrived in Tahiti with his mutinous crew of the *Bounty* he discovered that the Polynesian women were fascinated by the fair-skinned Europeans who washed up on their shores. Their descendants on Pitcairn Island, where they settled, now attest to the fact that the attraction went well beyond fascination.

It's ironic that the vanity element of sun worship, the bronze tan, has such blatant historical contradictions. *Gone with the Wind* is a good example. What fashion accessory was most notable among the fine women of Atlanta? The parasol! It was such an important defense against developing a tan that the name of a currently used sunscreen chemical, *Parsol*, may not be a complete accident. In the South and elsewhere until the turn of the century, having a tan was considered a sign of low class. A tan suggested that you were a laborer, someone who toiled outdoors, not a person of leisure and wealth. Scarlett O'Hara was not allowed to show her bosom before three o'clock so that she wouldn't get freckled. This value extends back in time to before the Victorian era, when the rough, sun-hewn skin of laborers was easily identified as a social nonstarter. But in our century something happened—through changes in fashion, advertising, and probably leisure time—a tan came to symbolize glamour, health, and wealth. The cartoon strip *Doonesbury*, for instance, got enormous mileage out of the actor George Hamilton's obsession with tanning. Month after month, *Doonesbury* wryly poked fun at the silliness of tanning, using it as a metaphor for vanity. Now we can add danger to that as well.

Here are some cold facts about radiation from the sun. Known to doctors and scientists as UVR, ultraviolet radiation from the sun is something we can't feel (it is *not* the warmth we feel from the sun), can't see, can't smell, and can't reach out and catch. But its power is inescapable.

On a day-to-day basis we may encounter many different types of radiation. There is ultraviolet radiation from the sun, X-rays used in CT scanning, and microwave radiation we use in cooking. Even radio waves are a form of non-harmful radiation. Ultraviolet radiation from the sun actually refers to two main types of UVR—UVA, or long wave UV radiation, and UVB, which has a shorter wavelength.

When radiation is emitted from the sun, it is transmitted to the earth's surface. When it is absorbed by the skin, it can prematurely age the skin or even lead to skin cancer. The best way to minimize one's exposure to UVR is to stay indoors for life. This is not only impractical—it would be harmful in other ways: it would prevent us from leading a normal social existence. It has been suggested that people may be at risk from low-intensity ultraviolet radiation emanating from the fluorescent or halogen lamps used in offices and homes. However, there is no scientific evidence that this exposure can lead to cancer. While medical history is filled with examples of new information developing down the road when better measuring techniques become available, I believe that exposure to normal indoor lighting is not a risk for skin cancer or premature aging.

The power of sunlight has become especially worrisome because many believe that thinning of the ozone layer, caused by the release of chlorofluorocarbons into the atmosphere, now permits more of the sun's radiation to reach the earth's surface. Therefore, more UVR rays reach our skin. While there is some debate about how quickly the ozone layer is depleting, and what its real impact is on UVR penetration, it is likely that the increased strength of these rays accounts in some part for the increase in skin cancer that we are seeing throughout the world. In fact, ultraviolet B (UVB), the cancer-causing rays, now reach the earth's surface in greater levels than ever before. It is estimated that for every 1 percent decrease in the ozone layer, there is a 6 percent increase in the incidence of non-melanoma skin cancer such as basal cell cancer and squamous cell cancer.

UVR has been linked to other health problems as well, most notably cataracts and depression of the immune system.

Too much sun can also damage our DNA, the essential building block of all life, which among other things directs our cells to make key proteins. When the sun damages your DNA, the ability of DNA to produce proteins is altered. Certainly repair of sun-damaged DNA is part of the body's biological repertoire, but this capacity is not endless. A few years ago, Douglas Brash, Ph.D., a researcher at Yale, and I studied tissue from my skin cancer patients. With the help of one of Brash's lab assistants, it was determined that UVR was the sole cause of a specific mutation in the cells of the top layer of the skin we studied. This mutation, in which the DNA was altered, could only have been caused by UVR. Cigarette smoke couldn't cause it, toxic waste couldn't cause it, bad thoughts couldn't cause it. By studying the skin cancers and pre-skin cancers of patients we also discovered not only that UVR from the sun caused this mutation in a gene called p53, but that damage to this change in the gene likely resulted, eventually, in the development of skin cancer. For the first time, we understood how the sun actually damages the skin and causes skin cancer.

> ### SOME MEDICATIONS THAT DON'T MIX WITH SUN
>
> - Doxycycline (Vibramycin, Monodox)
> - Furosemide (Lasix)
> - Tetracycline
> - Sulfonamides (Bactrim, Septra, gantrisin)
>
> There are others. Check with your doctor.

Having identified at least one important step in this process, it now has become possible to explore ways to reverse this damage and even, ideally, prevent it. Several exciting compounds are now being developed that will probably in time do away with the need for most surgical treatment of many skin cancers and, more important, provide a true sun protection, one that is more than a sunscreen or a sunblock. It could actually reverse the genetic injury before it has a chance to lead to skin cancer. I've called this agent the *morning-after cream*. Too much volleyball on the beach? Too much unprotected golf or tennis? Apply the cream that reverses the DNA mutations and you should be able to stop the development of skin cancer dead in its tracks. A medication that can accomplish this is now the goal of many skin cancer researchers, and active clinical trials are now in progress (see www.totalskinmd.com).

▪ SUNBURN

Minor sunburns are just that—minor. But if you are out in the sun for a long period of time your skin needs a lot of protection, including sunscreen, a hat, and adequate clothing. Without such protection, after hours in the sun you could end up with a burn severe enough to cause swelling and chills, necessitating a doctor's attention.

Severe sunburns often occur because the effects of the sun's rays do not appear for a few hours. Consequently, a person can't tell that he or she is getting a burn and continues to bask in the sun while the burn worsens. In fact, the full effect of sunburn is usually not felt until eighteen hours after the exposure. Because the sun doesn't warn us the way the heat of a flame does, the damage caused by sunburn can be as bad as, or even worse than, that caused by most minor heat burns. In addition, there are many medications that can make sunburn worse. If you are taking any medications, check with your doctor to find out whether what you are taking increases your sensitivity to sunlight; or see if they're listed in the box on page 95.

Symptoms of sunburn include red and tender skin, swelling, blistering, pain that worsens when the skin is touched, and increased sensitivity to any amount of heat. If the sunburn is severe enough, you may experience nausea, vomiting, dizziness, and flulike symptoms.

Obviously, the best policy is to avoid sunburn in the first place. However, even the most cautious of us sometimes make mistakes, so here is what to do if you or someone you are with is suffering from the effects of sunburn. First, cool off; since even a cool shower may be too painful, immerse yourself in a tepid to cool bath. Adding colloidal oatmeal (Aveeno) may be soothing. (Showering can make the sunburn more painful.) Second, treat the sunburn with an over-the-counter hydrocortisone cream to reduce the inflammation and encourage healing. You may prefer creams rather than ointments because they are moisturizing as well. The use of aloe vera gel is popular and it has a soothing effect. Commercial preparations of gel derived from aloe vera may help alleviate the discomfort. In some cases of severe sunburn, your doctor may prescribe oral prednisone, a form of corticosteroid, to reduce the pain and swelling. Non-steroidal anti-inflammatory medications such as Motrin (ibuprofen), may also help control the discomfort. Never use aspirin in children because of the risk of Reye's syndrome.

TREATING YOUR SUNBURN

1. Take a tepid bath with colloidal oatmeal (Aveeno).
2. Rest in a cool room.
3. Take aspirin (*adults only*) or ibuprofen to control discomfort.
4. Keep well hydrated.
5. Apply hydrocortisone cream 1% (over-the-counter) two to three times day.
6. Apply moisturizers liberally (make sure your moisturizer doesn't contain alcohol).
7. Promise yourself you will be more careful next time.

This list of simple tips should help keep your relationship with the sun healthy and damage-free:

- Whenever possible, avoid spending time in the sun between the hours of 10 A.M. and 4 P.M. The sun is most intense during these hours. Remember to correct for Daylight Savings Time.

- Avoid spending long periods of time in the sun. If it's possible to find shade or go inside for a few minutes, do so. If you're playing eighteen holes of golf and a little siesta indoors is out of the question, take shade breaks under a tree whenever possible.

BABY, THE SUN, AND YOU

It has been reported that the average person receives 85 percent of the sun exposure he or she will have in a lifetime by the age of eighteen. Children's skin is more susceptible to sun damage. For these reasons PROTECT YOUR CHILDREN FROM THE SUN. This point was driven home to me after we had our first child, who is very fair-skinned. His baby-sitter took him out for a stroll when he was about two years old. Later that night I noticed his lower shins were sunburned. I remembered the saying about the shoemaker's children going shoeless, and from that day on made sure that our children used sunscreen and avoided excessive sun exposure. Now my kids chastise me if I forget to apply my sunscreen.

- Wear a waterproof sunscreen with an SPF of 15 or more, depending on how fair your skin is.

- Make sure your sunscreen provides "broad-spectrum" protection, blocking both UVA and UVB rays.

- Wear your sunscreen in the winter as well, particularly if you engage in outdoor sports such as skating, skiing, or snowboarding.

- Apply your sunscreen prior to going out in the sun, and don't skimp on the amount you use. Similarly, you needn't overdo it. A thin, but thorough coating is sufficient.

- Don't forget your lips. Use a lip balm containing a sunscreen that protects against both UVA and UVB rays.

- Keep babies covered and in the shade. If there is no shade, bring a parasol or umbrella. Bonnets are a great accessory for infants and toddlers.

- Especially for children, consider special sun-protective clothing, especially a hat (see Appendix 4: Selective Guide to Skin Care Products).

- Never, never, never use a tanning parlor.

▪ PERMANENT SKIN CHANGES AND THE SUN

When the repair mechanisms in our DNA become unable to keep up with the pace at which ultraviolet radiation damage is occurring to the skin, we begin to see permanent changes in the skin.

For one thing, *actinic keratoses* develop. These are irregular, scaly patches of rough skin, which are usually pink to red. Liver spots or sun spots, tan or brown patches that appear most frequently on the face, backs of the hands, and other parts of the body, also develop. Other common signs of "photo-damage" (*photo* is Greek for light) include broken blood vessels, wrinkles, and in the extreme case yellow pebbling of the skin which resembles chicken skin.

Loss of elasticity is also a major factor that makes the skin look old.

SUNSCREENS VERSUS SUNBLOCKS

Sunscreens are different from sunblocks. Sunscreens contain active chemicals such as benzophenones (e.g., oxybenzone), cinnamates, salicylates (octyl salicylate). A few may even still contain PABA (para-aminobenzoic acid), a compound some people are allergic to. Sunscreens prevent sun damage by chemically absorbing the energy of the ultraviolet radiation before it can bombard the epidermis.

Sunblocks, such as zinc oxide or titanium dioxide, actually physically block the radiation, reflecting it off the skin. Blocks are less likely to cause allergic reactions and are sometimes called "chemical-free."

Because of UVA rays, excessive sun exposure causes the loss of elasticity in the dermis. In animals, just a few exposures of UVA, similar to that which a teenager might get on a tanning bed, blows important elastin tissue to pieces. Under the microscope, one can see the fragments of elastin tissue dispersed in a helter-skelter fashion. To simulate this, cut an elastic band into quarter-inch pieces and see how well it snaps back! Elastin tissue damaged in this way will never help the skin snap back into shape. And skin that doesn't snap back is wrinkled forever.

■ PROTECTION IN WIND AND COLD

Summer sun is not the only environmental danger to which we expose our skin. Cold, wind, and even winter sun can be damaging and take their toll on the health, appearance, and comfort of our skin.

Frostnip, the earliest stage of frostbite, is reversible. When frostnip occurs, the skin becomes white or icy to the touch and becomes less

PREFERRED SUNBLOCKS	PREFERRED SUNSCREENS
Neutrogena Chemical Free (titanium dioxide)	Ombrelle
	Sundown
Sundown Sunblock Ultra	Bullfrog
Baby Garde Sunblock Lotion	Waterbabies
	Presun

IS SPF JUST A NUMBERS GAME?

A product with SPF 15 blocks about 96 percent of UV rays. A product with an SPF of 30 blocks about 97 percent of UV rays.

The higher the SPF number, the less additional protection you get.

Use an SPF rated at least 15 and apply it regularly. Leave the bottle in a place where you'll be reminded to use it.

sensitive. Unlike frostbite, frostnip is easily treated. The best way to do this is to make sure the affected area is dry and then press it against an area of skin that is warm, such as under the arm, if accessible, or against the abdomen. If frostnip occurs on the toes, rub your hands together until they are warm and wrap the toes in your fingers. Most important, anyone suffering from frostnip should get out of the cold. Further exposure to the cold will cause the condition to deteriorate quickly into frostbite, which can cause permanent damage to the skin.

Frostbite occurs when the skin is exposed to extremely cold temperatures for long periods of time. Under these conditions, the skin and the underlying tissues actually freeze. The areas most commonly affected by frostbite are the nose, ears, feet, and hands.

Though 32 degrees F is considered the freezing temperature, internal body temperature must fall to a temperature far lower than that before tissues in certain areas begin to freeze. Frostbite is much more likely in people suffering from dehydration and lack of adequate food, clothing, or shelter. In addition, excessive exposure to wind or wet weather may hasten the onset of frostbite.

The skin of someone suffering from frostbite will look pale, and white patches that are cold to the touch may appear. Sometimes the affected area may be numb, but it may also ache. When the skin begins to thaw, the area will feel raw and there will be moderate to severe pain, depending on how long the skin has been frostbitten. As with many skin conditions, treating frostbite can be simple or difficult, depending on the severity of the condition. Obviously, the best chance of a full recovery occurs when the skin has been frozen for only a short period of time.

To begin treatment, allow normal body temperature to be restored. Never attempt to thaw frostbitten flesh until body temperature has been normalized. If frostbite is severe and it is possible to obtain emergency services, you should call EMS. If this is not possible, the current choice for treating frostbitten hands or feet is to submerge the affected area in warm water—do *not* use hot water!—to thaw the area rapidly. Temperatures that are easily tolerated by normal skin can burn frostbitten skin, so avoid using a heating pad. As the skin thaws, the frostbitten person should feel tingling and burning sensations in the affected area. This indicates returning circulation. If the area remains numb, you must seek emergency treatment. The time it takes skin to thaw depends on the depth of the freezing. The thawing process is complete when the area flushes, or reddens. In some cases, permanent scarring and chronic temperature sensitivity may result after frostbite.

▪ DRY SKIN

Everyone experiences dry skin at some point in life, some more than others. In the modern world, dry skin has become so prevalent that dermatologists even refer to it by the fancy name of *xerosis*. One nickname for dry skin is "winter itch," because it occurs most frequently in the fall and winter, when the humidity level tends to be low. Severe dry skin usually appears in areas where the number of oil glands is low, such as the trunk, arms, and legs. As we age, our oil glands slow down (like everything else!) and our ability to keep our skin moist is affected. So significant is the change in skin as we age that dry skin is a major problem in older patients. When dryness of skin is combined with the natural thinning of skin that occurs over time as well, scratching can lead to superficial skin infection. Preventing dry skin at all ages is important for comfort; in the older patient, keeping skin moist will also prevent a vicious cycle of scratching and infection.

In general, as the skin dries out, the dead cells of the epidermis harden.

FOR CHAPPED LIPS AND CRACKED SKIN

Aquaphor®
Vaseline (petroleum jelly)
Curel Skin Healing Stick
Bag balm: Used by farmers to treat irritated cow udders. Some people consider this product excellent for chapped lips. Contains lanolin.

With time, this harder layer of skin is likely to crack in places, causing the itching associated with very dry skin.

While dry skin may occur more frequently in the winter months, there are other contributing factors to the condition. For example, the excessive use of soap can deplete the skin surface of the fatty molecules that help retain moisture. People who wash their hands frequently—a health care professional, an artist who works with clay, or a homemaker who cooks most meals—may find they have extremely dry chapped hands because of frequent washing.

Excessive bathing may also dry out skin. Indoor plumbing (and the resultant ability to bathe daily) is a great mark of human progress, but as with all aspects of life you can have too much of a good thing. Bathing daily can cause skin to become drier and drier (and it's worse for people who exercise frequently and then take two showers a day, or a bath and a shower).

But that doesn't make sense, you say. Water is wet, the opposite of dry. How can bathing in wet water make your skin dry? Simple—think about the process of evaporation. As you towel off, room air helps dry you through evaporation. The added dryness from this process also saps the skin of its intrinsic moisture. Therefore, too much washing, whether it be in the form of showers or baths, results in dry skin.

What to do? Moisturize, moisturize, moisturize. While using a moisturizer on your face will not retard the aging process, using a good moisturizer on your body after your bath or shower will minimize dry skin. If you love to relax in a bath, add a bath oil—not bubble bath—to the water to keep your skin from drying. When you're showering just to get clean, make it fast. Don't use hot water. Not only will you minimize the chances of itchy dry skin, you'll be saving water, which will please your children and ardent environmentalists.

INDUSTRIAL-STRENGTH MOISTURIZERS

If you need extra-strong moisturizers use those that contain either urea or lactic acid.

Lactic Acid	**Urea**
Amlactin	Carmol 10 Lotion
Lac-Hydrin	Carmol 20 Cream

Avoid products with alcohol: they dry.

MOISTURIZERS FOR DAILY USE

. Avoid products with alcohol. For mild dryness, use creams; for very dry skin, ointments work well.

Neutrogena Moisture SPF 15
Eucerin Cream; Eucerin Plus
Complex 15
Moisturel
Purpose

Aquaphor (ointment)
Alpha-hydroxy acid containing
    moisturizers (may sting if skin is
    very dry or cracked)

If you wash your hands often and use an antibacterial soap, make sure it is a mild one. Lever 2000 or Dial are good products. Phisoderm is an excellent heavy-duty cleanser used by health professionals. Whatever you do, though, don't obsess about hand washing. You can take a little bit of a good thing too far.

10

Healthy Nutrition
and Your Skin

*I used to get terrible rashes on my arms but I
changed my diet and haven't had a breakout
since.*

—*Don, 39, maintenance worker.*

Good nutrition is good for you. While few would argue
with this statement, most of us don't live by it. Instead
we try to thrive by the idea that fast is good, the quick fix
is it. Add to this our equal and opposite obsessions with
food and weight, and you've got the recipe for unhealthy
nutrition.

Ironically, more of us than ever patronize health food
stores these days, hopeful that such places are meccas of
good health and even cures. The idea that we are what we
eat finds special emphasis in dermatology, where a per-
sisting misconception is that "chocolate causes acne."
While it is in some ways true that we are what we eat when
it comes to heart disease (too many low-density lipids and
too much cholesterol are bad, high-density lipids are
good), the same is not always true for other conditions and
aspects of health. Teasing out the facts about nutrition and
skin is especially important in a society where food has
become a fetish and good nutrition is expected to heal all.

Would that it were so. But there are many areas in dermatology, in both health and disease, where nutrition plays an important role, largely by contributing to general health.

The skin can hardly be unaffected by what we do to our bodies. Thus, it's clear that nutrition is important to the skin—although not in the ways some readers or vitamin pushers wish it might be. In other words, generally speaking, changes in your dietary habits *cannot* solve your skin woes.

The increasing role of nutrition in health reflects a general interest in macrobiotic diets and the use of diet to control high cholesterol, osteoporosis, and a whole host of conditions. However, many people begin to think what they eat can cure *whatever* they have. It can't. Exceptions to this include specific allergies and diseases that are caused by particular foods and manifest with skin symptoms. In the wide world of skin, while diet can help contribute to its overall health, it usually will not make a difference when it comes to a particular ailment. Take acne, for example—we now know that greasy foods, salt, and chocolate have little impact on whether or not an individual experiences outbreaks of acne.

There are basically three questions to consider when thinking about nutrition and the skin. In what way does the skin itself function in maintaining proper nutrition in the body? What few people know is that there are many processes that occur within the layers of our skin that are distinctly nutritional in nature. Second, under normal circumstances, can changes in diet influence the color, texture, appearance, or nature of our skin? Third, in conditions where the skin is not functioning properly (that is, when certain diseases have developed) can changes in nutrition prove beneficial? The rest of this chapter addresses these three questions.

▪ SWEAT, NUTRIENTS, AND THE SKIN

Under normal circumstances small amounts of nutrients are lost in sweat through the skin and in the horny layer of the skin surface that flakes off on a regular basis.

Human sweat is a weak salt solution, consisting of sodium, chloride, potassium, calcium, and even urea. The actual amount of salt lost in this way from routine sweating is really minimal and of no great significance (a young adult male will lose only 360 mg of nitrogen and 149 mg of calcium in a twenty-four-hour period). Where sweat loss is extreme, there can be enough of a depletion of sodium to produce a life-threatening situation.

This can happen when heavy sweating occurs in very hot environments or during excessive exercise.

Perhaps the most serious circumstance where there is a loss of nutrients through the skin is in burn trauma. The same dangers can occur in a few rare skin conditions, where the body forms blisters that simulate a burn situation. In both these circumstances, there can be massive loss of protein from the serum (the fluid or liquid part of blood). This highlights the fact that when the skin loses its normal barrier function, important compounds can escape from the body, thus creating a precarious situation. In general, however, it is important to realize that under normal circumstances when we sweat there is no significant loss of important nutrients through the skin.

▪ VITAMIN D, A NATURAL WONDER

A most fascinating and unexpected nutritional role of the skin is the one it plays in the metabolism of vitamin D, a very important nutrient for maintaining healthy bones, teeth, and skin.

It was only at the turn of the twentieth century that the role of sunlight came to be understood as important for health. The function of skin in vitamin D metabolism was discovered as a result of a major socioeconomic change that occurred in the preceding century, the Industrial Revolution. This revolution resulted in the mass migration of people from the country to the cities, where dense slums were hastily thrown up to accommodate the teeming population. These new urban immigrants worked long shifts and lived in dark buildings, looking out on sunless alleys. Factory workers received far less sun exposure than had been the case when they lived in the countryside and often worked outdoors.

As early as the 1600s observers noted that young working-class children in crowded areas in London and Manchester developed rickets, but it was the Industrial Revolution that made this disease a household word. Rickets is a bone-deforming condition that makes legs bowed, literally bow-legged. Muscle weakness is a serious symptom of rickets, which can deform other long bones as well. Amazingly, by the beginning of the twentieth century, approximately 90 percent of children living in cities of northern Europe were affected by this disease.

No one was quite sure what the cause was. Some believed it was an inherited disorder, others suggested it was caused by an infection, and still others thought that either a lack of activity or nutritional deficiency could explain it. In 1822, a Polish scientist had suggested that rickets was caused by the absence of sun, but his theory languished obscurely in scientific journals for about a century. Eventually, in a small experiment in 1921, eight children with rickets were regularly exposed to natural sunlight on the roof of a New York hospital; within several months their condition improved. Around this time other investigators zeroed in on the essential dietary factor, present in cod liver oil, that seemed to fix the problem of bowed bones. Interestingly, artificial light, in the form of the mercury vapor lamp, was able to simulate the effect of this compound and cure rickets in animals. Finally, in the 1930s, the element that was present in foods like cod liver oil and which seemed magically to get activated by the sun was identified: vitamin D.

As it turned out, vitamin D wasn't just vitamin D—it had many different variations. It also became clear that during and immediately after exposure to sun, events happened in human skin that led it to manufacture vitamin D. The complex chemistry of vitamin D wasn't worked out until the 1970s and 1980s: when vitamin D in the skin is exposed to ultraviolet light from the sun, one form of vitamin D promptly converts to other forms of the nutrient. Those other forms of the vitamin get into the circulatory system through blood vessels in the skin and play a critical role in the development and maintenance of healthy bones and teeth. These days, with the heavy supplementation of milk and food with vitamin D, the possibility of a vitamin D deficiency caused by little exposure to the sun is small. Combine a poor diet and no vitamin supplements with a life where the sun is always shut out, however, and the risk of vitamin D deficiency is real.

I need to point out that as far as doses of vitamin D go, this is a prime example of "more may not be better." Some people might think that since a little bit of vitamin D is good for bones, why not take a whole lot more? Or why not stay out in the sun and allow your body to manufacture more vitamin D than it might actually need? The problem is that vitamin D is a fat-soluble vitamin. Fat-soluble nutrients stay in the body for a very long time, building up when too much is ingested. In fact, you could develop toxic levels by taking too much artificial vitamin D supplement.

▪ CAN VITAMIN A AND ITS DERIVATIVES IMPROVE SKIN?

Another compound that has a close connection with the skin is vitamin A. When it was isolated from egg yolk in 1909, it was originally called fat-soluble factor A and known to be important for the normal growth of animals. Later, as its critical role in growth, vision, reproduction, and skin maintenance emerged, it was renamed vitamin A. As we now use the term, vitamin A refers to a whole host of compounds, not one specific chemical. Generally speaking, vitamin A derivatives have a counterpart in nature: carotenoids, so called because they are found in carrots, a natural source of vitamin A, as Bugs Bunny has known for a long time. In over-the-counter cosmetics one will often see the word *retinal* or *retinoid,* which refers to the entire group of naturally occurring and even artificially manufactured vitamin A–type compounds.

Vitamin A and its derivatives are extremely important in dermatology. They help treat diseases and they provide cosmetic benefits. Retin-A is a derivative of vitamin A that has been used to treat acne for decades and has become popular as an agent that is proven to reduce fine lines and wrinkles. Renova and Retin-A Micro are two brand names of this compound.

Isotretinoin, known as Accutane, is a vitamin A formulation taken by mouth that has proven extremely helpful in treating cystic acne but has the associated risk of causing birth deformities. Needless to say, no dermatologist or other physician should prescribe isotretinoin without carefully making sure the patient, if of child-bearing age, understands the risks and is willing to use an appropriate form of birth control. Blood lipids can rise when a person is on Accutane—anyone at risk for heart disease should be especially careful.

Very rarely a condition called *pseudotumor cerebri* can develop in those taking isotretinoin; persistent headache with changes in vision occur. The symptoms usually respond promptly when the drug is stopped. Even depression and psychiatric disturbances can occur in very unusual circumstances. Excess intake of vitamin A itself can lead to side effects similar to those of Accutane, including shedding of skin and hair loss. Overall, vitamin A products have been extremely helpful in managing skin diseases and are even more promising in terms of solutions to cosmetic needs of patients.

Vitamin A is stored in the liver and released to the body as needed. Vitamin A works on the skin cell itself in many ways. It may cause a whole range of effects, many of which are beneficial. Specifically, vitamin A derivatives are thought to control cells that might otherwise turn cancerous. Vitamin A compounds are very helpful in treating conditions such as psoriasis, where the skin proliferates very rapidly and thick scaly patches of skin can accumulate.

▪ VITAMIN C

The case for good nutrition as a key component of healthy skin is crystal-clear when we consider what happens when a key nutrient is absent from the diet. For centuries, sailors were subject to scurvy, a condition that produced skin and mouth sores that did not heal. The longer the time at sea, the more men wound up with swollen, discolored limbs, bleeding mouths, and loose teeth; some sailors eventually lost many of their teeth. James Lind (1716–1794), a naval surgeon, suggested supplementing the daily fare fed British sailors—meat, ale, and potatoes—with lemon and orange juice. Lind's idea proved a sound way to prevent scurvy; we now know that it was the absence of vitamin C, found in fresh fruits, that caused the disease. Soon the Royal Navy was issuing its men a daily ration of lemons or limes, which is how the British sailor acquired the nickname of "limey."

Many patients believe that extra vitamin C will help healing. In fact, vitamin C plays an important role in wound healing in normal amounts, but I do not usually recommend taking megadoses of vitamin C to enhance healing. Since vitamin C is water-soluble, what your body doesn't use is excreted in urine.

▪ ZINC AND YOUR SKIN

Minerals are the other micronutrients that are popular in health food culture. Human beings are made up of dozens of minerals. In fact, by weight—not counting the water that we mostly consist of—we would be mainly mineral, rather than animal or vegetable. While the role of many other minerals in growth and maintenance of our bodies is still being investigated, it is known that zinc plays a definite role.

Based largely on what happens in the absence of adequate zinc, it is now popularly believed that large amounts of zinc will assist in hair growth and skin rejuvenation. I must stress that it is not clear that an excess amount of zinc will regrow hair, fortify its strength and durability, or enhance the quality or nature of skin. Zinc has been recommended as an aid in wound healing, but there is conflicting evidence that zinc in amounts greater than normally consumed in the diet enhances healing.

▪ WATER AND YOUR SKIN

First off, let me say that there is no direct connection between drinking water—or spraying it on your face, for that matter—and healthy skin. There is, however, a relationship between good health and good skin. And adequate hydration is important for good health.

While water cannot "purify" or improve your skin, it does make up the majority of our body weight. It is better to be properly hydrated than dehydrated. As long as your kidneys are functioning well and you take in more water than your body uses in a day, your fluid status should be optimal.

▪ ALLERGIES RELATED TO FOOD

How often have you heard of someone who, having eaten strawberries, shellfish, or nuts, then developed hives? Perhaps this has even happened to you.

Some people develop hives when they touch certain foods rather than eat them. Individuals often complain of these symptoms in their hands when their work primarily involves working with foods or chemicals that are problematic. This is called *contact urticaria*. If you think you get hives or any other rash after eating certain foods, keep note of them and see your doctor. If you develop difficulty breathing, seek medical attention immediately.

MARGARITAS, SUN, FUN, AND RASH

An unusual but not uncommon skin rash can develop when a compound in limes, figs, and other fruits reacts with ultraviolet radiation from the sun. Interestingly, the rash is often seen on the hands of bartenders at tropical resorts. Limes, which they squeeze all day long, contain a compound called *psoralen,* which is activated by sun and can cause a sunburn or even contact dermatitis.

Psoralen is interesting for another reason. First used centuries ago by the Egyptians, it is currently an important part of therapy for psoriasis patients. They take the compound as a drug that, combined with artificial ultraviolet A radiation, can control the disease.

11

Alternative Medicine and Natural Therapy

Some time ago a patient I had been caring for began selling a line of skin products that contained extract from melaleuca—tea tree oil. She brought me glossy literature in which major claims were made about the benefits of this herbal product on skin. I couldn't scientifically evaluate all the claims, but evidence exists that tea tree oil does have antibacterial effects. There are many naturally occurring compounds that may provide benefit to the skin. The trick is in identifying the ones that work and knowing when to take advantage of them.

Alternative medicine, now often referred to as complementary medicine, has earned newfound respectability in conventional medical circles. Once an area of knowledge scoffed at by traditional doctors, it has now become an aspect of the healing arts in which the public and many physicians place increasing faith. Indeed, it has become such an important area of investigation that the National Institutes of Health (hardly a radical arm of the federal government) has established a division specifically devoted to the study of alternative forms of medical therapy. In my field, the *Archives of Dermatology*, the oldest scientific dermatology journal in America, recently devoted a whole issue to alternative medicine in dermatology.

When we talk about alternative medicine we are usually referring to herbal or natural therapies. Alternative medicine also includes a whole range of preventative and treatment strategies, from natural products to psychological interventions, such as hypnosis (which probably has a place in dermatology), and disciplines like yoga, massage, aromatherapy, and acupuncture.

A dynamic tension now exists in the world of medicine between those people who believe the only way to decide if a treatment works is through the scientific method and those who believe that other measures are adequate to determine the usefulness of a therapy. The scientific method involves testing a drug and measuring the results of its use. For example, to determine whether an acne medication works, a group of people apply a medicine in a rigorous program and the number of acne lesions are counted. If the number of lesions decreases in the study group compared with the people who use a placebo (in this case a plain unmedicated cream), this suggests the experimental treatment works. The proof of whether a medication works is in the comparison of the effects of the treatment with a group that is getting the placebo.

The burden of proof is particularly elusive in the realm of alternative medicine. Therefore it stands to reason that until enough trials are set up to test the medical value of particular remedies, the debate will continue regarding the true effectiveness of herbal and other therapies in medical treatment.

Because skin is so available, and because the medications and agents we use are frequently applied topically, a huge body of knowledge has developed over the centuries about a host of skin treatments. For instance, when we survey the liniments, poultices, and treatments used to treat skin disease since the time of the Egyptians, we discover that we are still using many of the same active ingredients, albeit designated by different names and often available in different formulations.

In fact, the world of medicine is rife with examples of herbal therapies. For example, digitalis, a mainstay of cardiac treatment (sold as the drug digoxin) is derived from the purple foxglove plant. Dermatology is more interconnected with herbal remedies or treatments than any other field of medicine. Self-medication is easier and more products are readily accessible than when treating the internal organs. Many people experiment or embrace whatever they can to improve their skin, and this includes all that the health food store or alternative medicine shop may have to offer—and new products appear there to tempt the consumer all the time. It's no wonder dermatologists must pay attention to the rise of complementary treatments.

Herbal remedies are a huge business in the United States today—

Americans spend over $12 billion annually on alternative medications and vitamins. Interestingly, more than half of all physicians comfortably recommend herbal treatments to patients and almost half of us admit to using some type of alternative therapy ourselves. The purchase and use of herbal treatments differs from conventional medication in one important way. The Food and Drug Administration does not require manufacturers to prove efficacy, safety, or adherence to production standards. If something proves dangerous to the public, as L-tryptophan supplements did in the mid-1990s, the FDA can pull the product from the shelves, but that occurs only after the harm has been done. In general, there is a much longer history of herbal therapeutics in Europe, and many well-established German companies have a reputation for the production of quality herbal remedies.

In the realm of non-melanoma skin cancer, a particular form of alternative therapy surfaces every now and then. Every few years I get a mailing from someone around the world or a patient comes in with a newspaper clipping about a natural compound alleged to cure skin cancer. It contains as its active ingredient a compound called *solasodine*. From my point of view, one of the problems with studies claiming that some agent cures skin cancer is that often no biopsy diagnosis is made prior to treatment. No controlled research studies are done. In the end, a particular salve or cream may be used successfully, but it wasn't treating cancer or precancer—it might have simply been curing a patch of dry skin. Be suspicious of any treatment that alleges it can cure skin cancer yet doesn't require a prescription. In addition, if you have a spot that doesn't heal, or matches the description of skin cancer provided in Part IV, get it biopsied and treated properly. Don't mess around with creams that are not proven to work and stay away from miracle cures you discover on the Internet.

▪ MEDICAL TREATMENT AND THE MIND

It has been common knowledge for a very long time that how we think affects how we feel and vice versa. Somewhere in the last fifty years, however, our romance with all things technological gave humankind a false sense of supreme power and control. We came to believe that with the use of our advanced procedures and our state-of-the-art technology, we could "cure" anything, as if medicine were a war, rather than a healing process.

Well, thankfully, our thinking is evolving. Some of us are beginning to see that to cure everything is impossible. The best medicine is practiced in partnership with the patient and with respect for the relationship between the body and mind. Thomas Edison, one of the greatest technology pioneers, predicted long ago, "The doctor of the future will give no medicine, but will interest his patients in the care of the human frame, in diet, and in the cause and prevention of disease."

Now, here we are in the new millennium. Where do we stand when it comes to alternative treatments and our health? There is no reason to eschew the many, very real strides Western medicine has made in improving the survival rates of those who suffer from cancer, heart disease, and diabetes, just to name a few major killers.

When it comes to skin disease, from cancer to Lyme disease or venomous bites, I need to state unequivocally that you should not go it alone. The treatment your doctor provides can save your life. In other situations that are not life-threatening, your own input at home and the use of alternative therapies may well solve your skin problem without additional investment of your time and money in expensive treatments that may be only partially successful. In addition, the sense of control you feel when you can take action yourself (after consulting with your physician, of course) can help relieve stress when coping with a serious skin condition—and relieving stress is always good for your overall health and the health of your skin. Psoriasis, eczema, and seborrheic dermatitis are among the common skin conditions that can be triggered by excessive stress.

In reviewing the most well known alternative therapies in dermatology, I'll try to cite evidence for what works, as measured in good studies, as well as any formal trials that have shown what doesn't work. If you are a devotee of alternative treatment, you will probably know about other options already. Please let me know your thoughts by email through the website www.totalskinmd.com.

▪ ACUPUNCTURE

Over five thousand years ago in China the practice of acupuncture became an important aspect of medicine. Acupuncture takes its inspiration from *qi* (pronounced chee). Qi is the vital life energy considered to be present in all living organisms; it must be kept in balance within the living system. Acupuncture aims to remove obstructions to the free flow of healing energy. In acupuncture, a fine needle is used to stimulate the body's healing process through body lines of energy. The needle is inserted at an acupuncture point, the exact anatomic location where that healing energy can be contacted.

It is believed that acupuncture works by stimulating immunity and the body's own endorphins, by affecting serotonin and adrenaline (two compounds that help transmit impulses in the nervous system), by constricting or dilating blood vessels, and by stimulating alternative pathways in the nervous system, which might close off impulses from other areas of the body. Acupuncture theory holds that there are twelve major energy pathways, or meridians. All of these are linked to specific organ systems and internal organs. On these meridians, there are thought to be over one thousand locations that can be stimulated through acupuncture to increase the healthful flow of qi.

One of the few skin conditions upon which acupuncture is thought to have a positive effect is acute urticaria, also known as hives. This condition, which affects 15 to 20 percent of the population, is usually a reaction to food or drugs, but it may also come from a viral, bacterial, or parasitic infection. In Western medicine, acute urticaria is treated with antihistamines or a short course of corticosteroids, but acupuncture evidently can help. In a study of psoriasis, however, no significant benefit was found for people treated with acupuncture.

▪ AROMATHERAPY

Aromatherapy has become extremely popular as a means of promoting health and improving our sense of well-being. Rooted in herbalism, aromatherapy involves the use of oils extracted from plants, which are usually massaged into the skin. Although many claims are made about the benefits of this therapy, few studies have been done to actually prove any psychological or physical benefits. Interestingly, though, the use of sandalwood oil has been shown to inhibit the growth of wartlike tumors in mice. Similarly, tea tree oil has an antibacterial and antifungal effect. On the other hand, certain essential oils can affect the surface of the skin and cause a contact dermatitis similar to that of poison ivy.

For over a hundred years lavender, thyme, cedarwood, and rosemary oils have been used to promote hair growth. Until a recent clinical research study, there were no scientific trials to prove that they actually are effective in this way. The specific research was conducted on 84 subjects with *alopecia areata*, a type of hair loss that occurs when the body's immune system attacks its own hair follicles (see p. 159). This condition affects about 1 percent of the population and is very distressing. Alopecia areata can result from stress and the course of the condition is unpredictable. In this aromatherapy study, the active group massaged their scalps with essential oils such as thyme, lavender, and cedarwood, while the other group used only a placebo oil. Of the patients in the active group, 44 percent showed improvement in their alopecia areata, compared with only 15 percent in the group who did not get the active oils. This was a significant finding, but actually raises some legitimate questions. Did these patients grow hair because there was an active ingredient in the oils? Or was it some other factor?

▪ VITAMIN THERAPY

These days we consume a bumper crop of vitamins, having been told they can do everything from cure disease to prevent aging. Our fascination with vitamins derives from an almost magical thinking that by consuming a special "missing" ingredient, we will enhance our health. The fact is that our notions about what vitamins do and which ones are good for us under certain circumstances derive from studies of conditions that result from deficiency of particular vitamins.

In so-called pharmacologic doses, which are sometimes thousands of times greater than what our bodies need, certain vitamins behave not as nutritional supplements but like drugs, to the extent that they can help alter a disease state rather than just restore a natural deficiency condition. For example, chemical derivatives of vitamin A are important anticancer medications, but excessive vitamin A itself can cause serious side effects.

A vitamin D derivative is used to treat psoriasis in a compound called Dovonex. Why? It turns out that psoriasis, a condition in which cells of the epidermis divide too rapidly, can actually be slowed down by forms of vitamin D. Excess vitamin D itself, however, can be toxic and cause illness.

A healthy person needs only small quantities of vitamins and minerals. Don't assume that if a little B-complex vitamin is good, a lot is better. In the case of vitamin B, any excess passes right through your kidneys and out of your body. By contrast, fat-soluble vitamins like A, D, E and K are retained in the fatty tissues of the body and can build up.

VITAMIN C

Vitamin C has antioxidant effects that are popularly thought to make it beneficial to combat skin aging. An antioxidant is a compound that sucks up or otherwise neutralizes the harmful oxygen molecules that result from normal chemical reactions in the body. It is true that in the test tube vitamin C can function as an antioxidant. However, claims of clinical benefit in skin are not based on any legitimate scientific studies. Many continue to be convinced that vitamin C is good for colds, although there is no hard evidence for that, either. True, the idea of smearing this vitamin on our skin in the hope that it will make us look younger does seem attractive in a simple sort of way. Nonetheless, the evidence is not there to support this use. A study done at Duke University on pigs suggested that adding vitamin C and vitamin E to sunscreens protected the animals against damage from UVB radiation (the kind that causes sunburn). But since there are enough effective sunblocks the added cost of vitamin C sunscreens or compounds doesn't seem justified. As to reversal of damage that has already taken place, I eagerly await scientific proof.

VITAMIN E

Vitamin E is widely believed to help improve scars and assist in general wound healing. It's a fascinating phenomenon: somehow the idea that vitamin E assists wound healing has become part of the conventional wisdom about health, and nothing can budge it. Since it generally can cause no harm and since massage of healing wounds may be helpful, I advise my patients to use it on surgical scars if they are so inclined. If the suture line is long enough I sometimes offer a friendly challenge: apply the cream to just half of the scar, but don't tell me which half. After six to eight weeks I then try to guess where they used it. In more than a dozen years of surgical practice, I've yet to be able to tell at the follow-up visit where they applied the vitamin E cream. There is also no evidence that cocoa butter helps healing but the associated massage may in time flatten raised scars.

If you do use vitamin E topically, however, keep in mind that it can cause allergic reactions. Early on, before the availability of creams, many patients would break open a soft gel capsule and massage the liquid into their skin. The type of reaction that could sometimes develop was similar to that of poison ivy: itchiness, redness, and oozing clear pimples. A hydrocortisone cream, along with cessation of the treatment was all that was needed to get back to normal. The true allergic potential of vitamin E was brought home very clearly in the early 1990s. A plethora of rashes caused by a new line of cosmetics occurred throughout Switzerland. When all the cases were reported, it turned out that at least 3 patients for every 1,000 units of cosmetics sold developed contact dermatitis. The offending agent was vitamin E linoleate, a mixture of tocopheryl esters. Symptoms developed anywhere from 1 to 160 days after people started using the cosmetics. Itching was severe and the rash took one to four weeks to disappear.

Some doctors have developed allergic contact dermatitis from using soaps and hand lotions that contain vitamin E. Also remember that vitamin E can accentuate the blood-thinning effect of Coumadin and aspirin. So patients who are on those compounds and who are about to undergo surgery need to stop taking vitamin E orally at least a week before surgery.

▪ WHAT CAN NATURAL THERAPY HELP?

Let's look at some specific skin conditions and the natural therapies that have been touted to treat them.

HERPES

The herpes simplex virus that causes the common cold sore and genital herpes can plague a person for a lifetime, which is reason enough to research alternative methods of treatment. There are superb antiviral agents. Denavir is a topical cream you can apply at the first tingling sign of a cold sore outbreak and Valtrex, an oral medication, is effective in reducing the duration of genital herpes as well. If you prefer not to use prescription medications, there is some evidence that certain essential oils are helpful. Lemon balm (*Melissa officinalis*) is an herb found in the eastern Mediterranean with the distinct odor of lemon. Its main ingredient is citronella. Lemon balm has been shown to have antiviral properties in the test tube. When lemon balm was used in patients with cold sores, healing time was faster than in a control group using a placebo cream. Still, prescription medications designed to block the virus remain the most predictable treatment for cold sores. Lysine and other natural remedies have not been proven to work.

LEG VEIN INSUFFICIENCY

Lower leg vein insufficiency can result in swollen legs and ulcers. Horse chestnut seed extract contains a compound called *escin*, thought to prevent the activation of white blood cells, which can be an underlying problem in lower leg vein insufficiency. A review of medical studies suggested that taking this extract orally was actually superior to taking a placebo. Using this alternative therapy for sixteen weeks was as effective in controlling the swelling effects of venous insufficiency as was wearing compression stockings.

WARTS

One area where alternative forms of therapy have been used for centuries is in the management of common warts. In one study, children with warts were treated with different homeopathic preparations, while another group received a placebo. When the results were compared, there was no difference in success between the group that received the pure placebo and the group that received the homeopathic remedy. (For more on warts see Chapter 25).

PSORIASIS

Hydrotherapy (treatment with hot or cold water or steam to restore health) at the Dead Sea is recognized as a good treatment for psoriasis. Dead Sea water contains a natural tar called bitumen. Elements in tar have been shown repeatedly to benefit psoriasis patients by slowing down the rapid turnover of skin cells, which is the hallmark of the problem. In addition, the ultraviolet radiation from the bright sun probably serves a therapeutic purpose as well. Dead Sea products are available to be added to your bath at home, but it is unlikely that this will simulate the effects psoriasis patients experience in the Dead Sea.

ECZEMA

In a research study in London a remarkable benefit was demonstrated in children with eczema who were treated in an alternative fashion. Using a combination of ten herbs, redness (an indicator of how active the eczema was) decreased 91 percent in children treated with the active herbs and only 11 percent in patients treated with placebos. There were no significant side effects from the herbal treatment.

ACNE

Witch hazel and oak bark are topical astringents that alternative practitioners recommend to patients, but there are no controlled studies showing effectiveness in this condition. Moreover, so many effective conventional treatments are now available that these should be used first to control what can, at times, be a skin condition that can lead to permanent scars.

DERMATITIS

Chamomile (*Matricaria recutitia*) is a member of the daisy family. It is used to treat dermatitis and other minor irritations of the skin. It contains compounds that appear to inhibit inflammation. In one study, it was found to be 60 percent as active as a topical corticosteroid cream. In a study of patients with atopic dermatitis, it was found to be about as effective as hydrocortisone.

WOUND HEALING

Pot marigold or common marigold (*Calendula officinalis*) is considered useful for burns, bruises, cuts, and rashes. German health authorities recommend it for topical treatment of minor wounds and leg ulcers, because it is believed to increase collagen metabolism, which aids in healing. It is most commonly used as an ointment or in cream form. In addition, a tea can be made for mouthwash or topical treatment. Although it is generally considered safe, ironically there are some rare reports of allergic reactions that can actually *cause* contact dermatitis.

▪ SOME COMMONLY USED NATURAL REMEDIES

GREEN TEA

The flower of the green tea plant (*Camellia sinensis*) has broad, linen white petals surrounding gently arching golden stamens. The leaves of the plant are used for the tea that is the national beverage of Japan. Green tea itself contains a group of compounds called *catechins*, which are normally destroyed when green tea is converted into black tea. Green tea has special value because catechins generally improve lipid metabolism in the bloodstream and can lower cholesterol. In dermatology its promise resides in its anticancer effects, since green tea contains compounds that have an antioxidant effect. The trick is to determine how to harness the anticancer effect verified in the test tube and convert it to useful application in human disease and prevention.

The promised health benefits of green tea have sprouted a range of products, including antibacterial soap, skin creams and lotions, shampoos, and even sunscreens. Although its effectiveness as a sun protection product has not been proven in human studies, the presence of antioxidants in green tea raises the possibility that products containing the active compound may be able to inhibit the cancer process initiated by the sun's ultraviolet B radiation. In one series of studies at Case Western Reserve University, administration of green tea resulted in a reduction of the tumors that occurred following exposure to UVB radiation.

WITCH HAZEL

Witch hazel has a long history in both traditional and alternative medicine in the treatment of hemorrhoids, burns, colds, and fevers and it has been an important natural compound for dermatologists as well. This astringent relieves itching and soothes all kinds of skin irritations. The active ingredients are *tannins*. In addition, there is an anti-inflammatory effect of witch hazel, a product which is available over the counter.

The popular astringent is derived from the witch hazel shrub (*Hamamelis virginiana*), which grows wild in the northeast United States. Native Americans brewed a concoction of witch hazel, leaves, bark, and twigs to help heal cuts and scrapes. The shrub, given its Latin name after a Greek word for apple tree, has many medicinal qualities. Witch hazel calms the pain of stings and has antiseptic qualities. The compound is now added to aftershave lotions and other products for soothing irritated skin.

As an astringent, witch hazel has drying qualities, so be alert to drying out your skin—especially in winter or if you live in a dry climate. Allergic reactions to witch hazel are uncommon, but if you use it regularly and develop a rash that doesn't go away it could be the cause. Witch hazel is an excellent example of a herbal remedy for which complicated scientific studies are not really needed. It is low risk, so the user can decide whether it helps or not. It is also inexpensive, which doesn't hurt either.

LICORICE

Licorice is a universally popular flavor, popping up in candies and after-dinner liqueurs alike and used in cooking as anise. Licorice root is a common compound used in traditional Chinese herbal medicine. The active ingredient is glycyrhizic acid. Evidence shows that licorice extracts can increase the skin's natural steroid hormones (cousins to hydrocortisone) and so may be beneficial in counteracting the irritation sometimes caused by other skin products. That is why some manufacturers of cosmetics and skin creams are now mixing it in with their primary skin products. Any other claims, such as an anti-wrinkle effect, have not been established. Because it has been found to increase the activity of topical hydrocortisone it may be helpful for skin conditions such as psoriasis and eczema, which normally respond to such corticosteroids.

FRUIT ACIDS

Alpha-hydroxy acids (AHAs) are a family of chemicals found in many fruits, hence the simple name "fruit acids." AHA products cause shedding of the surface skin cells, or exfoliation. The extent of exfoliation depends on the type and concentration of the AHA, its pH (acidity), and other ingredients in the product. It is also determined by the nature of your own skin. AHAs are derived from a wide range of fruit: malic acid from apples, tartaric acid found in grapes, citric acid from citrus fruit.

These acids are marketed as gentle skin peelers or astringents, and for general "anti-aging" uses. In addition to these claims, products with AHAs are sold to unclog and cleanse pores, fight oily skin or acne, and improve skin condition in general. Many people who use AHAs believe that they

---

LOOK FOR THESE AHAS IN
YOUR PRODUCT'S LIST OF INGREDIENTS

Glycolic acid	Alpha-hydroxycaprylic acid
Lactic acid	Hydroxycaprylic acid
Malic acid	Mixed fruit acid
Citric acid	Tri-alpha hydroxy fruit acids
Glycolic acid + ammonium glycolate	Triple fruit acid
Alpha-hydroxyethanoic acid + ammonium alpha-hydroxyethanoate	Sugarcane extract
	Alpha hydroxy and botanical complex
Alpha-hydroxyoctanoic acid	L-alpha hydroxy acid

(If your AHA moisturizer or treatment stings, it may be too strong for your skin. Consider alternative moisturizers that do not contain AHA.)

make the skin feel smoother and even look better. Studies have shown that products with less than 10 percent AHA are generally safe. In fact, it's important to realize that natural lemon has an "AHA level" of 27 percent. Most products contain AHA levels up to 10 percent. The exfoliation effect of AHAs can help even out the tan, blotchy discoloration that comes from sun exposure. There is no evidence that AHAs permanently reverse wrinkles or fine lines, but it is thought that by causing mild irritation, the swelling in the skin puffs up the tissue around the lines and wrinkles and minimizes their appearance. AHAs are available in many over-the-counter cosmetic products but are also used, in higher and more complex formulations, for chemical peels performed by your dermatologist (see chapter 7).

Because of the irritating effect of AHAs, some people report sun sensitivity. There is indeed some suggestion that their use may make some users more sensitive to UV radiation from the sun. If you are using AHA products, you must use sunscreen (SPF 15 or higher), wear a broad-brimmed hat, and avoid the sun during peak hours.

Two more things to be alert about: don't use AHAs on children and be aware that AHA concentration and pH value are generally not noted on all products, because the FDA does not require it. Consumers should report any adverse reactions such as irritation or sun sensitivity associated with the use of AHAs to their local FDA office, listed in the Blue Pages of the phone book, or to the FDA's Office of Consumer Affairs, 800-532-4440.

BROMELAIN

Bromelain is an enzyme derived from pineapple and sold in capsule form. Taken by mouth, bromelain is said to stimulate healing of soft tissue injuries, like sprains and bruises. In controlled studies bromelain has been shown to speed up the healing of hematomas (collections of blood that sometimes form after surgery). Prior to liposuction surgery, bromelain may help decrease bruising and hematoma formation. A few individuals have allergic reactions to bromelain. Discontinue it if you get any itching.

ONION EXTRACT

For centuries onion extract has been said to offer special health benefits. Recently, a popular new product has been promoted that is said to speed healing and improve the final appearance of scars. Marketed as Mederma, this topical cream contains onion extract.

In the test tube, onion extract has been shown to inhibit the production of collagen, the building blocks of scar tissue. Two controlled studies suggest that in this way Mederma may be of benefit, since it may aid the development of smaller, more flesh-colored, and thinner scars. Medically speaking, that's all that can be said to date

ALOE VERA

Aloe vera is one of about three hundred succulent plants found mainly in sunny climates. The leaves of such plants store large amounts of water. When cut, these leaves release a gel-like material that is thought to be soothing to the skin.

For sunburn, thermal burns, and any areas of skin irritation or inflammation, you can use the healing gel straight from fresh leaves. All you have to do is split a lower leaf lengthwise, score it with a knife, and rub the gel that oozes out directly on the affected skin area.

Since many of the products on the market that advertise aloe vera as a component actually contain very little of it, you may want to keep your own potted aloe vera plant by your kitchen window. There are many species of aloe, and many whose leaves are big enough to provide gel, but aloe vera, the "true" aloe, is the best choice. You can buy the plants at most nurseries. They are easy to grow (they are cactuslike, so do not require much water) and will multiply if properly cared for and given enough light.

12

"I've Got You Under My Skin":
Touch and Skin in Health

It is through the skin that we touch and are touched. This sense, like the skin itself, is so often taken for granted, but the role of touch in our lives is vital. When Michelangelo sought to portray God animating Adam, he didn't paint a bolt of lightning whitening Eden's sky, he chose an outstretched hand, reaching down from above—now an eternal symbol in our culture for the power of touch.

When Christa McAuliffe perished in the fiery *Challenger* space shuttle tragedy in 1986, President Reagan searched for the most meaningful way of capturing who she and her colleagues had been and what they had accomplished. He didn't talk about their military courage, their athletic prowess, their technical know-how, their vision, or even their boundless energy. Of all these strands of their lives at the moment they were shattered, the president chose to quote John Magee, a World War II Royal Canadian Air Force pilot and poet:

> *Oh! I have slipped the surly bonds of Earth . . .*
> *Put out my hand and touched the face of God.*

In one brilliant couplet, the primitive and the sublime, the horrific and the beautiful, the sum of their experience on this earth was captured with the image of touch.

Ever since the Tower of Babel, words and language have had their limitations as forms of communication, but touch—that most basic function of skin and of our nervous system—remains an unchanged universal link. But despite being a fundamental human sensory tool, touch plays different roles in different cultures. Imagine yourself at a party for the parents of children attending an international school in some very cosmopolitan city. The parents of the French girl rush up to greet perfect strangers with a kiss on each cheek. The English parents, backs stiff, heads upright, immediately extend their hands to give a firm grasping shake while protecting their personal social zone. The Italian parents, their bodies open with outstretched arms and their personal zone boundless, embrace others tightly. The Japanese parents bow courteously and smile imperceptibly.

The point is that in each of these cases, touch has played a critical role in initiating the social interaction. You might say, "Sure, but without vision, they couldn't see whom to greet or embrace." Actually, many people deprived of vision will tell you that the keenness of touch is what permits them to get through the day.

In chapter 4, I mentioned briefly the connection between the brain and the skin. But because we can't see the nerves and because their activity in the skin is constant and unremitting, it proceeds unnoticed. Unnoticed, that is, until we itch, sting, burn, tingle, or ache, or are numb, feel cold, or can't really tell what we are feeling. The panoply of words to describe the sensations we feel through the skin highlights how important this function is.

> To check authenticity, antique dealers rely on touch rather than sight. Repairs can fool the eye, but not the hand.

Holding a pen, swinging a golf club, and delicately applying mascara are obvious examples of the role of touch in life. But it turns out that the skin is of far broader importance than assisting in the activities of daily living. From shortly after we are born, the skin helps our intelligence develop, as it begins to define our emotional and physical world.

Years ago, the famous anthropologist Ashley Montagu studied the role of touch in development. He suggested that because of this function the skin was an arch through which all early experience passed, permitting integration by the brain and the development of patterns of sensation. When we stop for a moment to ponder touch, we realize that Montagu's idea is quite plausible.

Because the sense of touch is so important to health in general and skin health in particular, and because it is rarely approached from this perspective, I think it is interesting to explore how touch comes to be the gateway to our physical experience and how it helps us feel our way through the day.

▪ FIRST TOUCH

The birth process itself is an example of a primal, touching experience. The newcomer's slow journey toward and through the birth canal is a vital internal massage. While sometimes barely endurable for the woman in labor, her efforts stimulate the infant, who is about to engage the world for the first time. The contractions that move the baby through the birth canal massage the newly minted, well-protected skin. The press and release of each contraction assists circulation, sensitizes nerve ends, and prepares the skin of the newborn for the barrage of sensations, from temperature to pressure and texture, that he or she will encounter instantly in the brave new world.

First there will be the cool gusts of the delivery room air. Never felt that before. Doctor's latex gloves? Not nearly as smooth as skin. Cotton blanket? Who dreamed up this rough material?

Shortly after birth, it is touch that connects the infant to Mom and Dad and in turn to the world. Touch is nurturing. Touch is security. It is also one of the foundations of your child's healthy development.

▪ BABY TOUCH

Studies have shown that healthy touching—and lots of it—is important not only to a baby's emotional development and stability, but to learning in general. Babies that are held, cuddled, rocked, and carried tend to walk sooner and even speak sooner. Remember, the natural state for the infant is to be held by his or her parents. When this occurs, the infant experiences the swaying motion of the adult and hears the adult talking. This is where your baby's education starts: in the front seat you create with your arms, shoulders, and hands. Carrying your baby as much as possible is a wonderful way to add to the infant's sense of security and connection to the world.

When discussing human development, it is most important to note that in the years before a child can talk, touch is a loving as well as a learning

RUBBING IT IN

Since touch is good for you massage can't be a bad thing. Once there was the good, old-fashioned rubdown. Now, when you decide you want to try a massage, you have lots of options—so many that it may all seem a bit confusing. Here is a quick guide to some therapeutic effects of hands-on bodywork:

Choosing what's right for you will involve familiarizing yourself with the options; trusting your instincts regarding what type of touch you respond to best (some massage therapies can be rougher than others); making sure you know what your goals are (do you just want to feel good and reduce stress, or would you like to increase flexibility, improve posture, etc.?); and trying a few options before committing yourself to one technique.

Here is a brief rundown on five of the most common technniques:

- **Acupressure** is the needle-free cousin of acupuncture. Acupressure derives from Chinese medicine and is based on the concept that the circulation of the qi, or life energy, is at the heart of good health. A massage using this technique claims to treat the same 365 points present on the body's so-called meridians that acupuncture will.
- **Rolfing** came of age with mantras and self-help movements as an antidote to the effects of gravity, which over time does cause wear and tear on our joints and bones. The rolfer claims to stretch the body's connective tissue. Supposedly this technique can help to restore alignment and flexibility. Rolfing takes a series of ten treatments, so it is a sizable commitment of money and time. Some people who have experienced rolfing report that it can be painful. As with most forms of massage therapy, scientific support for benefit is hard to come by. Only you can tell if it is helpful to you.
- **Shiatsu** is a popular body massage technique. It derives, as acupressure does, from Chinese medicine. Shiatsu technique is more rigorous or forceful than acupressure and supposedly focuses on 600 points in the body.
- **Swedish massage** is the classic body rub, used mainly for relaxation. These days most practitioners of the gentle Swedish technique have added to their repertoires in order to compete with the ever-increasing massage options. Some masseurs and masseuses combine Swedish and shiatsu techniques, others use kripalu technique, an amalgam of Swedish massage, yoga breathing techniques, and energy stimulation that has become popular.
- **Trigger-point therapy** focuses on the tender areas present in the fasciae, the tendons, and the muscles. The therapist applies pressure to these tender areas with the fingers, knuckles, and/or elbows in an effort to "release" or free up the point where there is pain and tenderness. Then the muscles in the surrounding areas are stimulated deeply to avoid a recurrence of the problem. In addition to its use by massage therapists, chiropractors, physical therapists, and even some physicians use this technique.

tool. Simply put, the child who is stimulated by touch will learn more quickly.

▪ LOVING TOUCHES AND SECURITY

Cuddling, hand holding, hugging, a pat on the head all contribute to a healthy childhood and are directly related to the child's optimal social and sexual development later in life. Conversely, a child who has not been held and cuddled in childhood will almost surely suffer more during adolescence and young adulthood.

We live in a culture where we are more aware of abuse of children than ever. Our visceral reaction to news stories about the physical and emotional abuse of children, often mediated through touch, is inescapable. Because "mishandling" seems so prevalent, we begin to fear touching and equate bodily contact with harm. But appropriate touching is a way of communicating love, of connecting people, and of soothing and comforting people of all ages. It is an intimacy we cannot do without. When, for reasons of fear and indoctrination, we try to, things go wrong. Bad things happen. Children and teenagers act out. Violence can be a more frequent occurrence. And intimate, personal relationships can slam up against a brick wall. Nothing highlights the negative effect of isolation from touch more than the experiences of countless Romanian orphans reared in virtual isolation. Today, many experience psychological and social problems that are overwhelming.

▪ SOOTHING TOUCH

Even doctors, skeptics that we are when it comes to anything that hints of the touchy-feely, must grant that touch offers an irreplaceable form of emotional nourishment.

Touch can be a force of healing. In our Western culture, we feed people various medicines as if they were food, but we often forget to give the patient other important medicine—our healing touch.

Perhaps the most impressive demonstration of the power of touch is something I encounter daily. During the range of surgical procedures I perform under local anesthesia, anxiety and fear predominate in the patients. All the reassuring words in the world do not accomplish what the gentle squeeze of the nurse's hands can. More interestingly, our tendency to offer a hand to a worried or anxious patient is frequently met with a comment such as, "Oh, that was wonderful," or "Thank you for your hand. I hope I didn't break it!" Touch, in this setting, has no equal.

▪ TOUCH AND AGING

What the aging fear most is loss of control. They also fear not being taken seriously. What many suffer from, though, is loneliness. And if loneliness can kill, then lack of touch is its weapon.

We have a warehouse full of techniques to make the aging look younger, but that only goes so far. To the extent that looking younger makes people feel more attractive and thus more likely to engage in social activity, it yields an extra benefit. Often, this dividend of judicious cosmetic surgery is not always appreciated. The truth about aging is that while skin tone and quality change, the need for tactile stimulation does not.

While skin may change on the surface as time and weather pound away at it, we should remember that the nerve endings still carry the spirit of touch throughout the body. In fact, it is a cruel irony of life that while most of the other senses dull as we journey through life, the sense of touch can sometimes be the bane of an older person's existence. Itching from dry skin can be very bothersome and even lead to skin infection. Worse, the elderly are far more likely than younger people to suffer intractable, even disabling pain after a bout of shingles. Would that those painful nerves could degenerate like those of smell and taste and hearing!

▪ TOUCH AND DYING

Just as we cannot tolerate the withdrawal of physical support when we are infants, we need touch in our final days. The dying fear abandonment as much as they fear pain. Abandonment for a dying person is marked by the lack of physical presence of loved ones and those around them. If you are near someone you love who is ill and may be dying, never underestimate the power of your touch. Support for the dying can best be expressed through touch—whether it's a hand in a hand, a kiss, or a caress.

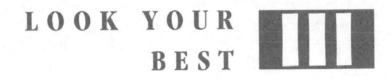

LOOK YOUR BEST

13

Medical Lasers: What Einstein Didn't Know

I saw Geraldo have laser surgery for his wrinkles on his show. It seems so simple.

—Susan, 41, hair stylist

Who hasn't heard about lasers? From *Star Wars* to the Wrinkle Wars, people everywhere are being inundated with the promise of medical magic at the end of the intense band of light the laser creates. What many may not realize is that there are many different kinds of lasers, in medicine and even in industry, not to mention the Pentagon. In medicine there are lasers to smash and vaporize kidney stones, sculpt the cornea so you won't need glasses, seal ovarian tubes, treat dental cavities, zap brain tumors, improve wrinkles, eliminate blemishes, vanish unwanted tattoos. The list goes on, and for virtually each purpose there is a separate $100,000 machine. In industry, lasers are used to cut steel, a patient who is a steel manufacturer informed me recently. I advised him not to try it on his sun spots.

In essence, lasers represent a class of instruments that have in common the development and controlled release of intense light for a particular purpose. There is no one laser to cure all medical problems. In fact, as time goes on, it is likely a greater variety of lasers, and variations on the current technological theme, will be introduced. This may confuse things even more for you. As we talk a bit about lasers, perhaps the most important thing to remember is that a laser is not magic, but in many cases, it is better than anything we've had before in dermatology for particular problems.

Technically, lasers are devices that generate beams of light that are directed to a particular target. In fact, the word *laser* is shorthand for "light amplification by the stimulated emission of radiation."

It was Einstein's work on the relationship between matter and energy that is the scientific basis of all lasers today. Lasers, simply put, are specialized light sources in which, through a variety of means, the light of a single wavelength is generated and magnified. Wavelength is really the signature mark of any laser and is a way we categorize all energy. For example, when you look at a rainbow or through a prism, the colors you see come from light that is broken up into all its visible wavelengths. That's why there is a Joseph's coat of colors. Lasers use just one wavelength of light that is then intensified. Because laser light is of one wavelength and is magnified manyfold, it is not only intense but remains highly focused as well. For example, if you shine a flashlight on a wall, the light waves splay out and form a bigger image on the wall than the circle of light that originates at the flashlight bulb. Laser light is highly focused, so it doesn't splay. This is critical to obtain the power and precision necessary for medical purposes.

Each beam of laser light contains energy, and for the laser to be effective in treating skin problems, a specific target must absorb that energy. Within the skin are several targets for laser energy. The targets most commonly used in the skin are water (we humans are about 60 percent water), hemoglobin (the molecule that gives red color to our blood), and melanin (the brown pigment that lends color to our skin). Certain wavelengths, or specific colors, of light are best absorbed by water, hemoglobin, and melanin. Lasers are designed so that they will target one of these molecules preferentially over the others. The other side of this very important coin is that with the proper selection of the correct laser, only what you don't want will be vaporized or destroyed, while surrounding skin that lacks the target color will be relatively unaffected. This specificity, called *photo-selectivity* because it is due to the specific "photo" or light wavelength, makes medical lasers especially valuable. Even though some lasers are not photoselective and depend more on the generation of heat alone, lasers represent a major advance over the red hot medical irons of the Civil War and before and even the electrosurgical devices of today that use electricity rather than light to alter tissue.

Despite the new frontiers that lasers allow us to explore, it is important to understand despite the fanfare and advertising, that the laser is just another tool. And any tool, whether a sculptor's chisel or a surgeon's scalpel, is only as good as the hand that guides it. While lasers can do many amazing things, you must have realistic expectations of what they can accomplish in order to achieve the greatest satisfaction from their use.

A wide array of lasers are available to treat a number of skin conditions. Before choosing to undergo a laser procedure, you should ask your dermatologist why one particular laser will be used over another to treat a given skin problem. In fact, you should be clear about what advantages a laser offers over conventional or traditional treatment.

▪ WRINKLES AND LINES

SKIN-RESURFACING LASERS

The hallmarks of aging skin include fine lines and wrinkles, especially those around the eyes and lips, and even on the cheeks. Liver spots, keratoses, broken blood vessels, and roughness are other marks of the ravages of time and years of sun.

In the past, chemical peels and dermabrasion had been used to "resurface" the skin—remove lines and blemishes and provide a smooth, more radiant surface. Dermabrasion was highly dependent on the skill of the dermatologist and the depth of injury was hard to control. Chemical peels are still widely used, and they are my treatment of choice for many symptoms of facial aging. However, a whole new world opened up in the early 1990s when the concept of using a laser to resurface was developed by Dr. Richard Fitzpatrick of California and others. They had the idea that if you could reduce and control the energy of the carbon dioxide laser (previously used by dermatologists for years to treat skin lesions), you might be able to simply strip off the top layer of skin, permitting regrowth of fresher epidermis along with some regeneration of the collagen in the second layer of the skin. Because fine lines and wrinkles result from natural aging and chronic sun damage to the collagen and elastin tissue in the dermis, stimulation of new collagen is thought helpful in tightening up the skin.

In the years that the resurfacing carbon dioxide laser has been in use, hundreds of dermatologists and other doctors have had the chance to learn where it works, how it works, and in what situations it cannot deliver what the patient hopes for. Another, newer laser used for resurfacing is the erbium: YAG laser.

Both the carbon dioxide and erbium lasers generate invisible light energy in the infrared spectrum. (We commonly know infrared radiation as heat.) The energy from these lasers is preferentially absorbed by the water within your skin cells. Since water makes up the majority of all our tissue, the laser light from these devices rapidly heats and vaporizes thin layers of skin. These two lasers will remove anywhere from 20 to 100 microns of skin at one pass. Keep in mind that 100 microns is approximately the thickness of one sheet of paper.

The main difference between these two lasers is that the erbium laser damages a thinner layer of skin with each pass so that more passes need to be performed to destroy the same thickness of tissue as the carbon dioxide laser. However, because the erbium laser light is more preferentially absorbed by water than even the CO_2 laser light, there is less surrounding tissue damage. These may be subtle differences, but the meaning to you is that the erbium laser results in more rapid healing time and a shorter period of redness on the face. On the other hand, it may require more

---

KEY POINTS ABOUT RESURFACING LASERS

- The carbon dioxide resurfacing laser reduces fine lines and wrinkles by removing the epidermis and stimulating new collagen growth in the dermis. The erbium laser, which is gentler, also removes the epidermis, but does not have as much effect on the collagen of the dermis, essential for effective wrinkle removal.
- Fastidious wound care is critical after laser resurfacing.
- Common side effects of treatment include persistent redness in the treated areas that can last for months. This is usually easily concealed with green-tint makeup.
- Hyperpigmentation, or brownish discoloration can also occur after healing; it is also temporary. Bleaching creams may help.
- Because the healing process continues under the surface of the epidermis for many months, we see continued improvement in wrinkles even twelve months after treatment. Be patient. Repeat treatments are always possible but in general, should not be done until twelve months have elapsed since the first treatment.
- Have realistic expectations—there is no machine on earth that can make your skin look like it did when you were sixteen, but the resurfacing lasers can certainly do more for you than any previous technology in dermatology.

resurfacing treatments to achieve the same results as the carbon dioxide laser.

Other conditions that can be treated by the carbon dioxide laser include xanthelasma—the collection of yellow cholesterol deposits that typically occur on the upper and lower eyelids. Various benign tumors that arise from the hair or sweat glands can also be smoothed out with these. These often appear as clusters of white bumps or pebbles around the eyelids. Warts and precancerous spots known as actinic keratoses can be successfully treated with these lasers as well, but in many cases, these conditions can be treated with simpler techniques first. In the latter two cases, laser offers no advantage, in my opinion, over less expensive methods.

WHO'S A GOOD CANDIDATE?

The best candidates for resurfacing lasers are those who have realistic expectations. No doctor is going to be able to make you look as you looked at twenty. Any expectation of painless "erasing" of wrinkles is more the result of hype than reality. I take extra pains to make sure that prospective patients understand the medical information I provide rather than put stock in what they hear on talk shows or infomercials. The ideal resurfacing candidates also have fair skin and typically do not tan easily. Such people generally do well because the risk of darkening of the skin from the inflammation of healing is less in fair-skinned patients.

Although one treatment with the laser may accomplish the desired effect, sometimes multiple treatments are required. The process of new collagen production that occurs in response to the resurfacing laser continues—as most skin healing does—for at least twelve months. Touch-ups typically should *not* be done until that period ends. For one reason, improvement continues over this yearlong period. People who are unhappy with the immediate results on the upper lip where they would like their verticals lines to disappear completely usually feel quite differently at six months, when they observe continued improvement. As with all things cosmetic, good things take time.

PREPARING FOR THE PROCEDURE

Before undergoing laser resurfacing, preparation is critical. While the particular program will vary from doctor to doctor, preparation clearly improves final results. I use a regimen that includes pretreatment with Retin-A (tretinoin), which seems to stimulate regrowth of the epidermis. A depigmenting cream containing the active ingredient hydroquinone may also be used to help prevent darkening of the skin after healing occurs.

Even if you don't have a history of cold sores or previous skin outbreaks of the herpes simplex virus, disruption of the epidermis caused by the laser light may reactivate a cold sore. It's best to take antiviral medication before and after surgery to be on the safe side. An antibiotic is also prescribed to be taken before and after the procedure in order to prevent bacterial infection.

THE PROCEDURE

Laser resurfacing is an office procedure and does not require hospitalization. Laser resurfacing is in essence a controlled burn so it cannot be done without anesthesia. When limited areas are treated, such as the lip region, or lines around the eyes or cheeks, local anesthesia with lidocaine is effective and intravenous sedation is usually not required. If full-face resurfacing is planned, intravenous sedation, under the direction of a qualified physician, is necessary. Some doctors prefer to treat the whole face even if just a few areas have lines and wrinkles, believing that an effective result might otherwise leave a patchy appearance. That has not been my experience, but you should follow the advice of the doctor who is going to do the procedure. My goal is always to perform the simplest procedure that will achieve the desired result.

If undergoing laser resurfacing in the office setting with local anesthetic, eat a normal breakfast on the day of the procedure, and take your routine medications. If you have been on aspirin or similar medications such as Advil or Motrin your doctor will likely ask you to stop taking them a week to ten days prior to surgery.

When I perform laser resurfacing, I first review the procedure with the patient emphasizing what can and cannot be accomplished. With the patient holding the mirror in the upright sitting position (your face looks different when you are lying flat) I ask her to note the areas she would like treated. I then mark these with a marker, and we then anesthetize the skin with lidocaine injections.

The patient then lies down on the procedure table and goggles are placed over the eyes for protection. Wet towels are draped around the areas to be treated to prevent tissue damage to skin that will not be treated.

HOW DO I KNOW WHICH LASERS WILL WORK FOR MY PROBLEM?

With so many lasers available and the media hype about them, it is hard to know where to turn. Don't worry about the particular lasers listed here—your doctor will select what is best for you, since several different lasers may be available to accomplish the same goals. Here's a simple guide to give a broad idea of the range of lasers in use. I've marked (in parentheses) how effective I think laser treatment is in each case.

Wrinkles
Carbon dioxide resurfacing laser, erbium laser, pulsed neodymium: YAG **(very effective)**

Red Spots
Broken blood vessels, rosacea, hemangiomas including port wine stains, cherry angiomas, red noses, starburst vessels, spider veins on the face
Vascular lesion lasers including the pulsed-dye laser **(very effective)**; *KTP laser* **(effective buy may require more treatments than the pulsed-dye laser)**

Brown Spots
Liver spots, freckles, nevus of Ota, café-au-lait spots, melasma
Ruby laser, neodymium: YAG laser, alexandrite **(effective for liver spots, freckles, nevus of Ota; less effective for melasma)**

Tattoos
Removal of tattoos can be effective, but different lasers are required for certain colors. In general:
Ruby laser, alexandrite laser **(effective for most colors)**
Neodymium: YAG laser **(effective for yellow and orange)**

After confirming by touch that all areas to be treated are numb, I proceed with laser treatment. One nurse holds the vacuum suction which takes away the vaporized particles. This makes a fair amount of noise so you should know to expect sound. Another assistant stands ready to provide the wet gauze that is used to wipe away the surface skin that has been treated. During the firing of the laser you will hear a rapid, relatively high-pitched buzz. How deep I go—that is, how many additional passes I make—depends largely on experience, the nature of the lines and wrinkles, the person's own skin qualities, and the risk I am willing to take to get the best result. In elective cosmetic cases, the rule of thumb is to be conservative. I believe we can always touch up an area that needs additional treatment; however, if you wind up with scars because the injury caused by the laser was too deep, neither you nor the doctor will be satisfied.

In my experience a cautious approach to laser resurfacing is best. Unfortunately, as this procedure explodes in popularity, a small number of doctors are not exercising good judgment and are combining it with other elective cosmetic procedures. In one case I consulted on, the surgeon had combined laser resurfacing with a neck lift. Scars resulted. When resurfacing your face, remember that you are asking a lot of your skin. Don't overdo it and don't rush the changes. When pursuing aesthetic elegance it is best to be conservative and cautious and realize that it took your mother nine months to make your face, and it probably took you an additional forty years of sun to get it where it is today. Take your time nudging it back to a fresher-looking state.

After the laser treatment is finished, a dressing will be placed on top of the treated areas. Some of my colleagues prefer a self-stick thin foam dressing that stays on for several days. I prefer a dressing that is changed daily. There is no right or perfect wound care regimen. The only thing that is important is for you to follow your doctor's instructions to the letter.

Burns and cuts heal best in moist environments. The key is to keep the skin that has been treated by laser moist and prevent any buildup of a crust or scab. This will help to achieve healing more rapidly.

Immediately after the procedure, the treated areas will look quite red and may be somewhat swollen from the anesthetic. Swelling will diminish

WHAT'S NEW IN SKIN RESURFACING

In 1999, colleagues at the University of California at San Francisco, University of Minnesota, and I studied a new technique for removing facial wrinkles. Based on the principle that removing the epidermis may stimulate new collagen in the dermis that will tighten up the skin surface, the method uses sophisticated electrical current rather than laser light to take off the top layer of skin. Early results are very promising with the method, known as *coblation*. For more information about this new therapy as it develops, check www.totalskinmd.com.

within a day or two. The redness may last for weeks or several months, depending on the type of laser used and the number of laser passes that were made over the skin.

You just experienced a controlled burn so *there will be some discomfort*. Pain medication is rarely needed for more than a day or two, and ice packs help a great deal.

Keep in mind as well that a resurfacing laser is used to surgically create a controlled scar. The skin responds to the laser injury by healing and new collagen is formed and remodeled. This takes many months, even though your surface skin or epidermis will be completely healed in about a week. So a key word for you is to be patient. The time it takes to heal completely and appreciate the full benefits of the surgery may be up to a year.

COMPLICATIONS

Potential complications of laser resurfacing procedures include scarring, increased pigmentation, and prolonged redness. You may need multiple treatments. You should not be afraid to ask your doctor how he or she plans to avoid or minimize these potential complications. If you are concerned about any changes that don't seem right, contact your doctor right away. As a physician, I can be of help only if I know what's going on.

▪ AGE SPOTS, BIRTHMARKS, AND TATTOOS

Lasers are now available that will treat dark spots on your skin. A whole range of lesions can be treated, including those with the colors brown, black, dark blue, and dark green in them. These lasers go by the names of Q-switched ruby (also known simply as "ruby"), Q-switched neodymium:YAG, and alexandrite. Each variety can generate a color of light that is preferentially absorbed by the melanin pigment in your skin or by the dye of the tattoo.

These lasers do not alone destroy the pigment. Rather, they fire bursts of light that are incredibly short, lasting a tiny fraction of a second. When the pigment absorbs the light energy, a shock wave is created and the pigment actually fragments into minute particles. Unlike the carbon dioxide laser, where the residue is scrubbed away with gauze, the body's own waste disposal system comes along and digests the miniscule fragments of pigment. Even though the laser has reduced the pigment to bite-sized pieces, at least for your body's cells, it still takes a couple of months for this process to reach maximal effect. So don't expect to see your tattoo disappear instantly.

The pigmented lesion lasers work well on the brown spots that develop on the backs of the hands and on the face after years of sun exposure. Many people call these age spots or liver spots. In fact, medically they are known as solar lentigines. Typically, one treatment can remove these lesions, but I always tell patients to expect a second treatment or more for complete removal.

Other kinds of pigmented lesions often require multiple treatments before they vanish. These include café-au-lait spots, which are light brown flat patches that are present from birth, and nevi of Ota, congenital dark blue or gray patches on the sides of the face which are common in Asian people.

Great caution should be exercised before treating other pigmented conditions, especially moles, with lasers. Although the vast majority of moles are benign, lasers cannot provide tissue for analysis in the process of removing the mole so there is always the very small chance that a malignant or premalignant mole may be removed partially without knowing it.

Any number of tattoo types may be treated with pigmented lesion lasers. Some colors—especially black and blue-black—respond better than others. Other colors can be treated, though a series of lasers with different wavelengths may be needed to get all the red (or yellow) out.

WHO IS THE BEST CANDIDATE?

The best candidates for treatment with pigmented lesion lasers are people with lighter skin. Unfortunately, the pigmented lesion lasers are not very bright instruments. They can't tell the difference between pigment that is from your own skin versus pigment that is in an unwanted lesion. Therefore, if you have a dark complexion, you will unfortunately be at higher risk here for an overlightening of the skin. Recently there has been some progress in developing new lasers that address this technical problem, so if you are dark skinned and would like to be treated, ask your dermatologist about it.

For most dark lesions, you should expect to need multiple treatments. To remove 90 percent of the color of a tattoo or a nevus of Ota, it may require eight to ten treatments.

THE PROCEDURE

If the area being treated is close to the lips, your physician may ask you to use an antiviral medication before your procedure to prevent cold sores. You may also be given a prescription for an anesthetic cream, such as EMLA or ELA-Max, that you apply at home about one hour prior to the procedure to decrease the discomfort associated with the laser treatment. Many people tolerate the laser surgery quite well without anesthesia, comparing the pain sensation to that of the snap of a rubber band or a mild grease splatter.

Prior to the procedure you will be given goggles to protect your eyes from any stray laser light. You may feel a slight buildup of heat in the treated area, and this sensation may linger for several hours afterward. For up to an hour immediately after the procedure, the area treated may appear white or grayish. Then, there is typically some redness at and around the site of treatment.

When the procedure is over, you will be given a dressing along with some antibiotic ointment to apply to help soothe the area. You should continue to dress the wound with an ointment for at least a week or so after surgery, or as your doctor advises.

Occasionally, areas of intense pigmentation, or areas that were treated with high levels of laser energy, will blister. The blisters will heal in approximately one to two weeks.

COMPLICATIONS

Potential complications of pigmented lesion lasers include lightening (or darkening) of the skin beyond that which is desired and scarring, which is relatively uncommon but still possible.

▪ GETTING THE RED OUT

A number of lasers are now available that can treat the often unsightly red broken blood vessels that we acquire with age and sun exposure. These so-called vascular lesion lasers can also be used to treat childhood birthmarks called hemangiomas. Types of vascular lesion lasers are the pulsed dye laser, the KTP laser, and the neodymium: YAG laser. Each of these lasers emit a color of light that is absorbed better by the hemoglobin in red blood cells than by the tissue in surrounding skin. The laser light comes out as a circle as

EASY ON, NOT SO EASY OFF

The ruby laser and others like it have provided great relief to many who would like to reverse previous indiscretions or have just had a change of heart about their tattoos. While these lasers are quite effective at removing most of the tattoo, it does require multiple treatments. In dark-skinned people, there is a risk of loss of pigment, resulting in small white spots. Have reasonable expectations and remember that it's unlikely a tattoo will vanish 100 percent. Individual variation in ink color, depth of pigment in skin, and location can all affect the final results.

small as a lead pencil eraser or as large as a dime. The larger the spot size, as it's called, the bigger the area covered, and the faster the treatment.

Numerous other conditions can be treated successfully with these lasers, including port wine stains, which appear as a deep red or violet areas on one portion of one side of the face; cherry angiomas, small red spots that develop with age, and usually appear on the trunk; and red scars. A new generation of these lasers is available that can be used to treat varicose veins, especially the smaller ones.

WHO IS THE BEST CANDIDATE?

As is par for the course in most laser therapies, the best candidates to undergo procedures with vascular lesion lasers are those with average to fair skin. While the wavelengths of light in these lasers do their best to avoid any damage to other skin pigment, they may not entirely leave the melanin in your skin alone. In fact, results are so much better on lighter skin that we typically tell patients not to come in for treatment if they have a tan. Broken blood vessels (spontaneously or as part of rosacea) typically respond after one or two treatments, while a port wine stain may require dozens of treatments to significantly lighten. People with such birthmarks may reach a point at which further treatment provides no additional benefit. (I assure them that, the way things are going, in a few years there are likely to be new lasers that might eliminate the balance of the growth.)

Pulsed dye lasers will cause black-and-blue marks at the site of the broken blood vessels or hemangiomas, and that is a drawback to their use. On the other hand, this kind of laser has been in use the longest, so we have the most experience with it. This purplish bruise will last five to ten days. It's important to be aware of this time lag before treatment so you can plan your activities. You may not wish to venture outside much until it clears up. Newer versions of this laser cause less bruising.

The KTP lasers, on the other hand, do not cause bruising, especially if they are used with a cooling tip but may require more treatments for a particular area.

THE PROCEDURE

In preparation for treatment with any vascular lesion lasers, avoid aspirin for about ten days beforehand.

During the procedure itself, your eyes will be shielded with eye goggles. As the laser is fired you will feel a rubber band–type snap at the site. One of the new pulsed dye lasers actually fires a burst of cold air so discomfort is significantly reduced. Some physicians may give you a prescription for a topical anesthetic cream to apply at home beforehand to lessen any discomfort. The procedure will probably last several minutes, unless you have an exceptionally large area to be treated.

COMPLICATIONS

Potential complications of the vascular laser vary by laser type. The pulsed dye laser is exceptionally safe. It has a very low risk of skin pigment changes or scarring, but it generally requires multiple treatments. The KTP laser can cause a hive-type reaction around the treated area, with itching, redness, and swelling; this will slowly disappear over the next day. KTP lasers may also leave marks somewhat like cat scratches, which typically heal without problems. Both types of vascular lesion lasers have the risk of temporary skin darkening that can last three to six months.

▪ HAIR REMOVAL LASERS

As lasers seem to be helping us in so many other areas of life, people have eagerly awaited the laser that would permanently get rid of unwanted hair. Now there are several lasers available to remove hair: the alexandrite, ruby, and diode lasers. There is even a "non-laser" laser called the PhotoDerm, which uses intense waves of multiple wavelengths of light. All these lasers emit a light color that is absorbed by dark pigment in the roots of the hair.

At present, it appears that two or three treatments spaced a couple of months apart will achieve a significant thinning of hairs in an area. The hairs that remain will not grow as quickly. When these hairs do grow back, they are typically smaller and of lighter color than they were before.

These new lasers haven't been out long enough for us to ascertain whether hair removal is permanent, so right now, permanence is defined somewhat arbitrarily as two years without hair growth after treatment.

Multiple treatments are required because of the natural way that hair grows. Every hair on your body goes through growing and resting phases (see chapter 14, "Hair"). The hair that is most susceptible to damage from laser treatment (in other words, removal) is growing hair. Unfortunately, the hair in places where people often want no hair, such as the lip, the ears, and on the legs, is in the resting phase. As a result, at its very best, laser therapy can remove half the hairs permanently in these areas with a single treatment.

WHO IS THE BEST CANDIDATE?

The best results with these lasers can be expected in people with light skin and enough pigment in the targeted hair to absorb the laser energy, but little pigment in the surrounding skin to absorb energy that shouldn't be absorbed.

THE PROCEDURE

Before treatment, I ask people to shave the hair in the targeted area and to avoid any additional tanning.

I provide a prescription for topical anesthetic cream to apply to minimize discomfort. In my experience, hair removal lasers are less painful than any of those that are used to remove pigment. Many of these lasers now emit a cool blast of air or have a cool tip that is in contact with the skin. These cooling devices prevent damage to the epidermis and prevent blistering.

You will don your protective eye apparel and be placed in a comfortable, reclining position. The length of treatment will be based on the size of the area and the diameter of the light beam that the laser emits. Some

DERMATOLOGISTS AND LIGHT

More than any other specialty, dermatologists have a deep respect for light. We tell patients to avoid it (sun), we use it to treat psoriasis (ultraviolet booths), and we harness it in lasers. The first medical laser, a ruby laser, was developed in the early 1960s by a dermatologist named Leon Goldman.

of these lasers now have two- to three-inch-wide attachments, in which case a large area such as the back can be treated in ten to fifteen minutes.

COMPLICATIONS

Potential side effects and complications of this treatment include changes in your normal skin pigmentation, blistering, and prolonged redness. There is also a small risk of scarring.

Because of adjustments in the wavelength of light, the duration of each light burst, and various cooling devices, damage to the pigment that is part of normal skin occurs less frequently these days. As the development of hair-removal lasers has progressed, darker-skinned patients can now be treated successfully with a corresponding reduction in the potential side effects or damage.

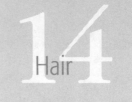

Hair 14

*I'm losing more hair every day. My father is bald
and I don't want to be like that.*

—*Kevin, 24, law student*

When it comes to hair, we all seem to want what someone else has. Hair may have little real value, except
to protect the scalp from the sun. Nevertheless, the huge
industry devoted to optimizing the amount of hair we
have and the quality of the tresses we bear attests to its
social, aesthetic, and emotional importance. We invest a
great deal of time and money to remove hair if we have

WISE OLD MAN

Hair is important in every walk of life. It plays a role in the first
impressions people make of us. The tale is told of a scholar who was a
child prodigy. He was named head of his academy at a very young age, but
the students and the faculty were concerned that he was not old enough
to have acquired the wisdom for such an important responsibility. God
heard these concerns, and one morning the scholar awoke with his hair
turned white. He was then accepted as the leader of the academy.

too much; add hair if we have too little; and bleach, color, straighten, and curl hair to help us be who we want to be.

The dermatologist's work does not end at the hairline, nor does the health of your skin. What happens to your scalp and the hair that grows there affects your overall health and appearance. How each of your hairs grow is not necessarily a matter of fate. Understanding the science behind these skin appendages will help you maintain them in the best possible shape.

▪ WHAT IS HAIR?

Strictly speaking, hair is just another fiber. It is alive when growing in the hair follicles just a few millimeters beneath the surface of your scalp; once it has emerged from your scalp to be visible, however, it is no longer living. This is why damaged hair is so hard to treat.

There are about 100,000 hair follicles on the scalp alone. Additional hair follicles are found all over the body, present in every area of the skin except the palms, soles, and lips. From an evolutionary point of view, hair on humans is fur on our mammal cousins. Both coverings emerged to provide warmth.

The hair itself consists of several layers of protein called keratin. The outside of the hair shaft is made up of overlapping layers, like shingles on a roof. There are no nerve endings in the hair shaft, which makes getting a haircut painless.

▪ HOW HAIR GROWS

To learn how hair grows, which is so important to understand all the problems that can develop with your hair, imagine that you are sliding down your hair shaft like a fireman slides down the firehouse pole. In this descent, you come to the hair follicle, which is located just below the dermis in the fatty layer. The follicle consists of a swelling at the very end of the hair shaft, which surrounds a group of capillaries that nourish the hair. This is the area where the hair is actually produced before growing out through the skin. Attached to the hair unit is a sebaceous gland, which supplies the sebum (oil) that gives healthy hair a glossy appearance. (Similar glands in water fowl, such as ducks, produce an oil that is amazingly waterproof and keeps the birds from getting waterlogged.)

At any given time, 90 percent of the 100,000 hairs on the average scalp are growing and 10 percent are resting. The growing hairs continue to do

BIRDS OF A FEATHER

An amazing discovery in a remote Chinese province, late in the twentieth century, demonstrated that the need for warmth in small dinosaurs, which actually were warm-blooded, resulted in the development of feathers. These dinosaurs with feathers were actually ancestors of birds. You might say that feathers, fur, and hair are all birds of a feather. The need to insulate the body against piercing cold weather made an extra covering essential, but for humans, hair no longer serves that important purpose.

so for two to five years, at a rate of about half an inch a month. Scalp hair growth in women is slightly faster than in men. At the end of this growing phase, which is called anagen, the hair is shed. For the next three months, the follicle goes into a resting phase, called telogen. At the end of that time, the hair follicle produces a new hair that starts the growth cycle all over again. So it is normal to lose 50 to 100 hairs every day, because when the hair follicle goes from growing (anagen) to resting (telogen), hairs are shed. But remember, the same follicle that has lost a hair will start to produce a new hair three months later.

If you're concerned about how many hairs you are losing, always brush over a sink and count the hairs you find. Also count the hairs you find in the shower, on your pillow, and on your clothes. Do this daily over a week and you will have an idea of whether your hair loss is within normal limits.

Hair follicle in growing (left) and resting phase (right). Notice the attached oil gland and band of muscle responsible for goose bumps.

Have you ever wondered why your eyebrows and eyelashes don't grow as long as the hair on your head? It is because their growth phase is shorter. There are seasonal variations in hair growth as well. Spring is the time when hair grows most rapidly, and fall is when hair growth is slowest. As we grow older, our hair growth rate slows down. Contrary to popular belief, shaving has no effect on the rate of hair growth.

▪ FROM UTERUS THROUGH ADOLESCENCE

Before birth, there is a wave of shedding of scalp hair. By the time of delivery, most newborns have already regrown a full head of hair, although some babies have absolutely no hair at birth. In this situation, the hair cycle is slightly altered and the wave of hair loss *in utero* occurred just a little late—all the hair has not grown back yet, but it will. Two to three months later, infants often have a noticeable patch of baldness on the back of the head. Although this is usually blamed on pressure from lying in the crib on the back in one position, it is just a natural shedding of hair that was never shed before birth, and it also will regrow in a few months.

Before puberty there are two types of hair on the body. *Vellus* hair is fine, usually nonpigmented, and usually not longer than a quarter of an inch. *Terminal* hair is longer, coarser, and often pigmented. In childhood, terminal hair is limited to the scalp, eyebrows, and eyelashes. At puberty, terminal hair replaces the vellus hair, starting in the pubic region. Somewhat later, terminal armpit hair develops in both sexes, and facial hair appears in boys. Subsequently, terminal hair development continues to include the arms and legs of both sexes and the back and chest of men. All of this hair growth is dependent on the increased hormone production associated with puberty.

▪ "DOC, I'M LOSING MY HAIR!!!"

Our hair, like our health, is something we take for granted—until we start losing it, which can be psychologically devastating. I know this from the people who come to my office concerned about hair loss: men—young men still in their twenties—who have noticed their hair thinning or that

HAIR AND RACE

Hair color, texture, and curliness are all genetically determined and vary by race. Asian hair is the thickest and is perfectly circular with a straight hair follicle and hair shaft. African hair is oval, the follicle is curved (helical), and the hair shaft is curly. Caucasian hair is a combination of the other hair types. Asian and African hair is always black, while Caucasian hair varies from blond to black. Blond hair is finer than black hair, but blonds actually have greater numbers of hairs on their scalp.

their forehead is beginning to look higher; women worried about general thinning of the hair or an increased amount of hair in the brush after brushing; parents with a child who has come home from school crying because a classmate has made fun of bald spots that have recently appeared.

Dermatologists often begin to determine the cause of hair loss by taking a good case history. How long has the hair loss been noticeable? Is it the same every day or does it vary from day to day? Is the hair loss localized to certain areas of the scalp or is it more diffuse? Are the hairs actually being shed or are they breaking off? Are there bald spots or just areas that are thinning? Does the scalp look normal or is there redness or scaling?

Is there a family history of hair loss? A detailed history also includes questions about any significant weight loss, medications, recent illnesses, emotional stress, menstrual irregularities, or pregnancy.

▪ COMMON BALDNESS

The most common type of hair loss is referred to as male-pattern baldness (when it occurs in women it is called female-pattern baldness). The condition is known medically as androgenetic alopecia: *andro* is short for androgens, which are the male hormones present in both sexes; *genetic* means this is an inherited type of hair loss; and *alopecia* is a term from the Greek meaning "hair loss." In men it can start as early as the late teens or early twenties in the form of a receding hairline or a thinning spot on the crown of the head. Recently, such hair loss has been associated with a possible increase in heart disease in some men. Over time, different patterns of hair loss develop, which eventually can lead to a bald scalp with a permanent fringe of remaining hair.

Hair loss in women usually occurs after menopause. It can begin at an early age, with most thinning usually occurring in the frontal and mid-part of the scalp. Significant hair loss in young women may be a sign of hormonal abnormalities related to excessive androgen production or to a thyroid imbalance. Every young woman with significant hair loss should have a complete checkup to rule out an underlying medical cause—abnormalities of the ovaries or the adrenal or thyroid glands need to be ruled out. Associated symptoms that suggest that such hormonal imbalance may exist include irregular periods, acne, and excessive facial or body hair.

Since androgenetic alopecia does not occur without the presence of androgens, the problem does not exist until after puberty. Many older medical textbooks say the inheritance of common baldness comes only from the maternal side, but in fact baldness can be inherited from either side of the family. The actual gene that controls this type of hair loss has yet to be discovered (researchers have identified other genes that control less common hereditary types of hair loss).

The specific androgen, or male hormone, responsible for this type of hair loss is dihydroxytestosterone, or DHT, which is found in the scalp of all individuals with androgenetic alopecia. DHT has no effect on normal hair follicles but only on those hair follicles that are genetically predetermined to be susceptible; "normal" hair is immune and will continue to grow as described in the section above. Over time an affected hair follicle becomes weaker; its growing phase becomes shorter and shorter. Each hair shaft that emerges becomes finer and finer, and the color becomes lighter and lighter. *Miniaturization* is the term used for this process in which affected hairs become shorter, finer, and lighter with each growth cycle. Keep in mind that the hair just doesn't fall out all at once, leaving the person suddenly bald—the process takes many years and is very gradual.

In androgenetic alopecia, the hair on the back and sides of the head is never lost, because this hair is genetically programmed to grow for a lifetime. The persistence of this rim of hair led doctors to wonder whether, if the only reason people lost hair on the top of the head was genetics, hair moved to the top of the scalp from elsewhere might take and thrive.

The first such "hair transplants" were performed in the late 1950s. They proved that these donor hairs would continue to grow when moved (transplanted) from the back or sides of the head to the bald areas on the scalp. These days there are several treatment options for common baldness.

MEDICAL TREATMENT

At the present time two drugs are approved by the FDA for the treatment of hair loss:

Finasteride (Propecia) is a prescription oral medication that specifically reduces the production of DHT by blocking the enzyme necessary for its formation. The pill, which is not approved for use in women, appears to be effective only in men: studies have shown that over 80 percent of men taking finasteride do not show evidence of further hair loss, and about two-thirds actually experience increased hair growth. The drug must be taken daily and, if stopped, the hair loss will eventually resume. Impotence is a possible side effect (in less than 2 percent of men), but it is completely reversible upon discontinuing the drug.

Minoxidil (Rogaine) is a topical solution that is applied to the scalp twice daily. It is sold over the counter in both 2 percent and 5 percent solutions—the latter strength is approved for use only by men. Minoxidil is effective in retarding hair loss and promoting hair growth. Like finasteride, if successful, it must be continued indefinitely. Side effects, which include itching or scaling of the scalp, are more common with the stronger solution.

Both minoxidil and finasteride are most successful in younger men who are just starting to lose their hair and are not completely bald. Both drugs treat the top of the head (crown) more effectively than the hairline (frontal). Minoxidil appears to be effective in treating frontal thinning in women and is particularly successful in menopausal women.

These drugs allow people who are losing their hair to take a proactive role in trying to prevent impending future hair loss. Nevertheless, it is still a losing battle for many people. More effective inhibitors of DHT will surely become available in the future.

Some dermatologists mix minoxidil with low concentrations of Retin-A and/or a low-strength steroid solution. Its additional benefit has not been proven, although I have seen some anecdotal improvement.

SURGICAL TREATMENT

Hair transplantation is now the most common cosmetic procedure performed on men. Originally invented by dermatologists, the technique has been refined from a relatively crude procedure to a highly sophisticated one that utilizes state-of-the-art microsurgical techniques. As mentioned, the procedure involves taking hair from the back and sides of the head, which is genetically programmed to grow for a lifetime, and moving it to the bald areas of the scalp where it continues to grow.

In the original method of hair transplantation, multiple hairs were removed from the back of the head in the form of small round cylinders called "plugs" and placed into round holes in the bald area, where the hairs would continue to grow. The procedure was done under local anesthesia. About fifty plugs per session were considered average, and it usually took four sessions to completely fill in an area and avoid a corn-row appearance. The bald areas treated could be adequately covered with hair, but the hairlines were aesthetically unacceptable, and people had to comb their hair over or forward to hide the evidence of the transplanted plugs.

In the past decade dermatologists have developed revolutionary techniques called micro- and minigrafting. The donor hair is divided up into groups of one to two hairs (micrografts) or three to five hairs (minigrafts). With this new technology, hairlines can be created composed entirely of single hairs. Because of the naturalness of these small grafts, which don't look "pluggy," people have good results after just one procedure. Some men can even comb their hair straight back, completely exposing their transplanted hairline. It takes less time to achieve adequate density in bald areas, since as many as a thousand grafts can be transplanted in a single session.

Recent improvements in how the grafts are taken from the donor site have further enhanced the procedure. The donor hair is now separated under magnification into naturally occurring groups of one to three hairs, called follicular units, allowing the hair transplant surgeon to achieve results that are almost undistinguishable from a natural head of hair.

HOW HAIR TRANSPLANTATION IS DONE

Hair transplantation is done as an office procedure. Local anesthesia is used, so that the patient is awake and can watch TV, read, or listen to

---

CHOOSE YOUR TRANSPLANT SURGEON CAREFULLY

There are many doctors in different specialties who perform hair transplantation, a procedure developed and refined by dermatologists. This procedure is highly skill-dependent, so choose your doctor carefully. Follow these guidelines:

- Check credentials—is the doctor board certified in dermatology or another medical specialty known for transplantation?
- How many procedures does he or she do a week? (A doctor who does only a couple a month is unlikely to have refined the process for optimal results.)
- Does the doctor do the procedure himself or herself? It is customary to have nurses assist in preparing the graft.
- Are the fees reasonable, given the level of expertise? Fees that are too low should raise suspicion, as should fees that are too high.
- Although advertising is now common in the hair restoration field, be cautious about "franchised" hair transplant operations in which no specific doctor is identifiable as the surgeon.
- If your dermatologist doesn't perform hair transplants, ask for a referral.

music during the process which, in the hands of a skilled transplanter, takes just a few hours.

Risks are minimal, and the most serious problems occur when physicians are inexperienced. *It is important that prospective patients choose their transplant surgeon carefully*—in order to avoid common mistakes such as improper placement of the hairline, wasting donor hair, and damaging existing hair.

Before any surgery is scheduled, you should be able to speak personally to the operating physician so that your goals and desires are clearly understood. You need to carefully research the credentials of your doctor, and if necessary speak to people who have had the procedure done by this doctor. An informed patient will always have the best results.

OTHER PROCEDURES FOR BALDNESS

Other surgical procedures available to treat androgenetic alopecia can be done individually or can be combined with hair transplantation.

Alopecia reduction, also known as scalp reduction, is used most often with patients who have extensive baldness involving both the crown and frontal parts of the scalp. In these patients it would probably not be possible to cover the entire bald scalp using hair transplantation alone, mostly because the amount of available donor hair would be insufficient.

The scalp-reduction technique is used primarily on the crown, combined with hair transplantation in the front. The two to three square inches to be removed are carefully marked out on the scalp and the area is surgically excised. The skin on each side is then separated from the underlying tissue, so that it can be stretched across the open area and sewn together, thus spreading the existing hair over a wider area. There may be considerable discomfort following the surgery and narcotic pain relievers may be required. Complications include scarring, thinning of the scalp, and reappearance of the bald area. The advances in micrografting have led to a decrease in alopecia reduction procedures.

Complicated plastic surgery procedures are also sometimes used to treat common baldness. Flaps of hair-bearing scalp are taken from the back and sides of the head and brought forward to replace the bald areas in the front. These procedures are done by relatively few surgeons and require a high level of skill. There are extensive possible side effects and complications.

NONSURGICAL TREATMENT

People who prefer not to have surgery or who have extensive baldness and want a full head of hair may choose to wear a hairpiece. Made of artificial or human hair, hairpieces come in many styles, thicknesses, and colors. Most of these hair replacement systems need to be adjusted every one or two months or they get too loose; they usually last one or two years before having to be replaced. There are many different methods of anchoring the hairpiece to the scalp—including glue, tape, snaps, or even stitches sewn into the scalp—or it can be attached by weaving it into the existing hair.

Complications do occur from wearing hairpieces. If the hairpiece cannot be removed, many people experience itching or irritation of the scalp since it is difficult to properly cleanse the area. If the problem persists, the hairpiece may have to be removed. Hairpieces that are sewn to the scalp often cause infections that may require antibiotics and removal of the stitches. Allergic reactions to the glue and tape are not uncommon.

Many people do not like the feeling of having something artificial attached to their scalp or are concerned about the hairpiece being noticeable. Others wear hairpieces for years without difficulty. It is important to choose a reputable facility because techniques and costs vary widely.

▪ OTHER TYPES OF HAIR LOSS

SHEDDING OF RESTING HAIR

If you woke up one morning and noticed hair on your pillow, then took a shower and the drain clogged with your hair, not only would you definitely be having a bad hair day but you would also probably be experiencing *telogen effluvium*. Because effluvium means shedding and telogen is the resting phase of the hair growth cycle, telogen effluvium is the excessive shedding of resting hair. It is characterized by the sudden onset of hair loss in a previously normal scalp. The hair loss is characteristically diffuse and does not cause bald patches. Usually a considerable amount of hair—about 50 percent—can be shed before the hair loss becomes noticeable. There is no itching, burning, or redness of the scalp.

The cause of this episode can usually be determined by a careful history. After a precipitating event, such as a severe illness with a high fever, surgery under general anesthesia, or severe sudden emotional stress, the hair suddenly stops growing and goes into the resting phase. In this condition a significantly greater number of hairs convert into telogen phase than the normal 10 percent, with the resulting loss of hair.

The actual diagnosis of telogen effluvium is easy when one takes a look at the individual lost hairs. If you pull the shed hair slowly through your thumb and forefinger, you can feel a little knob at the end of the hair shaft; examined closely, this knob looks white.

Hair loss following pregnancy is a classic example of telogen effluvium. After being stimulated by the increased hormonal activity of pregnancy, the hair roots are suddenly shocked by the stress of delivery. The result is an extensive shutdown of the growing hair follicles, with subsequent loss of hair one to three months later.

Crash diets resulting in significant weight loss can deprive the hair follicles of nourishment (as in protein deficiency states) and trigger telogen effluvium. Many drugs can cause this type of hair loss, including anticoagulants (Coumadin), beta-blockers, (propranolol), and antidepressants (lithium).

There is no specific treatment for telogen effluvium, because the problem is of limited duration and the follicles will revert to normal. All of the lost hairs will regrow since there was never any damage to the hair follicle, merely an interruption in the normal hair cycle. In those cases of hair loss caused by chronic emotional stress, malnutrition due to excessive dieting, or the continued use of drugs, the underlying specific situation needs to be corrected before the hair loss will clear up.

SELF-INFLICTED HAIR LOSS

Most of us have twisted our hair around our finger while watching TV or reading. But some people do more than twist their hair; they actually pull their hair out, leaving patchy areas of baldness and broken hairs. Although this can just be a very bad habit, in others it is a sign of significant emotional disturbance. Self-inflicted hair loss caused by such turmoil is known as *trichotillomania,* and is more common in children than in adults.

When the child denies pulling hair out it is helpful to go on a vigil to try to confirm that this is actually happening. The type and extent of hair loss depends on the severity of the pulling and plucking of the hair. It may be localized to a few selected patches on the scalp, mimicking alopecia areata (see below), or it may involve extensive areas. There occasionally may be some localized redness or flaking on the scalp. In the absence of a confession from the person afflicted or from the parent, diagnosis is still possible by studying the variation in the length of the remaining hairs in the affected areas. These sections can be completely bald if the hairs were recently pulled out, or there may be patches of very short hair as it regrows, but they are not long enough to be pulled out again.

The only treatment is to discuss the cause of the problem in detail, so that the person understands the nature of the hair loss and the fact that it could lead to permanent baldness. Psychiatric consultation might be necessary for some people.

WHEN STYLE AND HEALTHY HAIR COLLIDE

Have you ever worn your hair pulled back in a tight ponytail? Have you ever had your hair tightly woven in tiny braids? Either style may look attractive, but each can potentially inflict permanent damage to the hair roots. The constant pulling from tightly braided hair is a major cause of hair loss, particularly in African-American girls.

This type of hair loss is called *traction alopecia*. Typically, many children wear their hair in short tight braids, and as they get older they pull the braids back into a tight ponytail. As a result of this constant yanking on the hair roots, a particular pattern of hair loss begins to emerge. First the hair is lost in the temples, which can then extend to the front of the hairline. The hairs become shorter and finer, and after many years, a band of hair loss develops where the hairline should have been. This hair is so fine and short that the entire hairline area looks bald.

Traction alopecia can be caused by the constant use of tight rollers and can occur in any race. The process is gradual and takes years to fully develop. It is reversible, in the beginning, if hairstyles are changed. However, permanent hair loss can result after many years of constant physical stress to the hair roots. Many adolescent girls realize too late that their problem may be permanent.

ALOPECIA AREATA

Alopecia areata is a medical form of hair loss. It is a specific condition of follicles that usually occurs in several localized patches on the body or scalp and is limited in extent. In severe cases of alopecia areata, widespread hair loss may occur on the scalp (alopecia totalis). In those rare cases when all body hair is lost (alopecia universalis), the hair follicles that normally produce hair have become permanently dormant. It is said that

John D. Rockefeller suffered from alopecia. Rockefeller University, founded by him, conducts valuable dermatology research even today.

Alopecia areata occurs most often in children and is probably due to an immunologic reaction in the body to the hair follicle. In most cases of alopecia areata, hair growth begins again on its own within months of the first appearance of the bald patches. When this does not happen, there are treatments aimed at stimulating hair follicles to regenerate hair growth, but there are no guarantees. If hair loss is modest, corticosteroid may be injected into the bald patches or applied directly to the skin as a lotion to stimulate hair growth. Usually, hair begins to grow again within weeks, and the injections are repeated in about a month. Anthralin cream may also be applied to the hairless area; this irritant is used every day and rinsed off an hour later. The treatment usually stimulates hair growth within two to three months. Other treatments, designed to interfere with the offending immunologic reaction and involving other topical agents, promise some hope.

No treatments have proven effective in restoring hair growth when hair loss is total. If you are suffering from any variety of alopecia areata, you might want to contact the National Alopecia Areata Foundation (see Appendix 5).

SUDDEN HAIR LOSS

If hair loss is rapid or sudden, you should consult your doctor in order to rule out the possibility of internal disease, such as a thyroid condition, bowel disease, AIDS, or malnutrition due to anorexia nervosa. Insufficient protein from a vegetarian diet is another possible cause.

INFECTIONS AND DISEASES

Any rash or infection of the scalp can cause hair loss if it goes deep enough. The hair root itself sits in the fat below the upper layers of the skin and is generally not bothered by superficial irritation or inflammation of the scalp. There are diseases, however, that can strike the deeper layers of the skin and can cause scarring of the scalp with permanent damage to the hair root and subsequent loss of hair. Any severe bacterial or fungal infection of the scalp can potentially cause areas of baldness (see chapter 25).

Two specific diseases that can harm the scalp are lupus erythematosis and lichen planus. Lupus is a connective tissue disorder thought to be caused by antibodies that the body makes to its own tissues, so-called auto-antibodies. Lupus affects the scalp by causing inflammation around the hair follicles, usually in patches, which results in scarring of the skin and permanent loss of the hair. An area of alopecia caused by lupus is initially red and scaly; once the hair loss occurs the skin turns thin and shiny.

Early treatment with topical corticosteroid cream and local injections of corticosteroid into the patches may be effective in stopping the progress of the disease. Drugs that may be used to control the disease systemically, such as anti-malaria drugs or oral corticosteroid, may also help stop the hair loss. However, once scarring has occurred no effective treatment is available for regrowing the hair.

Lichen planus is an uncommon skin disease that can also affect the nails and hair. We don't know what causes this rash, which consists of itchy, purple, flat-topped bumps on the wrists, trunk, legs, and occasionally the scalp. There are scattered patches of inflammation that result in irregular areas of hair loss, scalp skin is firm, pink to purple, and may have a fine scale. The openings of the hair follicles may be enlarged. The patches are usually small but may merge to form larger areas of baldness. Treatment, which is most effective in the early stages of inflammation, consists of topical, injected, or, if necessary, systemic corticosteroid. Once the hair is lost, the roots are destroyed and regrowth is not expected.

After many years of inactivity, the bald areas in both lupus and lichen planopilaris may be treated with hair transplantation.

▪ HIRSUTISM

Just as balding may plague a man, hirsutism, or abnormally abundant hair growth, can be the bane of a woman's existence. Hirsutism is triggered by androgens, the male hormones. It may occur when a woman has an increased sensitivity to the androgens that are always present in her system in small quantities or when elevated levels of androgens are present in the blood. The hair grows excessively in areas dependent on androgens for hair follicle stimulation, including the mustache, beard, and sideburn areas of the face as well as the chest and upper back. Because some ethnic groups tend to have more hair than others, a diagnosis of hirsutism is reserved for women who have more hair in comparison to their mothers and sisters.

There are many temporary remedies that deal with unwanted hair, such as bleaching, waxing, shaving, and chemically dissolving the hair. The only permanent solution is electrolysis, although there is a great deal of excitement now about laser hair removal (see p. 145). Although hair-removal lasers do not permanently eliminate unwanted hair, they are rapid, relatively painless and effective at reducing the size of hairs, and thus its thickness. Laser hair removal is probably preferable to electrolysis for most people.

The purpose of electrolysis is to destroy each hair follicle so that it can't grow back. The best results are obtained if the follicle is zapped when it is in the active growth phase. Electrolysis is performed with a fine needle that is placed through the pore and gently advanced toward the hair bulb itself. Electric current, heat, or a combination of the two is used for a fraction of a second to permanently damage the complete hair unit. Electrolysis is a painstaking procedure that requires multiple visits making it less appealing than laser hair removal.

Women who undergo electrolysis sometimes complain about discomfort, so in areas that are especially sensitive, such as the upper lip, a topical anesthetic cream containing lidocaine can be helpful.

Electrolysis is not without potential side effects. It can worsen the appearance of broken blood vessels on the face and cause darkening of light skin, lightening of dark skin, or scarring. In the short term, some people get redness and some scabbing. The scars that might result are usually tiny circular areas of white that surround the pore where the needle has been placed.

▪ DANDRUFF

Dandruff is actually a low-grade form of seborrheic dermatitis (see p. 279). Symptoms include itching and scaling on the scalp, the evidence of which appears on clothing as flakes of dead skin. Dandruff is a more serious problem for some than for others, but it is a cosmetic problem rather than a real medical problem.

If you have dandruff, you should wash your hair daily. Proper washing will help to control your dandruff and cut down on outbreaks. Proper

BUBBLE HAIR

Bubble hair occurs from using excessively hot blow dryers or curling irons. The hair becomes brittle, and rows of tiny bubbles can be seen within the hair shaft under a microscope. The condition is completely reversible just by lowering the setting on your dryer.

shampooing will not dry out your hair or scalp and will slow the production and shedding of skin cells on the scalp that are responsible for those telltale white flakes on that beautiful black silk blouse or navy blazer. Many shampoos available over the counter contain an anti-dandruff ingredient, the most common of which is salicylic acid. Using an anti-dandruff shampoo controls most cases of dandruff. However, if your dandruff continues to be severe, you may want to consult your dermatologist, who can prescribe a stronger anti-dandruff shampoo, such as Nizoral, which has an antimicrobial ingredient. Tar shampoos are excellent for controlling dandruff as well—Neutrogena makes some excellent products such as T-gel Shampoo. Head and Shoulders Intensive Treatment is also very good.

▪ PERMS AND STRAIGHTENERS

Permanents, a.k.a. perms or permanent waves, add artificial curls and waves to the hair. The textures that result from the application of solutions in a permanent last longer than those obtained from setting hair with curlers. The active ingredient in these solutions is thioglycolate, an alkaline chemical that breaks sulfur bonds in the hair. After the hair is curled or straightened, another chemical is added to allow new sulfur bonds to form. The solution may be applied hot or cold. Cold lotions are considered safer than perms that depend on heat. The heat will not only singe hair but may also burn the scalp. If burning is severe, a rare occurrence, the price for your permanent may be permanent hair loss.

Sometimes these solutions may cause allergic reactions. If your hairstylist notices any scaling or redness when the lotion is applied, or if you notice persistent itching, you should forgo the rest of the permanent.

Hair straighteners are usually petroleum jelly–based and their effect is temporary. When these preparations get on facial skin, they can cause a specific kind of acne called pomade acne. Gums, paraffins, and waxes may also be used to straighten hair. A few hair-straightening agents depend on the same thioglycolate ingredients used in permanent wave solutions. These solutions can damage hair in the same ways that permanent wave solutions can.

▪ SUN AND HAIR

Too much ultraviolet light can turn healthy hair into dry, brittle, lusterless hair. Sun-damaged hair may even break when you comb or brush it. While some hair products contain a sunscreen, this sunscreen cannot protect the keratin in your hair. In addition, it's hard to apply any hair product evenly to every hair shaft. The best way to protect your hair from sun damage is to wear a wide-brimmed hat when you are going to be outside. Color-treated hair is particularly susceptible to sun damage.

▪ HAIR CARE AND GROOMING

Here are some practical points about hair care:

- Don't shampoo excessively—once a day is fine.
- Avoid the excessive use of chemicals for conditioning (conditioners just coat the hair shaft).
- Avoid excessive exposure to the sun.
- Do not wear tight braids. Tight braids, especially in children, can result in a form of baldness called traction alopecia (see p. 159.)

Nails

Fingernails and toenails are there for two reasons: adornment and function. The desire to dress up nails dates back to the dawn of time, and it also seems to start very early in life. For instance, my daughter first demonstrated a strong interest in her nails at the age of three. She would corral her mother and any available baby-sitter into painting her nails, and the more shocking the color, the more gleeful she became.

Nonetheless, these hard and durable parts of our hands actually serve other needs as well. For one thing, they assist in dexterity. One day, my five-year-old son decided he didn't need his nails anymore. To prove him wrong, we put small pieces of modeling clay under his fingertips, so it was as though he had no nails. My challenge to him: if he could pick up a dime with his fingers altered in this way, he could keep the dime. He failed several times, finally understanding how important nails are to everyday life.

Nails serve another important purpose, at least to doctors: they are a kind of external warning system because often it's there that the outward signs of internal disease may develop. Finally, in the world of dermatology, we are especially aware of the greatest importance of nails: scratching that pesky itch.

Nails are actually an integral part of the skin. The nail itself is made of keratin, the same material hair is composed of. Nails have no nerve endings. This is true for horses as well as human beings, which is why the farrier of bygone days and the horsemen of today are able to nail (pardon the pun) iron shoes directly into the hooves of the trusty mare or steed. Because fingernails are in constant contact with the environment around us, they are subjected to a great deal of minor and not-so-minor trauma. That's probably why nature made them so tough. Nails are torn, banged by hammers, and slammed by doors.

Nail growth is slow but steady—about an eighth of an inch per month for fingernails and a tenth of an inch per month for toenails. With age the growth rate slows and nails become more brittle. The apparatus that makes the nail sits just under the cuticle. It is called the nail matrix and functions much like a pasta maker, extruding new nail slowly but surely. For a detailed look at your nail see the illustration on this page.

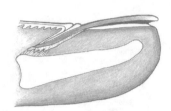

Cross-section of fingernail showing nail matrix where the nail is made

▪ NAILS GIVE CLUES

Many internal conditions or other bigger skin problems can show up in the nails. In fact, in psoriasis, the condition may be apparent only in the nails. From 10 to 50 percent of people with psoriasis have small pits or so-called oil spots on their nails. The same sort of nail pits, small depressions in the surface of the nails, are also sometimes seen in alopecia areata (see p. 159).

In people with AIDS, one may see brownish spots on the palms and soles. When this same discoloration occurs in the nails, it appears as a thin brown stripe. Brown stripes in the nail may be worrisome because occasionally they represent a melanoma growing under the nail. This is not very common but is important to know about and get diagnosed early, as there is a high mortality rate associated with this cancer. Although a dark line may develop from trauma (a bruise under the nail), any pigmented streak should be immediately evaluated by your doctor. This is especially true if the line has developed for the first time in a single nail in someone over fifty years of age. Pigment that is due to trauma under the nail will

NAIL CLUES

Nail changes can sometimes herald internal conditions and are therefore an important part of your regular physical exam:

Abnormality	Appearance	Internal Condition
Beau's lines	Horizontal grooves	Correspond to periods of severe illness
Splinter hemorrhages	Small dark brown or rust flecks	Bacterial endocarditis; trichinosis
Red lunula	Red discoloration in front of the cuticle	Rheumatoid arthritis, Lupus, alopecia areata
Clubbing	Curving of the nail with thickening of the fingertip	Lung disease
Spoon nails	Inward curving of the nails to resemble a spoon	Iron deficiency
Double white lines (Muehrcke's lines)	Transverse white lines that move out as the nail grows and occur in pairs	Liver disease; malnutrition

over time migrate out with the nail's growth, but the pigmented band of melanoma does not; in fact, it will sometimes get darker and broader.

In blacks, however, longitudinal or linear pigmented stripes of the nails, called *longitudinal melanonychia* (pronounced mel-AN-no-nick-ee-ah), are common. The condition is a result of increased pigment production by the pigment cells in the nail matrix. Both the incidence of these stripes and their darkness increase with the age of the person.

The challenge for the dermatologist is to make sure that the linear band in a nail does not represent an abnormal mole or a melanoma. Any line that is single, wider than a quarter of an inch, very dark, or has wide variation in pigmentation should be biopsied. If multiple lines are present on multiple nails and no one line stands out, it is much less likely that the band represents a melanoma.

Another important change you might see in your nails is *splinter hemorrhage*. This results from blood leaching out of the small blood vessels right under the nail, within the nail bed. If a splinter hemorrhage is seen closer to the lunula (the white, semicircular moonlike area of whiteness adjacent to the cuticle), it may be a sign of a bacterial infection of the

heart, called endocarditis. The most common cause of splinter hemor-
rhages, however, is trauma.

▪ PARONYCHIA

Paronychia is an inflammation of the skin around the nail. It is due to
infection and is characterized by reddening at the junction of the nail and
skin, swelling, tenderness, and pain. In addition, pus may be trapped under
the skin.

A paronychial infection is usually the direct result of a small break in
the skin. The break may be caused by trimming a nail carelessly or by a
cut or nick in the skin acquired during the day's activities. Acute paronychia is usually bacterial and caused by staph, strep, or other germs.
Chronic paronychia is often due to yeast such as candida and develops
when the fingers are very moist.

In general, infections of the nail are easily treated. If there has been
an accumulation of pus near the nail, it must be drained. This is not
nearly as terrible as it sounds, and the discomfort is often much less
than the pain the infected digit is already giving you. If you have infection in the nail unit, it is important to keep the area dry, especially if the
cause was candida. Sometimes, candida will clear up on its own just by
keeping the area dry. Yeast are like fish in this regard: they need water
to thrive.

▪ FUNGAL INFECTION

The most common fungal infection of the nail is onychomycosis. It
usually affects the toenails, but fingernails can be infected as well. Onychomycosis is characterized by a thickening of the nail, due to the accumulation of scales underneath. It usually turns the nail white and
eventually leads to the separation of the nail from the nail bed.

Taken orally, itraconazole (Sporanox) is one of the most common
treatments for this persistent fungus. Itraconazole has a cure rate of
approximately 70 percent; the course of treatment is two to three months.
A new antifungal treatment, terbinafine (Lamisil), has a similar treatment
cycle and an 80 percent cure rate. Before your dermatologist prescribes
either treatment, he or she may draw your blood to monitor for side
effects. After the fungus is eradicated, an antifungal cream may be prescribed to avoid a recurrence of the fungal infection.

▪ HANGNAILS

Hangnails are splits or projections in the skin adjacent to the nail, or tears in the edge of the nail itself. They can be painful and can become infected. (Paronychia infections can begin with hangnails.)

▪ SPLINTERS

Who hasn't had a splinter? It's true they are no calamity, but they should be attended to promptly. Most foreign objects that make their way under the nail are splinters of wood, but shards of glass, small nails, and even thin wires can also cause fingernail problems.

Fortunately, the skin of the palms, soles, fingers, and toes is thicker than on the rest of the body, protected by a thickened coat of keratin. Therefore splinters can usually be dislodged with a sterilized sewing needle, causing relatively little pain unless the culprit has penetrated deeply into the skin.

While most splinters cause no problems once removed, infections can arise at the injury site if the splinter is not attended to properly. If you can see the splinter, you can use tweezers to grab and remove it. Afterward, clean the area with antibacterial soap to prevent infection. If the splinter is not protruding, but hidden under the nail or otherwise hard for you to get at, you should call your doctor. Your doctor will remove the splinter with tools that are actually only slightly more sophisticated than tweezers. A topical antiseptic will then be applied, and an oral antibiotic may be prescribed to avoid infection or if the area is already infected.

▪ INGROWN TOENAILS

Ingrown toenails can become very painful. An ingrown toenail occurs when the nail (usually on a big toe) pierces the skin.

The best way to minimize suffering is to catch the problem early. If you notice the edge of a toenail growing into the surrounding skin, soak the skin immediately in warm water. If the problem is just beginning, try placing a tiny piece of cotton under the advancing nail edge to coax it into growing straight out.

Ingrown toenails are usually caused by improper nail care—in particular cutting nails too short. Try to prevent ingrown toenails if you can.

When all else fails, see your doctor. Left alone, ingrown nails can get infected, which is a real problem for people with diabetes or poor circulation.

If ingrown nails are a recurring problem, it is sometimes possible to fix them surgically in an office procedure. The toe is numbed with lidocaine (ask your doctor to apply a topical anesthetic cream first) and the edge of the nail matrix on either side, which is where the nail is made, is destroyed with a scalpel, a laser, or even a chemical called phenol. When the area heals, no new nail can be produced. End result: a slightly narrower nail that does not grow into the nail folds and cause pain.

▪ BRITTLE OR BROKEN NAILS

One of the most common questions I hear about nails is: "Is there anything I can do for my nails? They're so brittle." I am not aware that eating gelatin or coating nails with micronutrients like vitamins will help. If you remember, the nail is made by the little nail factory that lives just in front of the nail, near the cuticle. If brittle nails are caused by excessive dryness, applying a urea-containing cream like Carmol 20 will help.

▪ ARTIFICIAL NAILS

Many people prefer the cosmetic benefit of acrylic nails. These are fine unless you develop nail infections as a result of the irritation of adjacent skin. Also, some people may develop a contact dermatitis to the chemical in the adhesive or the artificial nail itself. The hassle of these complications may not be worth it, and the only way to stop them is to stop using artificial nails.

*I have these deposits of fat where I really hate
them, especially on my thighs. Dieting hasn't
helped.*

—Ginny, 34, secretary

U sing surgery to remove fat has long been a quest of
cosmetic surgeons, but the journey toward that dream
has been slow until recently. About twenty years ago,
physicians in Italy scraped out fat through a relatively
small incision using a sharp, circular-ended knife called a
curette. Because severe complications often resulted, this
technique did not gain widespread acceptance.

Seizing on that idea, doctors in France began using a
blunt-ended canula, a metal tube with openings along the
sides that looks a bit like an oversized straw, to remove fat
more gently while preserving the important connections
between the skin and muscle. This fat-removal method
minimized the chances of damage to surrounding tissue.
In a variation on the technique, doctors began infusing
into the fat small amounts of saline (salt water), which
was identical in composition to the water in our body.
This helped break up the fat globules, making them easier
to remove.

After the technique was introduced to the United States in 1982, liposuction rapidly gained popularity, though the potential for complications, many related mostly to the use of general anesthesia, remained. Three years later, American dermatologist Jeffrey Klein introduced tumescent anesthesia. The tumescent technique involves injecting low-concentration anesthetic solution (lidocaine) into the fat combined with epinephrine (to reduce bleeding and prolong the anesthetic effect) and saline. Large volumes of this solution are injected into the fat before surgery, thus swelling the area to approximately two to three times its normal size.

This numbs the fat completely, eliminating the need for and risks of general anesthesia. It also makes the fat very firm, so that it is easier for the surgeon to break up and remove the fat globules. With the excellent anesthetic effect and firming of the fat caused by the tumescent technique, the canulas used in liposuction have gotten smaller and smaller over the years, causing much less trauma to the fat and more rapid recovery as well.

As a result of these advances, liposuction surgery has become much more affordable and is reported to be the most common cosmetic procedure done in medical offices today. **Tumescent liposuction has an excellent safety record.** In the very few cases where serious complications developed, it was often because of inadequate physician training or a failure to recognize that the body's fluid status can be knocked out of whack if too much anesthesia is given or too much fat is removed in one session.

There are no clear guidelines on the amount of fat that can be safely removed in one surgical procedure, but the liposuction surgeon does well to be conservative when it comes to fat removal. When too much fat is removed, there is an increased risk of post-operative bleeding and "fluid shifting," which causes dangerous swelling in the affected areas.

Refinements to the tumescent technique continue such as the use of ultrasound to make it safer and more efficient at removing fat. In ultrasound-assisted liposuction, or UAL, the canula inserted into the fat vibrates rapidly. This constant, ultrasonic vibration liquefies the fat, allowing more rapid and even removal. The disadvantage of UAL is that the ultrasonic energy emitted from the canula makes it and the surrounding fat very hot, which can cause burning. The latest generation of ultrasonic liposuction equipment has incorporated cooling systems to allow the inserted tube to remain at a safe temperature while still imparting ultrasonic energy to the fat.

▪ AM I A GOOD CANDIDATE?

Most people mistakenly consider liposuction to be a weight-loss technique. It is definitely not. It *is* a way to change the body contour or outline. The best candidates for liposuction are not obese or overweight; they are people who have a stable body weight, exercise regularly so that their underlying muscle tone is good, and are at or near their ideal body weight. If you match that description and have small, localized deposits of fat that don't disappear despite diet and exercise, you will likely get good results.

Fat can accumulate in certain areas in disproportion to the rest of the body—the outer thighs (saddlebags), inner thighs, around the knees, the waistline in men (love handles), the chin, and the neck. These are the places most commonly treated by liposuction. People can expect a small weight loss, usually in the three- to five-pound range, but it's the overall contour of the body where the improvement can be quite dramatic.

Liposuction can be performed on larger body areas where more fat needs to be removed, but this larger-volume liposuction must be approached much more cautiously. As I mentioned above, there are limits to how much tumescent fluid can be infused into the fat at one time and how much fat can be removed safely during one surgical session. If a person has a somewhat larger amount of fat to be removed and is otherwise a good candidate for surgery, I recommend the fat should be removed in two to three separate liposuction procedures. This approach, serial liposuction, is safer than ultra-high-volume liposuction, and it allows fine-tuning over time to maximize the contour improvement.

In so-called ultra-high-volume procedures, large amounts of fat (twenty to forty pounds) are removed at once, often under general anesthesia. The infusion of massive amounts of tumescent fluid and intravenous anesthesia simultaneously increases the risk of dangerous complications. In addition, removing so much fat at once tends to leave the skin loose and floppy. This makes for slow healing and prevents skin from adhering to the underlying tissue. Additional surgery may be necessary later to remove the floppy skin. For contour improvement on the abdomen, however, some physicians who do moderate to high-volume liposuction will remove excess skin in a procedure called abdominoplasty, at the same time the fat is removed.

▪ YOUR LIPOSUCTION CONSULTATION

Many physicians who perform liposuction offer free consultations, and you may want to have consultations with several physicians before undergoing the procedure. This "shopping around" for a doctor is a good thing. It gives you the time and information you need to develop an informed opinion as to what can and can't be realistically accomplished. Liposuction is never an emergency procedure and you will live with the results for the rest of your life, so it behooves you not to rush through the process.

Your physician should be board certified in dermatology or plastic surgery, since these are the two specialties in which doctors have the highest level of training and expertise in liposuction. At a typical consultation your doctor should obtain a detailed medical history, including all current medications, allergies, and adverse reactions to medications or anesthesia, and past surgical procedures. You should also be asked about your pattern of weight loss or gain over the past six to twelve months.

Your physician should then examine you undressed, with specific attention paid to the areas being considered for surgery. These should be seen in several positions, including standing, sitting, lying down, and with your muscles both relaxed and contracted. Your underlying muscle tone, as well as the laxity or tightness of the skin overlying the areas to be treated, must be noted. In the case of abdominal liposuction, old surgical scars must be taken into account, and you should be checked for the presence of hernias both in the groin and around the navel.

At this initial consultation, your doctor will probably outline the procedure to be performed and go over what you will experience on the day of surgery and in the post-operative period. You may be shown before-and-after photographs of areas treated that are similar to those you are considering having done, as well as images of people in the immediate post-operative period, so you can see what the recovery process may entail. Such photographs should not be construed as guarantees of results in your particular case and are for illustration purposes only.

Finally, you should be given detailed written information to read regarding the pre-operative preparations, the procedure itself, and the post-operative routine.

I recommend that people take this material home, review it, and then write down any questions before returning for a second consultation. At that time, if the physician deems you a good candidate for liposuction and if you decide to have the surgery, pre-operative preparations should be reviewed. Routine pre-operative laboratory work will be ordered.

If you have significant health problems—including cardiac problems, taking multiple medications, or having blood-related conditions—you may still be a candidate for liposuction; you will, however require a physical exam and clearance for surgery by your internist, family doctor, or cardiologist.

Once the lab results have verified that you are an appropriate candidate for surgery, the liposuction will be scheduled. You will be asked to stop taking any aspirin-containing products for at least ten days prior to surgery, and the doctor will prescribe an oral antibiotic to take the day before the big event.

▪ THE PROCEDURE

On the day of surgery you will be weighed to establish safe doses of the tumescent fluid, and you will be premedicated with Valium, Percocet, or similar antianxiety and pain medications. Your surgeon will then design the surgical procedure, drawing on your skin with a surgical marker to make note of both the areas that need the most fat removed and the areas to avoid due to the relative absence of fat, as well as where the small slit-like incisions to insert the canula will be made. There is some flexibility in positioning the incisions, so feel free to discuss the choices with your doctor. For example, you might request that incisions be put in an asymmetrical pattern on the body so that they will be less noticeable as surgical scars and will appear more like traumatic or incidental scars or markings on the skin. In general, by approximately twelve months after the surgery, these small incision sites are often indistinguishable from normal skin, no matter where or how they were made.

Before the procedure, you will be photographed from several angles as a record of the appearance of the areas to be treated.

Your skin is then prepared with an antibacterial surgical scrub. The incision sites are numbed with a local injection of anesthetic, which feels briefly like a bee sting. The incision sites are pierced with a scalpel and then the tumescent fluid is infused into the fat through these slits. The initial amount of fluid placed into the fat may tingle and burn, causing mild discomfort. The fat and overlying skin, however, rapidly become numb, so you will usually be quite comfortable throughout the remainder of the surgery.

As the tumescent fluid is slowly infused into the fat, the affected area will swell to about two to three times its normal size. Once all this anesthetic has been infused, you'll be asked to relax for thirty to forty-five minutes until it takes full effect. The surgeon then inserts the canula into the fat through the same incisions that were used to infuse the anesthetic solution. By now the fat is entirely broken up and primed for removal.

The next part of the procedure may last an hour or two, depending on what parts of the body are being treated. Patients are generally quite comfortable during this time. After appropriate and symmetrical amounts of fat have been removed from the areas being treated, excess tumescent fluid will usually be milked out with gentle massage to reduce swelling in the post-operative period.

At this point, some surgeons suture the surgical sites closed and others leave them open, which is a subject of much debate in liposuction surgery. Suturing the incision sites closed stops the excess tumescent fluid from leaking out during the first one to two days after surgery, but there is evidence that this suturing technique leads to more swelling and bruising in the post-operative period. When the surgical slits are not sutured, there is oozing and leaking of fluid over the first day or two, which can be uncomfortable, but there is some evidence that this technique allows for slightly more rapid healing and less initial bruising.

If your incision sites are left open after surgery, absorbent pads are placed over them. The pads must be changed several times a day for the first forty-eight hours to absorb the tumescent fluid that seeps out.

Once the surgery and milking procedure is completed, an adherent surgical tape will usually be placed tightly over all the treated body areas, and a very tight binder, much like a girdle, is placed over it. The tape and "girdle" act in concert to hold the skin firmly against the underlying tissue, helping to start the healing process. They also decrease bruising and swelling and ensure that the skin adheres to the underlying structures for optimal contour.

▪ RECOVERING AT HOME

After liposuction surgery, the surgical tape is usually worn for four to five days, then you remove it yourself at home. The girdle binder is usually worn twenty-four hours a day for the first week after surgery and then twelve hours daily for another three weeks to a month. Don't even think of taking off your girdle before your surgeon says it's okay, since wearing it ensures the best contour when healing is complete.

Immediately after surgery your doctor should give you a list of post-operative instructions. You'll be told to drink plenty of fluids and to take it easy for the first day or two. After that initial period, you will usually be able to return to work and begin light exercise. Keep in mind, however, that all treated areas will be sore and may bruise significantly, with the bruising lasting up to three weeks.

Your doctor will want to see you for a checkup two to three days after surgery, and then again at one-week intervals for the first month. After that, monthly follow-ups to assess healing and skin retraction remain important.

Don't expect any improvement in contour for at least one month after surgery; in fact, the final results of a single liposuction procedure cannot be gauged completely for three to six months. It takes at least that long for all the swelling to disappear and for the overlying skin to completely heal and retract over the treated area. (You might say another criterion for judging whether you are a good liposuction candidate is your degree of patience—this is not a procedure for someone who wants overnight results!)

At three to six months after surgery, a touch-up procedure can be done if certain areas were not sufficiently contoured during the first treatment. This procedure is usually a small version of the initial procedure and may take sixty to ninety minutes.

▪ COMPLICATIONS

For the vast majority of appropriately selected people who are treated conservatively with the tumescent technique, there are no significant complications and the immediate post-operative period is a relatively benign experience. Indeed many patients have commented that the removal of the adhesive tape four to five days after the surgery was the worst part of the entire process!

Unfortunately, however, a variety of side effects and complications can still occur. It's a good idea for you to be aware of what can go wrong before choosing to undergo liposuction. The most common post-operative problems are:

- Swelling of the treated area and of adjacent sites (for example, liposuction of the abdomen can lead to swelling in the groin and pubic area)
- Bruising, numbness in the area treated, fatigue, discomfort, or soreness

• Scarring at the incision sites
• Minor irregularities or lumpiness in the treated areas

With time, all of these complications slowly improve. Other, less common side effects include persistent swelling in the treated area (this may take months to resolve), persistent numbness, hyperpigmentation (brown discoloration) of the skin overlying the treated area, and localized collections of blood or fluid called hematomas or seromas under the skin which may sometimes need to be drained. You will want to consult your doctor about these persistent problems, but given enough time, they do clear up. More serious complications related to lidocaine toxicity, fluid overload, and bleeding after surgery as mentioned earlier are rare in liposuction surgery.

▪ A WARNING

Liposuction is an increasingly popular procedure and is now being performed by an increasing number of physicians, some of whom are more experienced and more qualified than others. I stress that you must check the credentials of your dermatologist or plastic surgeon and ask as many questions as you can prior to surgery.

You should meet with your surgeon on at least two occasions before actually undergoing the procedure. If you have large areas that need to be treated but are otherwise a good candidate for liposuction surgery, I strongly recommend that you undergo two separate surgical sessions, to be done over a period of time, not one right after the other. This two-step process will likely minimize the side effects of liposuction, which are more common when the surgery addresses a larger area. In addition, the second time you undergo the procedure, you'll know what to expect and, therefore, be better prepared. While it may seem less convenient, I assure you that proceeding cautiously, over a period of time, is safer by far and offers better results.

What you might notice first about different marks and spots on your skin is the color. This atlas presents full-color photographs of common skin conditions and, in some cases, the results of treatment. If you notice a spot on your skin that you think may be skin cancer and is similar to photographs in this section, see your doctor promptly.

Use this metric ruler to measure your lesions of concern.

Seborrheic keratosis, a "barnacle of life," is a benign growth. Often, many are present on the trunk.

Because it is often tan or brown, *seborrheic keratosis* can be confused with melanoma. It can even become irritated, as in this case where the keratosis is reddened around the edge

Genital warts can be transmitted between sexual partners.

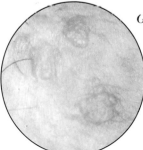

Wart around the fingernail, or periungual wart, should be biopsied if it has been present for more than ten years. Occasionally, these particular warts can change into skin cancer.

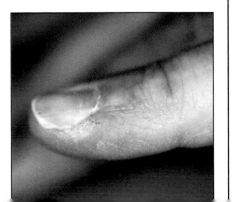

METRIC

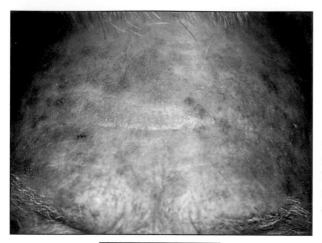

Sun damage in a fair-skinned individual showing broken blood vessels, redness, and rough sun spots called *actinic keratoses*.

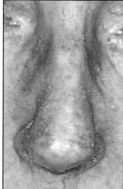

Rosacea of the nose is easily treated by laser.

Liver spots, or *lentigos*, are benign growths. If a change in color is noted and the spot has been present for a long period of time, it should be biopsied to make sure it is not an early form of melanoma.

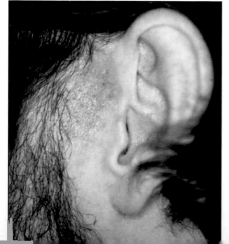

Superficial basal cell cancer can resemble eczema, so any rash of this sort that does not resolve with topical treatment should be biopsied.

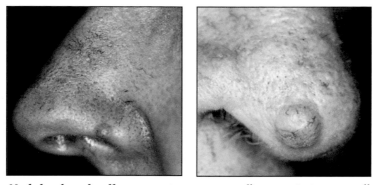

Nodular basal cell cancer starts very small, appearing as a small bump that bleeds occasionally or does not completely heal.

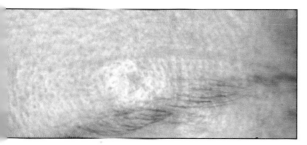

Morpheaform basal cell cancer, also called aggressive-growth basal cell cancer, has roots that extend under the surface of the skin. It is often larger than it appears on the surface and can be delayed in diagnosis because it resembles a scar in appearance.

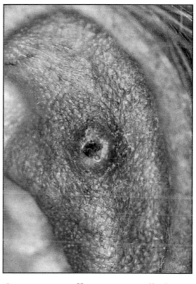

Squamous cell cancer usually has a slightly rough surface and, like basal cell cancer, may bleed.

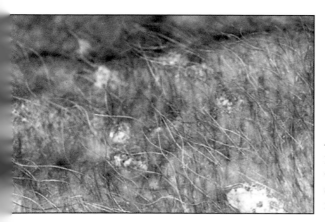

Actinic keratosis is a precancerous growth that occurs on sun-damaged skin. It is rough or scaly, raised, and usually red.

Normal moles.
Note regular borders
and even pigmentation.

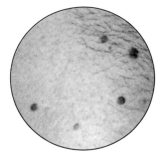

Atypical nevus, or mole, has
irregular pigmentation and border.

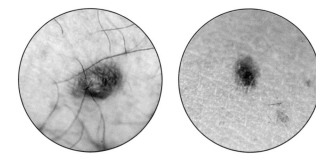

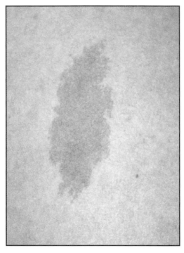

Café-au-lait spot, a non-cancerous
flat, tan growth, may be removed
with laser treatment.

Lentigo maligna.
Very early,
highly treatable
melanoma on the
face. Most often
seen in areas of
sun exposure.

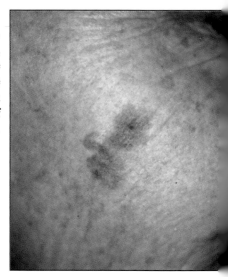

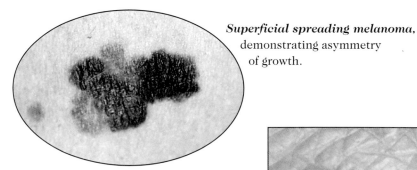

Superficial spreading melanoma,
demonstrating asymmetry
of growth.

*Acral lentiginous
melanoma* seen on the
sole, demonstrating
irregular border.

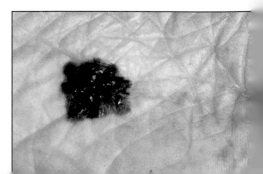

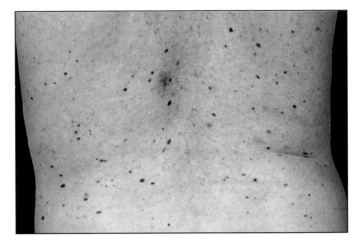

Patient with many atypical moles. Individuals with this many moles should be monitored closely by their dermatologist.

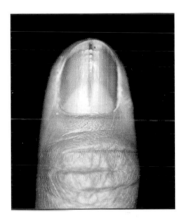

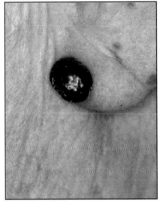

Nodular melanoma on the earlobe demonstrating very dark color (black in this case).

Brown streak in fingernail that could represent melanoma. Although such a streak is common in more darkly pigmented individuals, if you develop a pigmented band like this, see your dermatologist immediately.

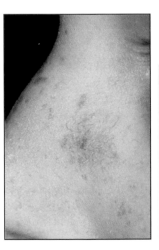

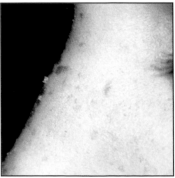

Same child, after treatment with the pulsed dye laser.

Broken capillary on the nose of a child.

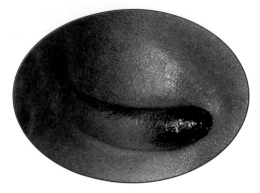

Growing *hemangioma* or blood vessel tumor on the eyelid of a child.

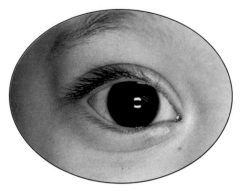

Hemangioma resolved after very early treatment with the pulsed dye laser.

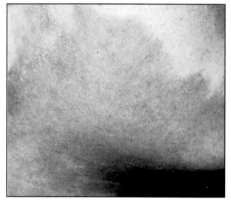

Port wine stain birthmark of the face

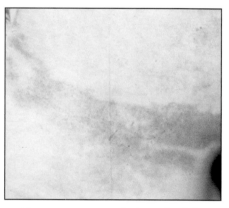

After treatment with the pulsed dye laser, showing disappearance of birthmark

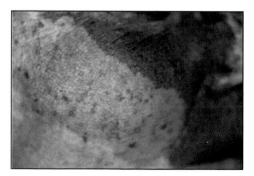

Port wine stain in an adult disappearing with laser treatment.

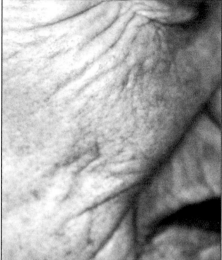

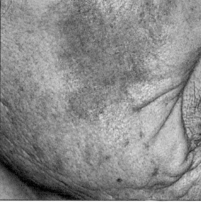

Wrinkles due to sun damage. This patient only wanted cheek wrinkles treated

Same individual two months after laser resurfacing. Note residual pink color that will resolve with time.

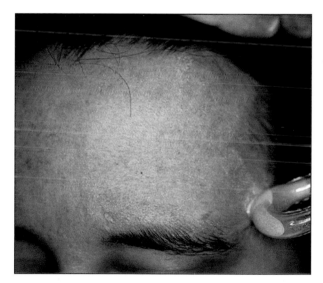

Micropeel freshens surface of skin.

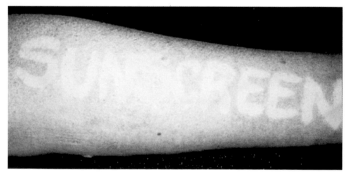

Sunscreen, used to spell the word here, is effective sun protection.

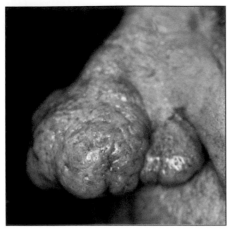

Rhinophyma, a condition in which the oil glands of the nose enlarge resulting in disfigurement

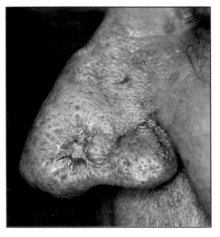

After sculpting with carbon dioxide laser.

Broken capillaries of **rosacea** can be successfully treated by laser.

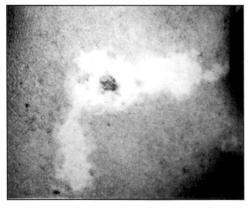

Vitiligo patch on face with small graft used in Flip-Top transplantation technique.

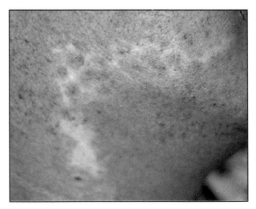

Same individual with increasingly normal pigmentation in previous area of vitiligo as a result of transplantation of pigment cells. The pigmentation will continue to even out.

17

Veins or Vanity: Who Needs Road Maps on Her Legs?

I want to wear shorts this summer. Do you think you can get rid of all these horrendous varicose veins?

—Paula, 59, schoolteacher

The five cosmetic problems that bother people the most are: facial lines, creases, and jowls; errant fat deposits; age spots; hair loss; and varicose veins and spider veins. Although there are many effective treatments for most cosmetic skin concerns, when it comes to treating varicose veins and spider veins, patience has to be the byword. Gravity is the major force working against any effort to eliminate the red, blue, and purple webs that course behind the thighs, along the calves, and even on the front of the legs. The pull of gravity would not map a network of small and large veins on our legs were we in the habit of sleeping upside down at night, like bats. However, we sleep on beds and walk upright, so gravity combines with certain factors in the anatomy of these veins to create a situation that keeps many women from wearing bathing suits and shorts.

As recently as 1970, spider veins were considered an unavoidable mark of aging, and most physicians cried "uncle" about the possibility of ever fixing the problem. Fortunately, lower extremity road maps of small and large veins can now be successfully treated with alleviation of associated symptoms. To understand how this is now possible, let's look at the normal anatomy of veins.

▪ WHY DO I HAVE THESE VEINS?

The main purpose of your veins is to return blood to the lungs so that the blood can reload with oxygen and go on to help your body perform its next task, whether that's smashing a tennis ball back across the net, finishing an important report, or keeping up with your toddler until the end of the day. The refreshed blood flows out from the main pump (your heart) via arteries to supply cells throughout the body with nutrients and oxygen. Once the oxygen molecules are snatched from the hemoglobin, the empty molecules return through the veins to repeat this endless cycle. Without veins, in other words, your heart would wait forever for blood.

In your legs, there are basically two systems of veins, which are connected to each other as two sides of a ladder are connected by its rungs. The superficial veins, which lie right under the skin, are one side of this ladder, and the deep system of veins that runs through the muscles is the other. The rungs that connect the deep veins to the superficial ones are known as perforating veins. Blood normally flows up from your lower extremities through both of these vein systems (the deep system does the lion's share of the work). In the superficial veins the blood usually goes through the perforating veins into the muscle, then up the deep veins toward the lungs and heart. The superficial veins have valves in them, which allow blood to proceed upward only or from the skin deep into the muscle—the valves are there to keep blood from flowing backward (if they weren't there, our feet would swell enormously and we'd all have to wear clown shoes).

When the veins are working properly, the amount of excess pressure in the veins is controlled and there is no reason for the abnormal spider veins or large varicose veins to form. Gravity is just one force that your body must fight in getting blood back to the heart; the fact that we walk upright, and indeed spend much of the day standing or sitting, is equally pernicious. The pressure exerted on your veins as they fight gravity to do their work is enormous. For example, if you are five foot seven, you are effectively exerting 67 inches of water pressure on the veins in your legs. Now imagine taking a garden hose that length, filling it with water, holding it over a patch of sand, and then releasing the water. Can you see the crater it creates? The pressure that made that crater is what the veins in your legs must contend with every minute of every day. Is it any wonder that, sooner or later, the valves and walls of these veins begin to surrender a bit to this constant pressure?

In face of the water pressure mentioned earlier, the veins in the legs can lose their elasticity, or stretchiness, and the veins may then bulge. When this happens, blood begins to pool in the stretched-out areas as it is pumped back toward the heart. This pooling creates what we call a varicose vein. In addition, the pressure stretches out the sides of the valves. Thus, a space around each valve will develop, and the blood will begin to leak backward toward the ankle and flow from the deep veins back into the superficial ones.

The change in blood-flow direction and the amount of blood in the legs can lead to various symptoms. You might experience pain, even when the only veins you can see are tiny spider veins. This pain occurs because of a tremendous backup in pressure that stretches these veins open. You may also experience aching in your legs, especially the calves, or swelling around the ankles. In a more advanced stage, when the swelling becomes too great, the oxygen going to the skin cells decreases and eczema may result, especially on the inside of your legs just above your ankles. With the swelling, blood leaks into the skin, and the pigment that gives blood its color may also give your skin a brownish red discoloration. Finally, if this goes on too long, ulcers may form just above your ankles; these are very difficult to eradicate. Some people also complain of cramping in the legs, especially at night, and a restless feeling in their legs.

SPIDER VEINS

Small "broken" blood vessels are known medically as telangiectasias; when they occur in the legs, they are referred to as spider veins. These surface blood vessels are visible to the naked eye and do not bulge out from the skin. Think of them as the little cousins of the deeper veins to which they are connected.

RETICULAR VEINS

Reticular veins are seen best from a slight distance. They are deeper and bigger than the spider veins that splatter the surface of the skin. Reticular veins are faint blue or bluish green networks of veins that run a little deeper beneath the skin than spider veins. They can be as thin as wrapping cord or as thick as a cooked strand of spaghetti. These reticular veins become visible because blood is leaking in the wrong direction, backward from the deep veins to the superficial ones.

VARICOSE VEINS

Some people develop large "ropy" varicose veins that look like little worms running beneath the surface of the skin. Up to one-fifth of adults may be affected, and although men get them, varicose veins are primarily a problem for women. (This is because female hormones like progesterone are known to weaken veins.) Two-thirds of those people destined to have varicose veins will develop the first one before age twenty-five. Often, they are first noted during pregnancy.

Advanced varicose veins can be dangerous. They can be associated with bleeding and blood clots in the superficial veins and, less commonly, blood clots in the deeper veins. These deep blood clots can cause serious health problems and can lead to other clots that travel to your lungs.

▪ WHAT DID I DO TO DESERVE THESE?

Once again, it's time to get out those family photographs and thank your ancestors. Approximately 70 percent of those who develop varicose, reticular, or spider veins do so because of heredity.

▪ FIXING VEINS

Despite the cosmetic problem caused by spider veins and varicose veins, they usually form in blood vessels that are not absolutely necessary for the healthy operation of our bodies; this allows for safe removal with the right technique. Our bodies are designed with great potential for duplication, probably because it was assumed that in the rough and tumble of daily life, we would damage a finger here, break a bone there, wear out a kidney at some other time, and so on. It's the same with the blood circulation system: if a little bit of it is removed, there is enough duplication that you can still function fine.

It is best if you get help from a physician who treats veins as a regular part of his or her practice. Dermatologists, vascular surgeons, general surgeons, and obstetricians-gynecologists often treat superficial veins; vascular surgeons and some dermatologists have special expertise in managing the larger veins as well.

A consultation is critical. During this first visit, the physician will take a medical history to see if you have any signs or symptoms of severe disease and will perform a physical examination to see if you have any other signs of venous disease beside the veins that are visible on the surface. Approximately 10 percent of patients who have just spider veins will have deep venous problems requiring more sophisticated treatment than surface sclerotherapy, the procedure used to treat superficial vein problems.

Some physicians will perform special tests using a small ultrasound device, as well as more sophisticated equipment, in order to check for changes in blood flow that indicate valve problems. However, not everybody who seeks treatment of small veins requires these tests, and sometimes they are merely an additional expense. If you are young and healthy, have no symptoms, and have no visible large varicose veins, these special tests are not required.

▪ EASY DOES IT—ALL GOOD THINGS TAKE TIME

Let's say that you make it through the examination phase, and your only problem is some spider veins on the surface that you don't like. What can you expect in terms of improvement?

First of all, you should not aim for perfection. None of us was born perfect, and the passage of time acts on our body much like weather does on a sparkling new copper roof. The worn patina may not shine like the original covering but it has developed its own beauty, a beauty of imperfection. Similarly, fixing a leg vein so that it looks better—not so that it disappears completely—is often improvement enough. In fact, with the standard treatment of sclerotherapy an improvement of 60 to 80 percent must be considered successful. Although different people and different veins respond in varying ways to the same therapy, it's unrealistic to expect more than that.

The smallest red spider veins resolve more slowly than the larger, more noticeable purple and blue ones. While larger, ropy veins may shrink away in only one to two treatments, small red spider veins will typically require three to five treatments, spaced two to six weeks apart. Any small spider veins that don't respond to a complete series of treatments are probably going to be resistant. Although you may be tempted to go at these cosmetic annoyances even more aggressively, this can backfire. Not only will these veins remain resistant to whatever you do, but your risk of developing new, smaller networks of veins, called mats, will increase greatly.

I'll tell you straight out: in the year 2000, there is no total cure for these vessels. Treatment can only control them. Even after a successful first series of treatments, you will require touch-ups every one to five years, depending on how rapidly you form new veins. Why? Remember gravity. Remember pressure. Remember how we walk upright. Until these circumstances change, we will always have leg vein problems.

In most cases insurance companies do not reimburse for treatment of the small veins, which they consider medically unnecessary. If you have large varicose veins and they are causing you health problems, you may be able to get insurance coverage for the procedure. However, the medical problems caused by varicose veins must be well documented.

▪ WHICH VEINS CAME FIRST?

Did the spider vein problem or the deeper vascular problem come first? It may not be as famous a quandary as that of the chicken and the egg, but the answer may help determine the course of your treatment. And the answer you get depends on the physician you see.

Some doctors are happy to treat your small spider veins first. Others will tell you that starting with the spider veins is treating the symptom rather than the underlying problem, that the spider veins are being fed by a deeper network of reticular veins that are not yet visible. There is no correct answer for everyone.

One approach is to treat spider veins only if you realize that you will probably have to return for additional treatments later. In a subsequent round, the underlying reticular veins or leaky perforating veins will probably need to be attended to. Alternatively, some doctors suggest that if the underlying large veins are treated first, the small veins on the surface may go away on their own accord, without further treatment.

▪ WHAT ARE THE DIFFERENT WAYS OF TREATING BAD LEG VEINS?

SURGERY

Surgery is required for leg veins that are more than 5 to 10 millimeters in diameter (a pencil eraser is about 5 millimeters wide). When the veins are more than 20 millimeters wide, tying them off, or ligation, is necessary. If there are leaky valves at the junction of large veins in your groin or behind your knee, surgery—by a qualified vascular surgeon—is also required to treat it before smaller vessels can be treated on an outpatient basis.

In a relatively new treatment called *ambulatory phlebectomy*, doctors can treat many vessels greater than 5 millimeters in diameter on an outpatient basis, using tiny slit incisions and local anesthesia to remove large veins. If you have large vessels and can find such an expert in phlebectomy, this procedure can be quite effective. Once the vein to be removed has been identified and marked, local anesthesia is instilled to numb the skin. Slits are made in the overlying skin and the vein is entered with a wirelike device. The vein is then partially pulled out and the skin is then bandaged.

SCLEROTHERAPY

Sclerotherapy is the technique used to banish most small veins. It involves the introduction of one of several different solutions into the tiny vein to cause irritation of the walls of the vessel, leading to scarring of the canal. Once the blood vessel forms a scar, it cannot contain blood and therefore you will not be able to see it. It essentially shrivels up.

The three most common substances used in sclerotherapy today are hypertonic saline (concentrated salt water), sodium tetradecyl sulfate (also known as Sotradechol), and polidocanol (also known as aethoxysklerol). Despite the fact that hypertonic saline stings and can cause brief cramping, it is proven to be safe for the treatment of these spider veins. However, it should never be used during pregnancy and it will not successfully treat any of the larger, deeper veins.

Sodium tetradecyl sulfate is relatively painless, usually does not cause cramping, and is also effective in treating both small and large veins. Outside the United States, the most commonly used agent is polidocanol, but the Food and Drug Administration still does not allow polidocanol to be used in this country for this purpose.

LASERS

Increasingly, lasers are being used to treat spider veins of the legs. Are lasers better than sclerotherapy? If you are needle-phobic, then lasers are the way to go. However, if you can tolerate needles, sclerotherapy remains a reliable method for eradication of spider veins, at least at the present time. Lasers have almost the same side effects as the sclerotherapy, except that they do not cause any cramping. In fact, a new modification of the laser used to treat leg veins allows instant cooling of the skin, which permits the use of higher laser energy for treatment. The results are promising.

▪ PREPARING FOR THE PROCEDURE

Let's look at what happens before, during, and after sclerotherapy, the most commonly performed procedure to treat leg veins. Prior to coming in for treatment, I may recommend that my patients buy and bring a pair of support hose with them. Information on specific brands, pressure, and lengths of support stockings or hose based on the particular problem is provided ahead of time.

Avoid aspirin or any aspirinlike products for ten days before treatment.

It is important not to shave your legs for at least forty-eight hours beforehand. That's because most doctors wipe the skin surface with alcohol to make the veins more visible, and the alcohol will sting if it is applied to skin recently abraded from shaving. Similarly, don't apply moisturizers to your legs the day of sclerotherapy—this makes the legs slippery, which makes it difficult for the physician to carefully inject the solution.

At the time of treatment I usually photograph the affected area, which helps me gauge progress over time. If, after several sessions, no progress is being made, we may try another approach or just fold the deck. Noting and marking veins in the standing position is also helpful. I also recommend that you eat a good meal before coming, to reduce the risk of fainting or becoming lightheaded or nauseated during the procedure.

Bring shorts that you can wear during the procedure to make it easier for the physician to have access to your veins.

▪ THE PROCEDURE

Some kind of soap or alcohol will be used on your skin to make it easier to see through the skin surface to the veins lying just beneath. A fine-gauge needle is used to inject small amounts of solution into the veins. The prick of the needle will sting, and some of the solutions do burn somewhat during treatment. If saline is used, you may get a brief cramp, like a charley horse, which resolves in minutes. Some doctors apply a cotton ball and tape over each site after injection.

Immediately after treatment, some physicians have an exercise bike available and ask you to pedal on it immediately. Others will ask you to walk for up to thirty minutes after a treatment. Immediate, regulated exercise gets your circulation going and helps to flush out all the solution from your veins. This may help you to avoid side effects. At the end of your visit, you will put on your support hose.

▪ THE POST-OPERATIVE PERIOD

I often recommend wearing support hose from three days to several weeks, based on the size of the vessel treated. There is no unanimity of opinion with regard to the use of support hose, and I also have patients in whom I use no compression. However, it appears that support hose does enhance results with even the smallest vessels treated, and they are certainly needed when large varicose veins are injected. There may also be restrictions on heavy lifting if you have had large vessels treated. In most cases, your doctor will want to see you at four- to six-week intervals, so that the effectiveness of the treatment may be assessed and retreatment performed, if necessary.

▪ COMPLICATIONS

Treatment of spider, reticular, and varicose veins may have side effects. Virtually all patients treated with hypertonic saline will complain of transient pain and cramping.

Between 10 and 30 percent of patients injected with the various solutions or treated with laser will have temporary brown pigmentation over the treated vessels or may develop what is known as matting. Matting results from the tendency of treatment to stimulate the body to form new, smaller networks of faint reddish-pink vessels. Matting is especially common in women taking estrogen or progesterone, occurs most commonly about eight inches above or below the knees, and in those who are overweight or have had many treatments with sclerotherapy. Aggressive treatment increases the likelihood of matting, so using lower-concentration solution in treatments spaced months apart is often the better way to go. As a rule, easy does it.

Some patients may experience hives. Treatment with the laser or with sotradechol seems to have the highest risk of causing hives along the treated areas. These hives will typically last up to twenty-four hours, but always go away. Physicians will typically prescribe a high-potency corti-costeroid cream immediately after treatment to decrease the symptoms of the hives. If tape is used to attach either gauze or a cotton ball over the treated areas to prevent oozing of a little bit of blood, a tape reaction, a blister or small red bumps around hairs, may also form.

A few people will have blistering or sores, especially around the ankle. This results from leakage of the solution into the skin around the vessel. When larger vessels are treated, there may be temporary swelling in the area and in some people bruising will occur after treatment. Rarely are there serious allergic reactions to polidocanol or sotradechol.

Superficial thrombophlebitis, inflammation of the inside lining of veins can occur, especially when the larger vessels have been treated. These tender, warm knots are actually small blood clots that rarely if ever spread elsewhere in the body. Physicians who treat large vessels anticipate this and schedule follow-up appointments so they can remove small clots if necessary.

▪ NOTED IN PRACTICE

Certain predictable events occur after treatment. Typically, a few months after the first or second treatment, you will look at the "before" photographs of your veins and be surprised at how your legs used to look. You might become quite eager to get rid of *all* your veins, even the ones you hadn't noticed before treatment.

Usually, you will be quite enthusiastic about your results after each of the first four or five treatments, but after that it will seem that you are getting less improvement with each session. This is the nature of sclerotherapy, and it explains why going for 100 percent improvement can be very frustrating, expensive, and, eventually, counterproductive. In the end, gravity and your own anatomy may lead to new varicose veins.

The good news is that you will generally find that your wardrobe will expand to include clothes you would not have considered wearing before your treatments.

18

Time (and Care)
Heals All Wounds

I'm just very self-conscious about these scars.
They remind me of the terrible acne I had as a
teenager.

—*Ellen, 35, social worker*

If you live a full, active life it is impossible not to acquire a few scars. Some of us see them as badges of honor. Some of us are simply embarrassed by them. How we feel about our scars often has a lot to do with how we got them. For example, a cluster of acne scars, even just one or two ice-pick scars, on an otherwise smooth cheek won't be met with the same acceptance that a scar acquired in a childhood accident might be. My older brother once pushed me off the top bunk bed, sending me to the floor with a new gash over my eyebrow. The scar is now faded and barely noticeable, but when I see it in the mirror, memories of childhood flash briefly in my mind.

A scar is the technical term for tissue the body makes to right a wrong. In the process an amazing number of events happen as though preprogrammed. A cut from a broken wineglass (don't retrieve them from the fireplace!), a scrape from the pavement, an incision from

"WILL I HAVE A SCAR?"

This is the most common question I hear when I talk about cosmetic procedures and reconstructive surgery. It is a smart question, but it took me a while to really understand what my patients meant by asking it. To a doctor, a scar, as this chapter explains, is a normal process for healing skin. To most people, however, the word connotes an unsightly, even deforming and distracting mark on the face or body. I now answer by saying that while scars are part of normal healing, using the techniques we have available, we will strive to hide it, making it as unnoticeable as possible. In the end, it's not how long the "scar" is but whether or not it is noticeable.

plastic surgery, all set in motion a cascade of finely tuned events in your skin.

When you get any kind of wound, however small, your body increases the production of collagen to mend the site. Collagen is the same material your dermis is made of but when the body churns it out to fix a wound, it is thicker and denser, to make sure it holds. As a result, at least early in the process, the scar may look and even feel thicker than the normal skin around it. Scars that result from a surgical incision are usually narrow and pale, unless you have a tendency to make excess scar tissue. Scars from accidents that are jagged may heal with a shape that reflects the original injury. How a scar looks in the end depends on what caused it, how it was treated, how your own body deals with it, and the patience you can bring to bear on the process. In general, like emotional trauma, time heals all wounds. But you can help.

▪ HOW A WOUND HEALS

Once you've been injured, whether by a scalpel, in an accident, or as a result of acne, the natural healing process begins. This process has three stages, which we'll get to in a moment: inflammation, proliferation, and maturation. Dermatologists also generally divide wound healing into two broad categories: primary intention and second intention.

Wounds that heal by primary intention are those that have been neatly sutured together in an effort to help the body form bridges of scar tissue that will remodel the skin. Sometimes surgical wounds that heal on their own, including some surgical wounds as well as deep scrapes and other accident marks, are in the second intention category; this natural healing is quite a remarkable process.

AFTER SURGERY

The inflammatory phase of healing begins about twelve hours after surgery and lasts for approximately five days. Don't worry if there is a little crusted blood around the incision. Adequate blood flow to the wound site is what ensures that the wound is healing. Blood is the magic potion that carries special cells, chemicals that first staunch the flow of blood by constricting vessels in the area, and platelets to plug up any leaks. In addition, brigades of specialized white blood corpuscles march to the area to fight off the germs that intact skin normally keeps out. If germs do gain a foothold in the wound, infection results. Infection is rare on the face or scalp where the blood flow is robust. In other areas, such as those farthest from the heart, like the legs and feet where blood flow can be more sluggish, the risk of infection is greater.

Proliferation begins about a day after surgery while the inflammation

---

JUST THIS ONCE, DON'T LISTEN TO GRANDMA

Wounds heal best when kept moist. It has been proven that moist wounds of the skin will heal up to 50 percent faster than wounds that dry out and develop a scab. Follow these simple rules, but don't try convincing Grandma to do it—old beliefs die hard. For scrapes, cuts, and surgical wounds, try the following:

1. Clean the wound daily with tap water. Don't use hydrogen peroxide. (The bubbles make it look as if something good is happening, but in fact, in the test tube, hydrogen peroxide can injure or kill cells.)
2. Apply a thin layer of antibiotic ointment such as Polysporin or Bactroban. Don't overdo it, since prolonged use of the former can result in an allergic rash.
3. After the first week, plain petroleum jelly (Vaseline) or Aquaphor works well to keep the wound moist.
4. Cover the wound with a Band-Aid or other nonstick dressing. Don't use gauze—the fibers can get in the wound.
5. Once the wound has healed and you can see new skin growing over it, you can discontinue the ointment.

phase is still in progress and continues for about a week. It is during this phase that fibroblasts divide rapidly in preparation for spewing out the bundles of new collagen. At this stage a variety of cells combine with collagen to build scaffolding upon which the more permanent scar tissue will be built.

Maturation refers to the slow process of remodeling the final scar. Although sufficient scar tissue forms within a few weeks, so that any sutures can be removed safely, the body continues to work hard laying cables of collagen and reconfiguring the scar. After two months the scar may still have a reddish, raised appearance, which can persist for a full year. The body's own natural refinement of scars continues, on average, for a full year, so in the world of cosmetic surgery and reconstructive surgery, we make no final judgments about the need to fix an imperfect result until the body has gotten its last licks in. In time, even the most thickened red or purple scars will become pale and flat.

AFTER AN ACCIDENT

Second intention healing is one of the skin's most miraculous defenses against an environment filled with sharp edges, hot barbecues, piercing thorns, and unkind tools. It is the body's way of saying: "Because I know you are sometimes a klutz, I will help." After a burn or a cut occurs, the body immediately begins its own remarkable campaign of rebuilding.

During this process, the wound begins to fill with fresh healing material called granulation tissue. Soon afterward the wound actually starts to contract, thanks to the work of specialized cells that make new collagen. As the collagen bundles remodel themselves over time and contract, the final scar can be much smaller than the original wound. Shortly after the wound has filled up with granulation tissue, the epidermis begins to grow over it. This allows the final healed wound to resemble the surrounding skin as much as possible. It is at this stage that you can help the body help itself. To speed successful healing and minimize any scarring at the end, keep the wound moist (See box on p. 191).

A young person's wounds will heal more quickly, but the risk of forming a raised (hypertrophic) scar is greater. Older people can take consolation in knowing that while their wounds may heal more slowly, there is less of a chance that the scar will be raised.

SLICK HEALING

In order to take advantage of the improved healing that comes with keeping wounds moist, several products are available that are waterproof, self-stick, and conform to the skin surface. By trapping the valuable wound fluid that develops in the first few days after injury, they help stimulate healing. The products include:

- Duoderm: (about $5 per four inch square), tan-colored, gelatinous
- Tegaderm: many sizes, clear plastic
- Vigilon: expensive, gelatinous, especially soothing if first stored in the refrigerator

Each of these products is available under different brand names. Each has been shown to decrease the stinging, pain, and burning that may be associated with skin injuries.

▪ HYPERTROPHIC SCARRING

Hypertrophic scarring is the term used for scarring that is raised, which happens when the body makes too much fresh scar tissue for the job at hand. Often this happens when the wound is under tension, such as a chest wound after heart surgery. This problem is different from a *keloid*, which is actually a tumor of scar tissue that grows on its own accord. Hypertrophic scarring almost always resolves, though the patience of Job may be required. Keloids never go away on their own. Hypertrophic scars resolve because an enzyme made by the skin called collagenase eats away at excessive scar tissue in the process of

> ### BAD SCARS
>
> Your own risk of developing hypertrophic scars or keloids should be assessed by your doctor based on information you provide. If you are at risk, this should weigh heavily in any decision to have elective surgery for cosmetic purposes.

remodeling it. Sometimes the raised scarring that occurs after surgery or an accident can be improved by the injection of corticosteroid into the scar. It is believed that this helps speed up the process of collagen remodeling, thus flattening a raised scar sooner than it would otherwise happen. This injection can be repeated at four-week intervals if necessary to flatten a raised or uncomfortable scar.

▪ KELOIDS

Normally the body makes scar tissue to fix an injury, but occasionally the body makes more scar tissue than it needs, to the point that the scar tissue becomes a tumor in its own right. Tumors of scar tissue are called keloids and they are a major problem in people of color and in others with a genetic tendency to develop the problem.

Keloids are darkened, thick, raised tumors that occur at the site of trauma or previous surgery. They are probably caused by a genetic abnormality that leads to the overproduction of scar tissue. It seems that in people prone to keloids, the fibroblasts, cells that produce the scar tissue collagen protein, don't slow down their production of scar tissue and keloids result. Unlike hypertrophic scars, which are also thickened bands of scar tissue, keloids will not get smaller with time.

Keloids can be itchy and/or painful and can be a source of great frustration and irritation to the patient. Although they can occur anywhere, the most common sites are on the central chest, the shoulders, upper back, and earlobes. Keloids, for some unknown reason, rarely occur on the face.

Treatment is extremely difficult (see chapter 26, "The Acne Family") and consists of injection of corticosteroid directly into the keloid, excision of the tumor, or excision of the tumor followed by a brief course of radiation to the surface of the wound. The use of silicone gel sheeting early on may be helpful. Applied to the surface of the healing area for 12 hours or more a day, this reusable thin, jellylike sheet can keep the tumor flatter. Despite all efforts, keloids still come back after treatment more than half the time. Keloids are made worse by stretching or tension. If one can keep pressure on the site of a healing wound, the scar tissue will not have a chance to overproduce, thus limiting the chance that a keloid will develop.

▪ SCARRING AFTER SURGERY

From a cesarean section to open heart surgery, from a stitched leg wound acquired in a motorcycle accident to a scar resulting from the removal of a cancer, most people would rather have the scar than the alternative. However, in some situations, such as emergency surgery, a scar may be jagged or unsightly, and you may wish to improve the appearance of a hastily done job of stitching—particularly when the scar is on the face or neck area. Surgical excision or the pulsed-dye laser may help improve the look of scar tissue. If there is persistent redness, lasers are quite effective at normalizing color. There is no good evidence that lasers can permanently flatten a raised scar in someone who is prone to healing poorly.

When traumatic scarring is impossible to avoid, improvements in surgical techniques have made it possible to repair major wounds, leaving behind minimal evidence. For instance, as little as twenty years ago, a woman who underwent a cesarean would have not only a beautiful baby but also a whopping scar stretching from the pubic area to the belly button. Cesareans now involve making a horizontal incision a few inches long below the bikini line. By the time the new baby is beginning to crawl, the surgical scar is all but invisible and you can be back in your bikini (in order to swim, not sunbathe, of course).

Hernia surgery is another example of how improved techniques can minimize scarring. The same hernia operation that would have left a diagonal scar running from pelvic bone to the flank can now be accomplished with a two-inch incision at the bikini line. Most recently, the increasing

---

CAN YOU HELP HEALING NATURALLY?

Here are a few products that are popular with comments about whether they really work.

Vitamin E cream: Although scientific evidence doesn't support any benefit, so many of my patients swear by it that I defer to them in its use. One cautionary note: there is a risk of contact dermatitis, so if you itch or the skin turns red stop immediately.

Calendula is thought by some to aid healing but can cause an allergic rash called contact dermatitis.

Silicone gel sheets are popularly marketed as a cure-all for scars. A sheet will help flatten some scars but only as long as it is used. Rejuveness is one brand that is widely advertised.

Mederma is an onion-based compound that some believe improves the final result of scars (try it and let me know what you think at www.totalskinmd.com).

use of laparoscopic surgery is reducing the need for extensive surgical scars.

▪ WHAT YOU CAN DO AT HOME

You can do your part to help a wound heal and soften the scar tissue on your own. Massaging a new scar from an incision or even a recent burn may help level a raised scar. Bland lubricants such as petroleum jelly can help make it easier for you to rub the area, which may still be tender. Proper technique involves pressing down on the scar in a circular fashion, against the hard undersurface of the underlying bone. Imagine that you are kneading bread, because in fact you are helping to break down bands of dense scar tissue. Do not overdo it and certainly wait until the surface of the wound is completely healed before you begin.

▪ FACIAL SCARRING

One of the most common and frustrating problems that I encounter in my practice is facial scarring. There can be many reasons for facial scarring, but the majority of people who come to see me about the problem experienced acne as adolescents or young adults. Pockmarks from the chicken pox virus used to be common too, but with the new vaccine, these scars will soon be a thing of the past.

Any facial scarring is upsetting, but I find that many people are especially bothered when it's the result of acne. Acne scarring seems to cause embarrassment even to the most un-self-conscious people. It may be because the scars arose during adolescence and serve as a daily reminder of how having acne increased the suffering of the person during an awkward period of life.

Depending on how severe your adolescent acne was or your adult acne has been, your acne scars may be a minor irritant or a more serious impediment to the quality of your life. If you want them attended to, there are more options than there were a generation ago, but the solutions can't provide a quick fix. The first step is determining what kind of scars are present. There are different types of acne scars. They can be small, deep ice pick scars, which are difficult to repair. Typically they measure 1 to 2 millimeters in diameter, and have a sharp edge with a "punched out" appearance. Another type of acne scarring is a shallow depression; such a mark can be anywhere from a few millimeters in diameter to half the size of a

THE SIX O'CLOCK NEWS, M.D. \

Beware of news reports that promise that lasers can magically remove scars. They can't. First, scars are a permanent part of healed skin. Second, although lasers can smooth out raised scars and lighten the redness or brownish discoloration of healed areas, they can only do so much. There is not yet a scar-erasing laser.

penny. Often people with these depressed scars complain that the scarring gets worse as they get older. What's really happening is that the skin relaxes and sags with age through the loss of active elastin tissue, and in the process the depression in the scar becomes more accentuated.

All such acne scars occur because the surface of the skin is bound down by the tissue that developed where the acne cyst once raged. The puckered or depressed look of an acne scar is much like the effect of a button on the back of your sofa: the thread holding the button corresponds to the vertical band of scar tissue that pulls down the surface of the skin.

In the past, the most common treatment for acne scarring was dermabrasion. In this procedure, a device was used to shear off the top layer of the skin. By stripping off the skin to the level of the upper dermis, a controlled scar would develop. Ideally, this would smooth the imperfections in the epidermis. Dermabrasion is less popular now because laser resurfacing can usually accomplish the same results with more precise control and with fewer risks.

The laser used to help acne scarring is the same one that is used to treat fine lines and wrinkles related to aging (see "Skin-Resurfacing Lasers," p. 135). In my experience, multiple treatments are necessary and satisfaction is not great unless the person has reasonable expectations. Patience is critical as well: the acne scars didn't develop overnight and they won't go away in forty-eight hours. People with acne scarring need to remember that even when resurfacing and other treatment helps, they will never have the skin they had when they were eleven or twelve. Nonetheless, we can make the scars less noticeable and easier to cover with less makeup.

Depressed acne scars can be treated by injecting Zyderm or Zyplast collagen into the skin just under the depression in order to raise it up. Collagen injections are not permanent, so repeated treatments are usually

---

ACNE SCARS: TOUGH ALL AROUND

Zoe, a twenty-four-year-old graduate student in economics, was extremely upset over the state of scars on her face. When she came to see me she had multiple depressed scars that were also hyperpigmented. The brownish discoloration made the scars all the more noticeable. Some fresh scars were still red and yet others were in the early stages, made worse by her constant picking. I promised that I could help only if she followed these rules:

1. Don't pick.
2. Wash only once a day with nonsoap cleanser.
3. Apply anti-acne medication as prescribed.
4. Use sunscreen.

I also advised, as sensitively as I could, not to expect perfection. I told Zoe that when all her acne has quieted down, we would address ways to fix each of the different types of scars she had. It doesn't pay to paint part of the house if big areas are still peeling.

---

necessary to maintain a good result. The dermatologist needs to break down the bands of scar tissue because these bands are causing the retraction in the first place. You must be skin-tested with the collagen before use to ensure you have no allergies to the material, and if you have collagen-vascular disease you should not be treated with this approach.

For ice pick scarring and chicken pox scars, among the most difficult acne scars to treat, a different technique is used. Under local anesthetic a small device that looks like a cookie cutter is used to punch out the scar. The small wound is then stitched with very small sutures to convert the scar into a smooth surface scar that is just a few millimeters in length. After this has been done on all affected areas, it is then possible to resurface with the laser to blend the area together and obtain a better result. There is a low risk with the punch excision technique of a worse cosmetic result depending on skin type.

If your bouts with acne are not in the distant past, you need to be cautious before proceeding to surgery for any scars. No surgery should be done until your acne is completely under control. Even then, waiting a bit is advisable, since any surgery that is done could stimulate a flare-up of acne or be complicated by any residual acne that might recur. The use of sun-

screen to prevent hyperpigmentation from the sun as well as proper moisturization and care of the skin is extremely important.

No surgery should be performed if you have been on Accutane in the
preceding twelve months. Evidence suggests an increased risk of scarring
after dermabrasion, and even if other methods are used, it is best to play
it safe and wait a full year after your Accutane course has been completed.

▪ SCARRING FROM COSMETIC PROCEDURES

Vanity has its price and no more so than when dealing with cosmetic
procedures and surgeries so many people are eager to pursue. Abnormal
scarring is the most obvious risk of cosmetic surgery, especially for those
who don't heal well. Some people know they don't heal well if previous
surgery has resulted in hypertrophic or discolored scars.

Some patients tell me that they don't heal well and point out a wide
scar on their belly or shoulder as evidence. In fact, these are areas where
it is difficult to get a great result, no matter who does the work or how the
surgery is performed. The final appearance of a scar has as much to do with
its location and movement of the body at that site as it does with the technique used.

If you chose your doctor for cosmetic surgery well, your physician
should advise you before the surgery about possible scarring. If the doctor
tells you, "Don't worry, that never happens when I do the surgery," get out
of the office as fast as you can! Find a doctor who will be very clear about
the relative risks and who takes the time to make sure you understand
what you are getting into.

SKIN CANCER IV

19

Cancer and Your Skin: What You Must Know, What You Can Do to Protect Yourself

I never had any doctor examine my whole body for
skin cancer. No one even suggested it. Why doesn't
the public know they should ask for this?

—*Bob, 70, retired salesman*

Just a few decades ago, skin cancer was not a subject of much discussion, perhaps because it was something that affected only older people. And, since it was usually not life-threatening, it could hover in the background as something that was not fully understood. Since then, however, the incidence of skin cancer has climbed steadily and it is now the most common cancer in humans.

As an active skin cancer researcher and dermatologic surgeon, I believe that the increases we are seeing in melanoma, a serious form of skin cancer, and non-melanoma skin cancer such as basal cell cancer and squamous cell cancer, will be met with improved diagnosis, better public education, and treatments that are less invasive. In the future, treatment will be more keyed to our understanding of the genetics of how cancer develops.

Because skin cancer, including melanoma, is so easy to diagnose—all you really need are a good pair of eyes—I also believe early diagnosis alone will lead to improved survival and less disability from these very modern diseases.

> **WARNING SIGNS OF SKIN CANCER**
>
> • A spot that bleeds
> • A sore that appears, heals up, and comes back
> • A mole that changes in color, shape, or texture
> • A mole or other spot that begins to itch
> • A new mole

- # FEARING CANCER, FEARING FEAR ITSELF

Once a patient hears the word *cancer* the first and most visceral reaction is fear. For centuries no word has conjured more fearsome images than cancer. It has always been a diagnosis that has fallen on patients' ears like a death sentence. The term itself, originally coined by Hippocrates, refers to the crablike appearance of dilated veins on the distended bellies of terminally ill cancer patients. Cancer has, in our culture, been equated with wasting, suffering, and certain death, and as such continues as one of the most frightening medical conditions we encounter. One of the more potent images of cancer is that of

> *Let me assert my firm belief that the only thing we have to fear is fear itself.*
>
> —*Franklin D. Roosevelt, first inaugural address, March 4, 1933*

insidious growth, so the word has taken on meaning even outside the examining room. During Watergate, White House counsel John Dean spoke of a "cancer on the presidency," reaching for the dread disease as a metaphor for the corruption of the body politic.

Our grave cultural fear of cancer is such that it persists even in an era when such a diagnosis is no longer necessarily a death sentence. Sadly, this fear often grows greater once a cancer is diagnosed, and this very human emotion sometimes blocks us from seeking to get the diagnosis made in the first place. Beliefs rooted in fear die hard, and when cancer does strike at a stage when it is no longer curable, it reinforces the fright that accompanies the diagnosis.

We also seem to be hearing about cancer all the time; it seems to be everywhere we turn. Researchers tell us nightly on the news that foods and activities that provide us with joy also contain the seeds of cancer risk; the same researchers also say that if we eat this or that, we may avoid cancer.

This omnipresence of cancer in the media perpetuates the unconscious fear that it lurks behind every small pleasure, as well as the hope that there might be a magic bullet in one innocent piece of fruit or homeopathic medicine. Both attitudes contribute to public confusion and fear and create an unusual dichotomy that keeps many from seeking treatment. On the one hand, cancer is the dreaded danger, hiding around every corner; on the other, the false promises of miracle cures lead many otherwise intelligent people down a potentially dangerous path.

It is our fear of cancer that makes the disease all the more deadly, because that fear inhibits us from facing abnormalities that may be cancerous and from calling the doctor before the cancer has advanced.

But what exactly is cancer, this all-encompassing word that is now so much part of our lives, our language, our daily culture? In reality cancer is an umbrella term for a whole collection of diseases.

A cancer is a malignant tumor. A tumor is an abnormal growth that may be benign or malignant. Some people equate the word *tumor* with cancer, others believe a tumor is a noncancerous growth but only "malignant tumors" are indeed cancerous. In a malignant tumor, the normal tissue cells have lost the control necessary to grow in a orderly manner. These cells, which begin to divide in an uncontrolled fashion, are cancerous and can interfere with the activity and functions of the rest of the body by crowding out the normal tissue.

The term *skin cancer* itself encompasses several different malignancies. Skin cancer may be the most common cancer in humans, but it is also the most easily cured. Because we know so much about skin cancer's causes, and because we believe we know how it starts, we can in many ways prevent it from starting early in life.

Understanding how skin cancer develops helps us understand how to prevent it and how to treat it effectively. Because there are several different kinds of skin cancer, each with its own unique features, it is helpful to understand the ways they differ and the ways in which they are similar, as well as whom they generally affect and the parts of the body where they commonly occur.

▪ THE SCOPE OF SKIN CANCER

Precise figures on skin cancer are hard to find. The data on melanoma is extensive, thanks to tumor registries run by states and other organizations that require doctors to report the diagnoses. However, there is no requirement that diagnoses of basal cell cancer and squamous cell cancer be reported to these registries. In general, though, we do know that each year there will be more than 1 million cases of non-melanoma skin cancer. Of these, there will be approximately 2,000 deaths, primarily from squamous cell cancer. Melanoma is a far different problem. Of the approximately 45,000 expected new cases each year, there will be about 7,500 deaths. It is now estimated that 1 in 75 Caucasians will develop melanoma in their lifetime. Recent data suggests that melanoma is also the most rapidly rising cancer in women in their twenties and early thirties.

Skin cancer is very rare in people of color because of the natural sun protection factor, roughly equivalent to an SPF of 13, that their pigment provides. Nevertheless, because there is such a wide range of coloration in individuals of color, skin cancer is still a possibility. For instance, I have seen basal cell cancer in lighter-skinned African-Americans and in Latinos from Puerto Rico who have grown up under the very harsh sun.

African-Americans, Asians, and others of color can burn in the sun, and it is appropriate to make sure that proper sun protection is observed, even when you can say to yourself, "Hey, I'm dark already. What can happen to me?" My advice is always, "Sun damage doesn't discriminate." Be guided by your own experience in the sun.

Interestingly, two-thirds of squamous cell cancer in blacks occur in areas not exposed to the sun. Just as with individuals with type I or type II skin (see chapter 5, "Frequent Questions"), squamous cell cancer can develop in long-standing traumatic scars, especially those that result from a burn, chronic irritation or inflammation, chronic ulcers, previous radiation, or in people with a long history of discoid lupus erythematosis. If you notice a nonhealing area, it should be biopsied by your dermatologist immediately.

The key to detecting skin cancer in time so that it can be treated successfully is skillful observation. This means you should get to know all your skin (as well as you do the proverbial back of your hand), check yourself regularly, and know what you are looking for. The chapters in this part of the book will describe the signs and symptoms of skin cancer so you can be an alert detective and help identify a possible problem before it becomes a major threat to your health.

While self-examination has become de rigueur in the early detection of breast cancer, the same cannot be said yet of skin cancer. Many people avoid looking at any new skin spots or changes just when they should be paying attention. In fact, men have a higher mortality rate than women when it comes to skin cancer, largely because they avoid taking skin conditions seriously and don't seek treatment. Any new growth on your skin or any ulceration that does not heal deserves a trip to the doctor. In a very real sense, it is usually not skin cancer itself that kills; neglect and procrastination are the culprits.

Of the three most common types of skin cancer, melanoma is the most dangerous and pernicious. If it is not diagnosed until an advanced stage, it is ranked one of the most deadly of all cancers. Chapters 22 and 23 deal with melanoma and non-melanoma skin cancer, respectively, to help you know what to look for and what you should do if and when you discover a suspicious spot on your skin.

Happily, nature is of help in our crusade to identify skin cancer early. Both melanoma and non-melanoma skin cancer can be heralded by *precancers*. In the case of non-melanoma skin cancer, a lesion called an *actinic keratosis*, a small, red, slightly rough growth that occurs in people who have had a lot of sun exposure can often be a harbinger of the risk for developing basal cell cancer or squamous cell cancer. Some of these lesions, if neglected, do in fact evolve into true skin cancer. Similarly, while common moles pose no risk of turning into melanoma, a mole called an *atypical nevus* (formerly called a "dysplastic nevus") is thought to be an indication that the bearer may be at risk for developing melanoma. In some cases, severely atypical or abnormal moles or nevi can transform into melanoma. Although a lot remains to be learned about the biology of these "precursor" lesions, they serve an important function: they are the foghorn, the red flag, the glaring lighthouse beacon that tells us to pay attention to the hazards that may be brewing on our skin.

▪ PREACHING TO THE CHOIR?

In the field of cancer prevention, one of the most effective tools we have is public education. It is now a matter of scientific fact that smoking causes lung cancer. But it has taken extensive programs in public education to drive that point home and, more important, to change behavior. Interestingly, some believe that the dramatic change in smoking incidence in this country only occurred once the public education programs shifted their focus to children. This had at least two effects: it helped prevent many kids from starting to smoke, and it got the newly educated kids to put pressure on their smoking parents to kick the habit.

Finding the right way to get a public health message across is critical. When it comes to skin cancer, repeating the message regularly, articulating the risks clearly, and explaining what you can do about it are essential

for success. There is evidence that we are making progress. How often do
you see tan models now? How often do your kids remind you to put on
sunscreen lotion?

I have given many presentations on skin cancer and made it a policy
early on to speak to any group that was willing to hear a health talk. Once,
shortly after I started at Yale Medical School, I got an invitation to speak to
a sorority at Southern Connecticut State University. I realized that regardless of the turnout this was exactly a group I wanted to reach. I showed up
on a rainy night in March, and after making my way through the empty
pizza boxes and Diet Coke bottles strewn about the dormitory common
room, proceeded to have one the best experiences ever on the skin cancer
speaking circuit. The women were attentive and asked questions that
demonstrated their clear understanding of the need to take precautions
against skin cancer. How many then hauled off to Fort Lauderdale for
spring break and roasted in the sun I cannot tell, but the will to know was
there, and that is the first step in any health education program.

I am firmly convinced that talking about skin cancer saves lives. Many
of my academic colleagues avoid the media, afraid they might be mis-
quoted. My view is a bit different: you can misquote me all you like, but if
you get the core message right, I will be satisfied. That message saves lives.
Every time a magazine runs an article on skin cancer, especially when it is
accompanied by photos, the phones in our office and those of many dermatologists ring in response. This form of public education works well.

Throughout this part of the book, I hope to show you how to recognize
skin cancer, understand what it is, and know what you can do about it. Ideally, this information will help you to break through the fear that might
keep you from making that phone call.

20 Getting Past Denial, or How to Deal with Something You Really Don't Want to Deal With

I had this blood blister on my arm for about two years. It was dark, so I've been wearing a Band-Aid on it because I didn't like the way it looks. But you know, Doctor, I think it's getting raised now.

—Madeleine, 54

Madelcine's growth was biopsied on the spot because of concern that it was melanoma. When the biopsy sample confirmed the diagnosis, the patient returned for complete removal of the cancer in the office. She has done well since but would probably have had a better prognosis if she had sought attention when she first noticed the dark spot. Believing the growth was a blood blister and covering it with a Band-Aid is a typical example of denial.

Denial takes many forms. President Clinton denies sex is sex. Politicians deny their views are partisan. Even children deny they have to go to the bathroom when they do. Nowhere is denial more of a real problem than when it comes to health. The crux of the issue is that to deny is human. To procrastinate is natural. To avoid the unpleasant is one way we get through the daily grind.

In many cases denial can be a helpful strategy. There

is only so much we can handle in our complex lives, and by sorting through what we can and cannot deal with at a certain point in time, we are sometimes better able to deal with problems we can actually solve. However, denial also has a bad side—it can prevent us from getting the medical help that can make the difference between living and dying. The trick is to find a way to get through that very clever roadblock that pops up in our minds when we see a growth on our skin that we know we should get checked out.

I devote these pages to the subject of denial because I have seen so many cases where people would be better off today were it not present. Denial plays a special role in dermatology because the evidence that something is wrong, that something really should be checked out, is as plain as the wart on your nose, so to speak. Unlike the vague symptoms related to diabetes, or fleeting chest pain that may or may not indicate a heart problem, there is a daily reminder in your mirror that something is awry. This presents special opportunities for directed medical care and a solution to a small problem before it becomes a bigger one. In short, if we could get everyone who is at risk for melanoma to recognize the growth in its earliest stages and promptly seek care, the death rate from melanoma would plummet. If we could get everyone who develops other forms of skin cancer to get them diagnosed when they first appear, the incidence of bigger problems that can stem from them would drop as well.

> *After the biopsy turned out positive, I didn't go back for my surgery. In fact, I walked out of the doctor's office. I tried treating my melanoma homeopathically. I'm in real trouble now.*
>
> —*Patty, age 40, fighting advanced melanoma*

In general, I find that men deny symptoms more than do women. I don't think this reflects a broader gender disposition (though my wife might disagree), instead, it's that women are more in touch with their bodies. This has been shown time and again in broad-based studies. Women go to the doctor more frequently. Women will get new symptoms checked out more often than men. In fact, women are more likely to take note of symptoms that might indicate a change in health. Often men cannot even give good histories about their medical problems. For example, here's a common exchange with men:

"When did you first notice the growth?" I ask.

"I don't know."

"Was it ever treated before?"

"I don't remember."

I think men really don't know the answer to these questions. Men as a group simply are not focused inwardly on their bodies. As a result, I think denial is more common in men than in women. The tendency of men not to seek out medical care is also highlighted by one of the most common scenes I encounter in the examining room:

As the man is sitting on the examination table, I ask him how long the growth on his cheek has been present.

"About a month," he says.

Sitting frustrated in the corner is his wife or significant other, her hands crossed in her lap, shaking her head in disagreement. I turn to her and say, "So how long *has* it been present?"

"At least a year," comes back the more accurate answer. This is usually followed by a shaking finger and the words "I told him to go to the doctor when it first came up, but he just said it was nothing."

After this requisite point-counterpoint, we are able to move on. This scene, which gets played out again and again, highlights not only gender differences in seeking health care but the fact that denial can often be overcome—or at least dealt with when there is a caring family member to help.

I think that anxiety is the underlying propellant of denial. The sad irony is that fear of the unknown, when it comes to melanoma, for example, will only make things more unpleasant if the cancer goes undiagnosed and is allowed to spread.

Soon after I started practice, I initiated the Yale Skin Cancer Detection Program with Dr. Jean Bolognia, Yale's pigmented lesion and melanoma expert. This effort, modeled after the national skin cancer screenings promoted by the American Academy of Dermatology, was designed to identify skin cancer early and to educate the public about its risks and how to prevent it. In addition, we wanted to understand how best to get people to take advantage of early cancer diagnosis programs.

At screenings run by the program, full-body skin exams were conducted. Melanoma can occur anywhere—from the top of your scalp, hidden in the dense forest of your hair, to the bottom of your feet, and even under your nails. So to do a proper exam for melanoma, such a full-body exam is necessary: *anything less is inadequate.*

Each patient who attended the free screening was asked to fill out a lengthy questionnaire. This helped us establish all sorts of information about attitudes toward health, safety, and acceptance of medical risk. For example, a question was included about the use of car seat belts because data about this already exists and gives an indication about what level of health risk a person is willing to take.

As part of the research we conducted, we tried to determine what the barriers were to a full-body skin exam. The group that was most resistant to a full-body skin exam was older women; we determined that concern or shame about body image was the inhibiting factor. Knowing this, we approached these patients differently, so we could better provide them the care they needed.

A man who came to one of our early public screenings provided a memorable example of fear and denial. The full-body skin exam revealed a textbook case of melanoma on his right shoulder. We explained to the gentleman the need for biopsy and treatment, and recommended he see a dermatologist immediately. He did not have one so we offered him a chance to come Monday to our office (the screening was done on a Saturday morning). He made the appointment but didn't show up for the biopsy. We called him several times and even followed up with a letter explaining the need for biopsy and treatment, but he never followed through with us.

What is both interesting and sad is that this man came to a skin cancer detection screening because of this growth. Once his suspicions were confirmed, he was able to choose how he wanted to handle it. It's regrettable, to say the least, that he didn't return for biopsy, but the incident illustrates how, ironically, knowledge can play an important role in denial. Many times people want to know what the problem is, then some deal with it by denying it. Of course, when it comes to melanoma there is really only one thing to do. It must be treated promptly. The challenge for the doctor is how to present the information to the patient in a way that does not cause unwarranted fear. A doctor who, through miscommunication, scares off a frightened patient and thereby precludes proper treatment, has not done the patient a favor.

If you fear that you have a potentially serious medical problem, take a deep breath and remind yourself that many others have gone through it before and done well. I actually think it is best to break down the problem into small, manageable pieces, the way you would if you heard an annoying noise in your car. You know that the noise means something is wrong and that it probably is something simple. You make time to take the car to the repair shop. So make time to get yourself to the repair shop. Similarly, if you are worried about something on your skin, get thee to a dermatologist. If the doctor is concerned it is a skin cancer, let him or her do the biopsy. It is quite a simple procedure that only takes a few minutes. Don't worry about it. Focus on getting this simple procedure done. If the results of the biopsy indicate melanoma or other skin cancer, you will have addressed it early; therefore the odds are excellent that it will be curable. That's all there is to it. So take a deep breath, make the appointment, and get it done.

▪ WORRY

People who are at special risk for skin cancer, or are especially worried about getting skin cancer, I follow very regularly, or whenever they have concern about a new lesion. This provides a measure of security that minimizes their worry and in many cases allows us to diagnose cancers and precancers early. It is interesting that in this group of patients, after their initial skin cancer, they rarely have to be treated for large or complicated tumors because they are diagnosed at such an early stage.

Worry, the opposite of denial in my universe, can sometimes be medically helpful. In my experience worriers rarely transform into avoiders, but avoiders can sometimes be converted to healthy worriers. For example, there is a common growth that we develop as we age called a seborrheic keratosis. This growth is usually tan or brown and slightly raised with a bit of a rough surface. It can occur anywhere. Often one keratosis can have a variety of colors, which make it resemble pictures of melanoma. People often worry about this growth, which I call a "barnacle of life," and come to see me concerned that it might be a melanoma. While I am usually able to reassure them that it is not malignant, not uncommonly a real skin cancer is diagnosed at the time of the visit. This second growth may not have concerned the patient, but because he or she came in for the other problem, I had the chance to diagnose, treat, and educate.

TIPS ON OVERCOMING YOUR OWN RESISTANCE

- If you're the shy or squeamish type, have a family member or friend give you a full-body skin examination and do the same for them. This is especially helpful in examining hard to see areas like the scalp and soles.

WATCHING THE CANCER GROW

Several years ago an accomplished artist came to see me about a growth on his trunk. I took one look at it and made a "doorway diagnosis." This is what we call a lesion so obvious that you can tell what it is from the doorway. The patient proceeded to tell me that he had been watching this spot grow and had been carefully measuring it every few months. I convinced him to let me biopsy it. It was melanoma and we removed it easily in the office, addressing his fear of doctors and procedures. He would have been better off if he had watched it less and seen a doctor sooner. The only explanation I have for his behavior, which continues to bewilder me, is fear. Getting past that barrier is sometimes the biggest step in taking good care of yourself.

- If you are at any heightened risk for skin cancer or if you are more than forty years of age, find a dermatologist who comes highly recommended and whom you will trust and see him or her twice a year.
- You should consider yourself at increased risk for skin cancer if you:
    are fair-skinned
    have blue, green, or gray eyes
    have blond or red hair
    have a family history of melanoma
    have a history of skin cancer
    have many moles
    had a lot of sun exposure throughout your life
    had blistering sunburns in childhood
- If you think you've noticed something, but aren't sure and are afraid to look, have a family member take a look. Have him or her help you make the doctor's appointment and even go with you. This type of support is often very helpful.

THE EARLIER YOU TAKE CARE OF A PROBLEM, THE LESS OF A PROBLEM IT WILL BE

It's important to remember that treatment for skin cancer is quite simple. The sooner a problem is identified, the easier it is to fix. The longer you wait, the more problematic it can become. Don't let your imagination run wild. Don't visualize yourself in a tragic story akin to those you may have heard about others who have had cancer.

No two people are the same. Even when you get information firsthand from skin cancer patients, it may not be medically accurate. It often simply serves to cause needless worry that leads to denial and avoidance. If you are the type of person who follows the Sergeant Schultz school of medical care (remember *Hogan's Heroes*?) and want to "see nothing, hear nothing, and know nothing," go to your doctor and let your doctor take care of things. If you are more comfortable knowing everything about what the growth is, how it should be treated, and what the prognosis is, make sure your doctor accommodates you as well. Regardless of your level of tolerance for medical information about yourself, make sure that that changing mole or that spot that bleeds on and off, gets checked out as soon as possible.

After you read the rest of this section, mark the page, turn this book over, and proceed to do a full-body self-exam or, if you do have a spot you are worried about, call your dermatologist and make an appointment. You'll be glad you did.

21

Warning Spots of Cancer and Moles

The bad news about skin cancer is that it is on the rise. The good news is that in many cases, people who are prone to skin cancer get advanced warning. In this chapter I describe several growths that are considered precancerous. They are important to know about and to recognize because they are easy to treat and may help in the prevention of melanoma or other skin cancer. When it comes to melanoma, certain moles may be a precursor to the cancer, but the vast majority of moles are not. Because many other precancerous spots may appear similar to totally harmless growths, some of the more common benign skin growths are discussed in this chapter as well.

Since nature raises red flags for cancer on our skin, it is prudent to take advantage of them and become familiar with those common growths that might herald the development of the malignant growths.

▪ ACTINIC KERATOSES

An actinic keratosis (pronounced actinic ker-ah-TOE-sis, also known as AK) is a precancerous growth. AKs are very common in fair-skinned individuals, especially those of northern European descent who have had a lifetime of

---

ACTINIC KERATOSIS

These precancerous "sun spots" can sometimes be felt before they are seen. There is a wide variety of them—most are visible to the naked eye and can appear in any of these forms:

- Rough spots on the surface of the skin noticeable only by touch
- Small reddened area, narrower than a pencil eraser
- Visible rough spot or patch, up to the size of a dime
- Faint, flat pink spot
- Occasionally bleed, with small scabs forming

---

sun exposure. The cause of actinic keratosis is sun exposure. Several years ago, our skin cancer research group at Yale was able to identify how ultraviolet radiation likely begins the process in the skin that leads first to these precancerous growths and later to squamous cell cancer itself. Although AKs are precancerous, we don't really know the rates at which they may convert into invasive squamous cell cancer.

While it is true that only a small percentage of AKs turn into invasive cancer, combining data about ultraviolet radiation mutations with the appearance of the abnormal cells under the microscope, makes clear that AKs are the earliest stage of a skin cancer. AKs have atypical cells—large, dark nuclei, for example, and a disordered appearance under the microscope, indicating their tendency to divide more rapidly and more chaotically than the normal epidermis around them.

Practically speaking, if you have AKs they should be controlled. Some tiny ones may bear watching, but from a medical point of view any lesion that is big enough to be seen easily and felt doesn't belong on your skin, represents an abnormal process, and should be removed (see box).

Because people who have one AK usually have many more, at least over a lifetime, they should be treated. I've observed that patients with AKs on their face and scalp (these are the most common locations) usually come in at the end of the summer with many more lesions than they had at the end of May. Similarly, after a sunless winter or good sun protection, the number of AKs seems to decrease to some degree. This highlights, again, the value of good sun protection.

▪ How to Treat an AK

If an individual does not have many AKs, the simplest treatment is to gently apply liquid nitrogen with a cotton tip applicator or Q-tip. A versatile chemical used by plumbers and metalworkers as well as dermatologists, liquid nitrogen can selectively destroy precancerous cells. The normal cells surrounding the keratosis are relatively resistant to the freezing and survive. The treatment stings briefly, the skin then looks red for a day or two (like a bug bite) and occasionally a small scab may form (this is the dying tumor).

As with any surgical procedure, the skill of the physician determines the final results. It is important that lesions not be overtreated, because that may result in small permanent white scars. Any actinic keratosis begins in the epidermis, the top layer of skin, so it is rarely necessary to destroy below that level. Nevertheless, because it is impossible to always predict the AK's depth, the risk of scarring must be viewed as an acceptable risk—a little white spot may be preferable to what you would have if a skin cancer developed at the site.

Depending on the size of the AK, which can range from the size of a couple of grains of salt to that of a dime or quarter, other techniques may be used. If the growth is large, more aggressive treatment such as scraping and burning may be warranted. A larger AK may be closer in its actual behavior and appearance under the microscope to squamous cell cancer. The scraping method should be done cautiously.

Freezing or scraping and burning AKs are good techniques for people who have just a few keratoses, but may not be suitable for those with multiple lesions of all sizes on sun-damaged skin. This skin usually already bears the mutations that foretell the growth of new AKs. More extreme measures may be called for here.

One of these options is to apply an anticancer drug called 5-fluorouracil (5-FU) in cream form to the skin. Known best by the brand name Efudex, 5-fluorouracil is a mainstay of colon cancer therapy as well. Normally the cream is applied twice a day for four weeks. During that period, the skin becomes red and irritated, especially where AKs are present or even unknown AKs are brought to the surface with this treatment. The use of a topical steroid cream such as hydrocortisone 1% helps with the irritation as do open wet dressings (see page 274).

The irritation caused by Efudex can be a problem. Sometimes, if I really feel my patient would benefit from this medicine, I treat small sections at a time or control the irritation by using it only three or four days a week. Some dermatologists also add Retin-A to the four-day-a-week regimen or variations of it. The most important precaution when undergoing this treatment is to be prepared for the side effects. If you need it, you need it, but your dermatologist can probably customize a regimen for you that is acceptable.

Another treatment for AKs, when they are extensive, is the medium-depth chemical peel (see page 66). In this approach, the skin is first cleansed with an agent that removes oils and scale. No anesthetic is required. Next a pharmaceutical-grade acid such as trichloroacetic acid is gently applied with a Q-tip. The brief stinging or burning that occurs as a result is easily controlled with ice packs. At completion of the peel your skin may look a bit frosted. This indicates that the acid has been effective, destroying cells in the top layer of the skin. Over the ensuing 3–4 days, the skin appears red as though you had a sunburn; during that period, moisturizing assists in healing. By the seventh day after the procedure the skin is almost completely finished peeling off, just as skin peels after a sunburn (not that you would ever get one!). The dermatologist may do several peels, every eight to twelve weeks. After the process, a smoother, fresher appearance to the skin is often noted. In my experience, over time there is a decrease in keratoses, especially if the person follows sun precautions.

▪ MOLES

There probably isn't a human being alive who doesn't have at least one mole. It is, in fact, a small tumor and the average Caucasian adult may have twenty to forty of them. As we learned in chapter 2, dermatologists refer to moles as nevi. The word *nevus* (pronounced NEE-vus) comes from the Latin word for blemish. Nevi are small tumors of pigment-producing cells of the skin; in very fair-skinned people, they may appear flesh-colored or pink, rather than brown or tan. Moles are different from other pigmented spots such as freckles or seborrheic keratoses. Moles reside on the surface of the skin and in many cases extend into the dermis. Moles, which have a wide range of appearances, can be especially important warning signs if they become abnormal. Such atypical moles may be melanoma precursors.

One of the most common reasons for patients to see a dermatologist is concern about a particular mole. While the vast majority of moles are non-cancerous and never turn into cancer, it is important that every patient with many moles be evaluated at least once a year so that any mole that has changed or appears irregular can be evaluated for the possibility of melanoma.

That some moles can turn into melanoma is a well-established scientific fact. The problem for doctors and patients is knowing *which* moles turn into cancer (and which ones don't). Based on training, a dermatologist can, within reasonable limits, decide which moles should be removed because they present a risk for melanoma. Such atypical moles usually have irregular or very dark pigmentation or have recently undergone a change in size. The advantage of diagnosing such moles is that if they represent melanoma in its precancerous state, complete removal in the doctor's office is a simple, relatively pain-free way of eliminating the chance that melanoma will develop in that mole. It is important to note that not all melanomas start in a mole and that this form of skin cancer can develop spontaneously.

After a full-body skin exam is performed, your dermatologist will identify which moles are of concern and will likely perform a small biopsy to remove them. A biopsy is usually just a partial sampling of the growth in order to determine what the best treatment, if any, is. Often, the "biopsy" may remove the mole completely. If the mole that was biopsied was not completely removed but did show signs of abnormality, total removal is now called for.

SHOULD YOU HAVE A FULL-BODY SKIN EXAM?

Monitoring your moles is an effective way of screening for melanoma. Use the following guidelines to determine if you would benefit:

- You are over forty.
- You have a family history of melanoma.
- You have fair skin, light-colored hair, blue, gray, or green eyes.
- You freckle easily.
- You have had blistering sunburns or chronic sun damage.
- You have many moles.
- You've had previous atypical moles diagnosed.
- You are concerned about any mole.

If any of these apply to you, see your dermatologist and request a full-body skin exam.

If the biopsy indicates that complete removal of the mole is necessary, the margin, or the area removed around the mole, should be no more than a quarter of an inch. The actual size of the mole and the margin around it determine the length of the scar you will have. Make sure your doctor is familiar with the proper margins and does not overdo it. Remember, atypical moles are not cancerous so conservative removal is sufficient.

About 2 to 8 percent of the population has at least one atypical mole. If it is determined that you have atypical moles, you should go to your dermatologist for regular skin exams. Many university dermatology departments have *pigmented lesion clinics* where dermatologists who are experts in moles can monitor you on an ongoing basis or provide second opinions. Despite media announcements about computers that can diagnose melanoma, it remains the case that the only way to be sure whether a mole is precancerous or not is to use the best medical computer we know: the dermatologist's skilled eyes and brain. If a mole is questionable he or she will perform a biopsy and the mole will be evaluated under a microscope. Under high magnification atypical moles have cells that are very large, sometimes forming little nests, and also have very large nuclei. Large nuclei are an indication that the DNA is very active and that the cell has the potential for dividing rapidly. (Cancer, as we learned earlier, is a condition in which cells divide rapidly and out of control.)

In most pigmented lesion clinics or in your dermatologist's office, patients who are at risk for developing melanoma—because they have a large number of moles, atypical moles, or a family history of melanoma— may be photographed so that the moles can be monitored on a regular basis.

A new examination technique that is gaining interest is called *epiluminescence microscopy*. In this case, a small amount of oil is placed over the mole and a magnifying scope similar to an otoscope or an ophthalmoscope is placed over the mole so that it can be viewed in a magnified fashion. This method can even be enhanced by digitizing the image of the mole, and in the future it may be possible to correlate this pattern with the risk of the mole turning into melanoma. This may prove to be a means of minimizing the number of biopsies that are required to evaluate an abnormal appearing mole.

Until this method is refined, the general rule I recommend is: *When in doubt, check it out*. If after the biopsy is done, there is still some question about whether it is abnormal, and some of the mole remains, follow the dictum: *When still in doubt, cut it out*.

PATTERN RECOGNITION:
IS IT A MONET OR A REMBRANDT?

If you have many moles it's wise to learn how to perform a self-exam. Examining your own skin involves knowledge of your moles and a sense of which ones appear to be changing.

Two factors make it possible to learn to do this. First, identifying errant moles is really an issue of pattern recognition. You don't have to be a doctor to look at your moles and identify the one that stands out. I believe that if you can look at a painting and can distinguish a Rembrandt from a Monet, you will be able to identify a mole that is different from all the others.

The second factor is that you know your body the best. I believe that we all have an amazing intrinsic or innate ability to identify those things that are just not right about our own body. In fact, one of the most important tips I give residents is that "the customer is always right." By this I mean that even if a mole does not appear abnormal to me but the patient communicates that he or she thinks it is a problem—it should be biopsied

---

SO YOU HAVE A MOLE ON YOUR FACE
AND YOU'RE NOT A SUPERMODEL . . .

The majority of moles are benign. You might have a raised flesh-colored, tan, or brown mole on your face that you would like removed for cosmetic reasons. There are two options in this case. Laser is not one of them, in my opinion.

- **First choice:** Have a doctor shave off the raised mole flush with the surrounding skin. It will heal up in about a week. This does not result in complete removal of the benign growth, since cells will remain below the surface of the skin. The risk of this method is that you may get a small indentation, though this is likely to improve over several months. If the site does not heal as you would like, you can always proceed to:
- **Second choice:** Plastic surgery excision, but even with this approach, you will have a permanent fine line scar.

With the shave method (first choice), the mole may heal beautifully but pigment may come back or the mole itself could regrow since the procedure did not remove the area beneath the surface of the skin.

---

and studied. Too often I have heard of cases where a patient has brought a mole to the doctor's attention and even though the doctor was legitimately not concerned about it based on its appearance, subsequent biopsy demonstrated that it was atypical—or even melanoma.

I tell all my patients that if they have any concern about a mole they should bring it to my attention immediately so that it can be biopsied. The risks of biopsy are minimal. The site is injected with lidocaine solution so that it is anesthetized, and then a small shave of the mole is performed. Occasionally, a punch biopsy may be done (see Appendix 1 on dermatologic procedures). Your dermatologist will help you decide how closely your moles should be monitored. Perform a skin self-exam as described in the box on this page.

It is important to put things in perspective. You may have many lesions that are pigmented, but most often they are not melanoma and in many cases are not even moles.

Some people with atypical moles believe that covering the mole with adhesive bandages or sunscreen while they're out in the sun will minimize the risk of melanoma. Although it is generally a good idea to minimize sun exposure, there is no way to guarantee that this approach will prevent melanoma overall. Again, I must emphasize that the best way to

---

HOW TO EXAMINE YOURSELF FOR SKIN CANCER AND MOLES

1. Find a private, well-lighted room with a full-length mirror.
2. With the help of a hand-held mirror examine your neck, back, shoulders, and back of your legs.
3. Next examine under your arms.
4. Examine your neck, chest, front of your legs, and genital area.
5. Carefully study your face, including ears and hairline area.
6. Next, sit down comfortably and look at your soles, palms, and inspect between your toes and fingers.
7. As you examine your skin become familiar with any moles you have had for a long time so that you will be able to tell if any have changed.
8. To examine your scalp, one area that will be hard for you to see, enlist the help of a friend. Use a hair dryer set on low to blow away hair and permit better examination of the skin.
9. If you notice any new moles, moles that have changed, or spots that are bleeding see your dermatologist.

HOW TO USE SUNSCREEN OR SUNBLOCK

- Test the product first on a small area of skin on your forearm to make sure you are not sensitive to it.
- In children use sunscreen that does not contain alcohol and is creamy enough to better see where it has been applied.
- Apply liberally and massage into skin smoothly to avoid skipping areas, which will show up as streaks of sunburn after being outdoors.
- Be careful applying sunscreen around the eyes, especially in younger children who might rub the area. If the eyes get irritated, wash with tap water.
- Apply sunscreen about 30 minutes before going outdoors.
- Select a water-resistant or waterproof product and apply after swimming or outdoor activity.
- Use lip balm with sunscreen or sunblock in it.

---

deal with melanoma is to identify it early, when it is at a fully treatable stage.

▪ CONGENITAL MOLES

Aside from atypical moles there is another type of mole that some doctors believe has some potential to turn cancerous over a lifetime. These moles, called *congenital nevi*, are usually present at birth or shortly thereafter. They tend to grow over time and tend to be very dark in color. These moles often have hair in them, an almost universal sign that the mole is benign. However, in those congenital moles greater than 1.5 centimeters (there are about 2.5 centimeters to the inch), it is believed there is a small but measurable risk of turning into melanoma. As a result, many dermatologists believe that these large congenital moles should be removed on a preventative basis. How to take care of congenital moles is still controversial, so you should be guided by your dermatologist.

Another type of mole, the giant congenital mole, whose size is greater than about three inches in diameter, has a 4 to 6 percent chance of developing melanoma. Unfortunately, because of its size, removing these moles can be a problem. The question about whether to remove these growths often arises in childhood. Because of the large size, skin

---

NORMAL MOLES

- Symmetrical, round, or oval
- Border is sharp and well-defined
- Color is usually uniform tan, brown, or skin color
- Usually less than a quarter of an inch in diameter
- Develop throughout childhood and into early adulthood
- Normal, benign moles usually look very similar to each other.

---

grafting is sometimes the best approach, but careful consultation with your dermatologist, pediatrician, and plastic surgeon should be pursued to develop a plan that will be best for your child. In general, it is believed that if a congenital mole should be removed because of concern about melanoma, it should be completed before puberty.

When the decision is made to remove a congenital mole, one option for removal is the staged approach. In this technique, under local anesthesia, half the mole is removed in an office procedure. Three to six months later, the doctor goes back and removes the residual mole, thus limiting the total length of the scar and often providing the best cosmetic result. Be sure to discuss with your doctor the various options for removing moles that are large or are located in difficult areas. Not all large moles are amenable to the staged approach.

All moles that are removed should be evaluated by a competent dermatopathologist, a pathologist who is specially trained to study skin specimens. If you belong to a managed-care plan that requires that pathology specimens be sent to a general pathologist, you should insist that they be reviewed by a qualified dermatopathologist. Although you would not normally think to ask where your specimen is being analyzed, in this case it is appropriate and your dermatologist will likely welcome your interest in your care. Often, the dermatopathologist must consult with the dermatologist in order to get additional information about the mole, which is best accomplished when the dermatopathologist and the dermatologist have an ongoing professional relationship.

▪ FRECKLES

Freckles are harmless, and on many people they are cute. Unfortunately, some of those who have them don't feel the same way and seek to have them removed.

Freckles are superficial spots on the skin where the regular skin cells of the epidermis (not melanocytes) have increased pigmentation. Sun generally makes freckles darker, so if you don't like your freckles, your best strategy to minimize them is to use good sun protection. If you have some freckles that are of special cosmetic concern, they may be treated by laser.

22

Melanoma

*I noticed a new growth on my belly. It's been
there for about two months. I just didn't like the
way it looked so I asked my doctor to biopsy it. I
hate the thought of needles, but I was concerned.
It turned out to be an early melanoma. The needle
was no big deal.*

—Jeff, 33, art gallery owner

Malignant melanoma is the worst of all skin cancers.
It can kill. For reasons we don't quite understand, it
is occurring more frequently in women between the ages
of twenty-five and thirty-four. Melanoma is now the most
common cancer in women age twenty-five to twenty-nine;
it's second only to cancer of the breast in women thirty to
thirty-four. People over the age of seventy have more than
double the risk of getting it than people under fifty.

Another alarming fact is that the incidence of
melanoma overall is increasing faster than that of any
other cancer, having almost doubled in the past decade.

Read this chapter carefully, for the good news is that
this serious cancer can be—and should be—diagnosed
early, when it is usually completely curable. Knowing
more about melanoma in its earliest stage can save your

HOW COMMON IS MELANOMA?

In 1999 melanoma incidence in the United States increased 6 percent over the previous year. Melanoma diagnoses in 1999 totaled 44,200; 7,300 people died from it. Most of these deaths were likely preventable.

life or the life of a loved one.

To play it safe, please go back and read about denial in chapter 20. It explains how, although we often know all the warning signs of melanoma, human nature sometimes prevents us from confronting a problem when it is puny, putting us in the position instead of having to deal with it when it is pernicious.

While melanoma may not be totally preventable because of genetic factors we don't fully understand, it can be fully treated if diagnosed early. Regular total body skin checkups and skin self-exam help. In this chapter, you will learn enough about melanoma to become a lay expert. This too will help you deal successfully with the risk of melanoma.

▪ WHERE DOES MELANOMA COME FROM?

Melanoma arises from melanocytes, the pigment-producing octopus-shaped cells that line the bottom layer of the epidermis. There is about one melanocyte for every ten regular epidermal cells. Cells similar to these melanocytes make up the normal moles we all have.

Cancer researchers believe that atypical cells are on a journey toward becoming true cancer cells. Not all atypical cells finish the march. From the point of view of cancer prevention, the trick is to identify those cells or growths that are atypical and remove them before they do become cancerous.

Because some moles can become atypical, we believe they can actually turn into melanoma. However, this is not necessarily true for the vast majority of abnormal moles. It is also cer-

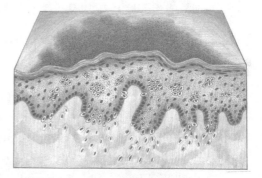

Cutaway view of malignant melanoma, showing pigmentation on surface and cancer cells extending into the second layer of skin

tainly known that melanoma often can arise on its own, without an associated abnormal mole (see chapter 21).

▪ WHAT DO YOU KNOW?

Sadly, general knowledge in this country about melanoma and how to recognize it is not very high. In a random telephone survey of 1,001 Americans, only 34 percent knew that melanoma was a skin cancer. Twenty-six percent knew that a new mole or a change in a mole were signs of melanoma, but fewer than half of this number ever performed skin self-examination. But the record elsewhere proves that public ignorance can be remedied. For instance, in Australia, where skin cancer is a major health problem and public education programs have been going on for decades, more than 90 percent of all surveyed—and a whopping 95 percent of adolescents—knew that melanoma was a skin cancer and were knowledgeable about prevention methods.

Although it is the least common of the three major skin cancers, the rising incidence of melanoma means it is reaching epidemic proportions in this country. The National Cancer Institute reports that more than 44,000 new cases of melanoma will be diagnosed yearly. The disease is more common in men, affecting 3 men for every 2 women.

There is one figure about which there isn't much debate: more than 7,000 people die from melanoma each year. Overall, this includes over 4,500 men and 2,500 women. Many of the victims are young.

Excessive exposure to the sun and sensitivity to the sun are considered risk factors that have contributed to the rising incidence of melanoma in this country, but sun exposure is probably not the whole story.

Researchers are becoming increasingly aware of the profoundly important role that inheritance, or genetic makeup, has to do with the risk of getting cancer. This is no less true for melanoma. Although environmental factors are clearly important for most cancers—tobacco smoke causes lung cancer and the sun causes other forms of skin cancer—carcinogens likely cannot do their harm if there isn't an inborn genetic disposition. One form of genetic disposition is skin type or complexion.

For example, in the case of melanoma, the gene called MC1R helps direct the body's production of the protective skin pigment known as melanin. Melanin, which is produced by the skin in response to sun exposure, probably protects the DNA in the nucleus of the skin cell from further damage from the sun. Fair-skinned people are at much higher risk for melanoma because their DNA is probably more "exposed" to mutation from the ultraviolet radiation of the sun. Researchers have in fact found that people who have abnormalities in the MC1R gene and have red hair and fair skin have a fourfold increased melanoma risk.

As with all new information about cancer genetics, this does not mean that you should rush out and have everyone in your family tested for this gene. At this early stage, this type of information is more useful for helping us understand what causes melanoma. If you have fair skin to begin with, you must be vigilant concerning your risk for melanoma.

The genetic story does have implications for early diagnosis and pre-

---

WHAT TO LOOK FOR ON YOUR SKIN

The ABCD method of checking for melanoma has been widely touted for public health purposes. The problem is that some of the changes described in it do not occur early, and we want to catch melanoma early. Nevertheless, I recommend you learn these ABCDs and know them cold. In addition, I include ways to become suspicious of growths even earlier, when the cure rate is potentially higher.

A *Asymmetry.* If you fold the mole over in your mind's eye, the halves do not match.

B *Border irregularity.* The edges of the mole are ragged, notched or blurred, not smooth like normal moles.

C *Color.* The coloration of the mole is irregular. There are shades of tan, brown, and black. Even red, white, and blue can add to the mottled appearance.

D *Diameter.* Any diameter greater than a pencil eraser (about 5–6 millimeters) should raise suspicion.

In addition to these broad guidelines, two more, a "C" and an "S":

Concern. Even if you don't know why, if you sense there is something of concern about a mole, insist your doctor biopsy it.

Suspicion. This is one time when it's okay to be suspicious. Doctors call it having a "high index of suspicion." I call it being vigilant. But whatever you call it, when it comes to melanoma, the best rule is "When in doubt, check it out."

vention, though. About 5 to 10 percent of patients diagnosed with melanoma have at least one family member with melanoma. Variants of cancer genes called p16 and CDK4 are associated with familial melanoma. The mutation that occurs is the kind caused by ultraviolet radiation from the sun.

Genes or no genes, it is important to understand who gets melanoma, what it looks like in its earliest stages (it's less helpful to diagnose any cancer after it has already grown and galloped away), and what can be done about it.

Approximately 70 percent of melanomas appear on normal skin, while 30 percent originate in a preexisting mole in which changes in color, size, and/or shape have occurred. Itching, bleeding, swelling, and pain may accompany these changes.

When caught in time, malignant melanoma is, in most cases, curable. Thus it is critical for me to note and repeat to you once again, that self-examination, early diagnosis, and immediate treatment can literally save your life. Learn the ABCD's of melanoma (see box).

Dermatologists classify people into six skin types when assessing any individual's risk for a range of skin problems (see chapter 5, "Frequent Questions"). If you are skin type I or II, you should become very familiar with the early signs of melanoma. Melanoma can occur in different sites and the location varies between men and women (see box below).

Happily, melanoma survival rate is also increasing. For example, the five-year survival rate has increased from approximately 50 percent fifty years ago to 85 percent in 1990. This is due to public education programs, stressing self-examination and early detection, and doctors now knowing far better what to look for than they did years ago. Incidentally, it may also

---

COMMON LOCATIONS TO DEVELOP MELANOMA

- For both men and women, the most common location for a melanoma to appear is on the back.
- Men are also highly susceptible to melanomas on the chest or abdomen.
- Women develop melanomas on the legs more often than do men.
- Both sexes may find that melanomas appear in areas not commonly exposed to the sun, such as under the arms, in the groin area, on the buttocks, and in women, on the undersides of the breasts.

be due to the increasing popularity of my chosen profession. In 1973, there were about 2,000 dermatologists in the United States. Today, there are at least 8,000 of us in the U.S., all the more of us to diagnose and educate about melanoma. But it will be best, if you can learn to help diagnose yourself as well.

▪ HOW WIDESPREAD IS MELANOMA?

Epidemiology is the study of the occurrence, distribution, and causes of disease. It tells us how big a health problem is and it can also give clues about which individuals are at risk. While it is true that statistics don't mean much for the individual, they do help guide our thinking about a medical problem.

Malignant melanoma affects men more than it affects women. Women tend to have a higher survival rate than men. This is probably attributable to the fact that women are more conscious—even self-conscious—about their skin and that men simply avoid going to the doctor.

According to the American Cancer Society, in 2000 the lifetime risk of being diagnosed with melanoma will be approximately 1 in 75. Compare this with the lifetime risk in 1980, 1 in 250, and you can see why we dermatologists use the word *epidemic* when discussing the disease. We mean it.

The incidence rate in Caucasians is at least six to seven times that of blacks in comparable geographic locations. Melanoma is also much less common among Asians than it is in Caucasians. Interestingly, the most common sites of the cancer differ among various races. Caucasians tend to

---

THE MELANOMA RISK FACTORS:

If you are a match for any of these, you are at risk for getting melanoma:

- Family history of melanoma
- Personal history of melanoma or atypical (dysplastic) moles
- Skin type I or II
- Tan poorly
- Sensitivity to the sun

- Freckles
- Red, blond, or light brown hair
- Green, gray, or blue eyes
- Excessive sun exposure
- New or changing mole

get melanoma distributed over the entire body surface, while both blacks and Asians tend to develop the cancer on the palms, soles, nail beds, and mucous membranes. Those Caucasians who burn easily and have fair skin, blue, gray, or green eyes, and blond or red hair also seem to be at greater risk for melanoma than other whites.

▪ WHAT TO LOOK FOR

My wife saved my life. I never would have gone to the doctor.

—Roger, 14-year survivor of malignant melanoma

As in all cases of cancer, the earlier the melanoma is diagnosed, the better. According to the *Journal of the National Cancer Institute*, people who check themselves for changes in existing moles or new growths and abnormalities are 44 percent less likely to die from melanoma. The obvious key to early detection is to know what to look for.

Traditionally, we talk about the ABCD's of melanoma (see box, page 230), which has served as an excellent means of educating the public about the need to check for melanoma. However, the truth is that we want to diagnose melanoma at its earliest stages and sometimes interpretation of the ABCD's can lead people to wait too long before seeing their dermatologist. Although the ABCD's are helpful, you should remember that any mole that doesn't seem right to you should be checked out.

Over the years the single most important thing that I have been able to teach residents is an approach that I learned myself early on. I call it the Wal-Mart approach to melanoma: *When it comes to melanoma, the customer is always right.* It is not uncommon for patients to come see me with a concern about a particular mole or mark. To my eye, and objectively speaking, the spot in question appears like a completely benign mole that would not under any other circumstances pique concern. The person can often not articulate why he or she is concerned about the mole, unable to say what is different. But the patient knows he or she doesn't like it. My policy: *Biopsy it.* I have come to believe over the years that patients have a sixth sense about their own bodies and listening to their concerns can only help the physician. Many times I have evaluated moles that appeared totally normal but proved premalignant or malignant when we biopsied them because it worried the patient.

If you have a mole you are concerned about and your dermatologist doesn't want to biopsy it, find another doctor. Having said that, however, I must also advise you to be cautious of the physician who is too eager to excise and biopsy multiple normal moles about which you yourself have absolutely no concern. Time and again I am confronted with cases where doctors have excised innumerable benign keratoses that never had any risk whatsoever of being melanoma or other skin cancer. Often such a doctor will tell the patient, "Don't worry, Mrs. Jones, we got it all." This is disingenuous because the lesion wasn't cancerous in the first place and didn't have to come off. Do yourself a favor: find a good dermatologist you trust and rely on him or her for special expertise in skin disease.

IS THERE A MACHINE THAT CAN DIAGNOSE MELANOMA EARLY?

There is much in the media now about new techniques for diagnosing melanoma. These include digital imaging of lesions, serial photographs, and a process called dermoscopy in which an illuminated magnifier, like the otoscope used to check for earaches, is placed on the skin to magnify the skin lesion. All these techniques are still being explored and show promise.

We are still a far way off from having technology that will allow us to place you in a machine and have your moles read like a supermarket bar code on a jar of apple juice. Technically, this should be possible because the diagnosis of melanoma by your doctor is based on pattern recognition. In time, we should be able to develop a database of information about the patterns of melanoma that will allow for sophisticated automated pattern recognition of skin lesions. The trick is making the technique reliable enough that we would want to trust our health to the artificial intelligence of a computer.

For now the diagnosis of melanoma only can be made under the microscope. Until the time comes when we are able to evaluate your skin cells at a magnification of 400 times directly, a biopsy will be necessary. A biopsy is removal of the growth to determine what it is. I am aggressive about diagnosing melanoma. Until the technology improves, if I am concerned that a mole may be abnormal or a melanoma, it must be biopsied. The risk of biopsy is negligible and the cosmetic result should be excellent. As a result of the biopsy we will know for certain whether or not you have melanoma at its earliest stages, when it is most curable by simple office

---

MELANOMA CHECKS

- Every adult over forty should have an annual full-body skin exam.
- Public skin cancer screenings at which only sun-exposed areas are examined ARE ABSOLUTELY UNACCEPTABLE if that is the only melanoma check you are getting. Melanoma can and does develop where the sun doesn't shine.
- If you are at high risk for melanoma you should perform a full-body self-exam on a regular basis.

---

excision. Nevertheless, there are some patients who have innumerable moles, many of them abnormal; it is impractical to perform biopsies on all these. These patients should be followed in a pigmented lesion clinic or by a dermatologist specially equipped for monitoring. A biopsy is just the first step in diagnosing and treating melanoma. If the biopsy shows melanoma, the area must be re-excised with margins of skin. (see After a Melanoma Diagnosis, p. 246)

▪ Having a Biopsy

When melanoma is suspected, the only acceptable approach is to perform a biopsy. This relatively simple office procedure accomplishes two important goals: it confirms whether in fact you have a melanoma and it helps determine how serious it is. Melanoma cannot be diagnosed without a biopsy and the type of biopsy done is determined by the nature of the lesion, its size and location, and the information that your dermatologist is seeking.

In general, when a melanoma is suspected, it is always best to remove the whole lesion and send it for biopsy. Because the actual thickness of the melanoma is the single most important factor in determining prognosis, or how well you will do as well as the need for other treatment, the biopsy must be complete and thorough.

The most rapid and effective means of biopsying relatively small, flat, pigmented lesions is by *tangential excision*. In this method the skin is anesthetized with lidocaine, a local anesthetic. The doctor excises the lesion in its entirety by cutting under it horizontally beneath the expected depth of the growth. This virtually guarantees that the complete lesion will be removed for analysis. In the method known as the *elliptical excision,* the lesion is outlined in the shape of a football, anesthetized, and then removed in its entirety. The wound is then sutured closed.

After tangential excision, the wound heals on its own. If no further treatment is needed because the biopsy proves noncancerous, the site will heal up with a round white scar. After an elliptical excision, there will always be a thin, linear scar.

Both methods are acceptable as long as the full depth of the lesion has been removed. A physician experienced in melanoma will likely be able to decide on the right biopsy approach.

Many people are under the impression that if you cut into a melanoma you run the risk of spreading it in the bloodstream. This is not true. Sadly, melanoma does not need our help to spread, and there is absolutely no evidence that cutting into melanoma facilitates its spread. It is far more important to get the diagnosis of melanoma right than to worry about an unsubstantiated risk of spread.

Once the biopsy has been performed, it is extremely important to wait for the results to see whether melanoma is present. Remember that melanoma can only be diagnosed by biopsy. For an accurate result, the biopsy specimen must include all or at least the majority of the growth.

When the results of the biopsy come in, a key finding is the *Breslow depth*. This measures the depth of the melanoma. The Breslow depth determines prognosis (how serious the melanoma is) and this figure helps

Melanoma Thickness Affects Survival

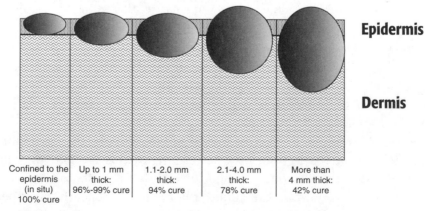

| Confined to the epidermis (in situ) 100% cure | Up to 1 mm thick: 96%-99% cure | 1.1-2.0 mm thick: 94% cure | 2.1-4.0 mm thick: 78% cure | More than 4 mm thick: 42% cure |

Epidermis

Dermis

The thicker the melanoma when it is diagnosed, the lower the cure rate.

QUESTIONS TO ASK YOUR DOCTOR BEFORE SURGERY

- How advanced is my disease?
- What is the level of invasion of the tumor?
- Are the lymph nodes involved?
- How long does the surgery take?
- Will I receive general or local anesthesia?
- What will I be given for pain?
- How big will the wound be?
- Will I need reconstructive surgery?
- Will I be incapacitated and, if so, for how long?
- How long will it take for the wound to heal?
- What type of scar will the surgery leave?
- How often will I need to come back to see you?
- Will I need to see an oncologist (a medical cancer specialist)?

---

guide your doctor's determination of what kind of additional treatment is needed. (The biopsy report may also include a measurement called *Clark's level*. This early method of gauging the seriousness of a melanoma also provides helpful information in certain situations.)

I must make two other critical points about biopsy. First, make sure that your doctor is sending the specimen to a board-certified dermatopathologist. Dermatopathologists are general pathologists or dermatologists who have had extensive special training in reading pathology of the skin. This is such a specialized and complicated area, especially when it comes to melanoma, that you must insist that your specimen be read by such a professional. Many managed care companies try to use general pathologists for this purpose, but insist on your right to have your specimen read by a dermatopathologist. Ask your dermatologist if he or she will be sending your specimen to a dermatopathologist that he or she trusts. Your dermatologist will be glad to have your support.

Second, although this might seem obvious, make sure your doctor actually sends the specimen off. In my career I have heard of cases (including one of a melanoma) where the doctor simply threw the specimen away because the lesion looked benign. It doesn't hurt to ask to see the specimen in the bottle if you don't find the thought too gross. It's your body!

▪ THE RESULT

I am always acutely aware of the anxiety that a patient experiences while waiting for the biopsy report, which generally takes about one week. If I am concerned about the possibility of a melanoma, I send the specimen through as a "Rush" and can have the results in about two days. We either call the patient with the result or send a follow-up letter. Regardless of the notification method used by your doctor's office, within ten days call for the biopsy results if you haven't heard. With something as potentially serious as a melanoma biopsy, don't assume no news is good news. Follow up!

After the results of the biopsy are known, more decisions can be made. There are several different types of melanoma, the most common being the superficial spreading melanoma. The actual type is less important, most of the time, than the Breslow depth. Other factors that may affect the prognosis of melanoma are its location and whether the patient is pregnant.

▪ TYPES OF MELANOMA

Just as there are many different models of Toyotas, so too are there different types of melanomas. These varieties have different cure rates. Here is a brief rundown of invasive melanoma. *Lentigo maligna,* also known as *melanoma in situ,* is not invasive but is discussed here as well. The color plate section includes examples of each type.

SUPERFICIAL SPREADING MELANOMA

A flat lesion characterizes superficial spreading melanoma (sometimes, however, the lesion may be slightly raised). When this melanoma grows out in the surface of the skin, like oil on water, it is considered in the earlier "lateral" growth phase. When it begins to get thicker, entering the "vertical" growth phase, the risk of spread in the body is greater. This type of melanoma can have many different colors in it. It is the most common type of melanoma.

NODULAR MELANOMA

Nodular melanoma takes its name from the nodule (see page 12). There is no lateral or sideways spreading in this variety, which constitutes about 15 percent of all melanomas. The nodule can be as small as a pea or even larger. Nodular melanomas are usually of uniform pigment that is generally dark brown or black.

ACRAL LENTIGINOUS MELANOMA

The rare cancer *acral lentiginous* (pronounced AK-rul LEN-tij-i-nis) melanoma is seen more often in blacks than in whites. It's also called palmar-plantar-subungual-mucosal melanoma, which refers to the areas of most frequent occurrence—the palms, the soles, the nail beds, and the mucous membranes of the nose, mouth, anal, and genital regions. It is often diagnosed after it has already progressed, so the cure rate for this dangerous form of melanoma is less than that for the more common forms. Full-body skin examination on a regular basis can help with earlier diagnosis and more successful treatment of this type of melanoma.

LENTIGO MALIGNA

Lentigo maligna, or *melanoma in situ,* is considered an early form of noninvasive melanoma. Appearing most often in older people, the tumor is confined to the epidermis, so it lacks access to the dermis, which would provide an opportunity for it to spread. Therefore it may be considered a pre-melanoma, even though it is made of the same abnormal melanocytes that could proliferate and grow into a true invasive melanoma.

It is my impression that increasingly these growths are being diagnosed in younger people. They appear often as tan or brown patches on the sun-exposed areas of the head and neck. Most often they are seen on the cheeks.

Patients often bring such spots to the dermatologist's attention because of cosmetic concerns. They wonder whether laser treatment might not eliminate the unsightly blemish. To the untrained eye, lentigo maligna can look like age spots or liver spots. When in doubt, I never treat such spots with laser until I determine by biopsy that they are not lentigo maligna.

Historically, lentigo maligna has not been of much concern; the feeling was that it had to be of long duration—say, approximately twenty to thirty years—before true invasive melanoma could develop. Moreover, the large size of many lentigo maligna lesions presents special challenges. They are usually treated only by excision, which can result in unsightly scars or the need for skin grafts.

The problem that dermatologists now have is that as lentigo maligna becomes more common, treatment can pose challenges and nonintervention could be a risk. While certain approaches such as cryotherapy in which the lesion is frozen or laser in which the pigmentation is removed by laser light have been explored, the concern is that incompletely treated lentigo maligna can develop into invasive melanoma. In addition, a melanoma on the head and neck may be more risky than elsewhere. This is because the rich supply of blood vessels and lymphatic channels in the head and neck area can potentially carry errant melanoma cells elsewhere in the body.

My approach to lentigo maligna is to make the diagnosis by biopsy and then, if feasible, excise it in a simple fashion, hiding the scar in the natural lines of the face. Whenever the lentigo maligna is too large to accomplish this, I use a staged excision rather than a single large removal (the latter would require a skin graft, which can be permanently unsightly).

In a staged excision, the initial procedure removes approximately 50 percent of the lesion; the patient returns in six to eight weeks to have the rest of the lesion removed, permitting me to hide the second scar in the original lines. Because lentigo maligna is very slow growing, this delayed approach poses no real medical risk.

Some dermatologists use Mohs micrographically controlled surgery (see page 262) for lentigo maligna, as they would for basal cell cancer or squamous cell cancer, but I do not believe there is sufficient data at this point to justify this approach.

OTHER PROBLEMS WITH LENTIGO MALIGNA

One problem that arises with lentigo maligna is making sure that it is really what it appears to be. The abnormal melanocytes can sometimes be confused under the microscope with cells that are just badly damaged by the sun but are not yet cancerous. Cells don't come with flashing neon signs that say, "I am cancerous," so it is left to the dermatopathologist to determine on which end of the cancer spectrum a cell sits. Moreover, that decision cannot be made in a vacuum, as one must look at the whole picture. If cells look suspicious for lentigo maligna but the face is severely sun damaged, with wrinkled skin that is blotchy from years of sun exposure, I would be less eager to make a final diagnosis of lentigo maligna. Furthermore, if after my initial excision the biopsy report suggests that there are still cancer cells at the edges, I would evaluate the patient before going

back to excise more tissue. That's because in some people with sun damage one can continue performing these excisions until an unreasonable
amount of tissue has been removed. Unlike nodular melanoma, which is
usually a single nodule, lentigo maligna may well behave like buckshot.
Multiple areas on the face could develop lentigo maligna and it would be
unrealistic, if not impossible, to excise all of the cells. In this case, unlike
other melanomas that are truly invasive, a balance between watchful waiting and conservative intervention will serve best. Where possible, though,
the goal is to remove the lentigo maligna in its entirety.

Recently dermatologists have been experimenting with the use of the
ruby laser to treat lentigo maligna. This laser is used to remove pigmentation in tattoos and other growths, so it seems reasonable that it might
be useful to treat other brown growths, such as lentigo maligna. Occasionally, the lesion is so large that surgery is not feasible. I did treat an
elderly woman with lentigo maligna that completely covered her right
cheek. A plastic surgeon was at a loss with what to do so we initiated treatment with the ruby laser. Although the lesion cleared completely, it
remained important to go back and monitor by biopsy, since the disappearance of pigmentation is not always a sign that the cancer cells have
been eliminated. Laser treatment for lentigo maligna cannot be considered standard care except in exceptional circumstances where there are
no other alternatives.

If you have a complicated lentigo maligna, make sure that your condition is checked by a doctor with extensive experience in the management
of this tricky condition.

AMELANOTIC MELANOMA

Although we think of melanoma as a pigmented growth, in the rare
form called amelanotic melanoma there is no change in color. This unusual
flesh-colored melanoma announces itself by some other change that the
doctor or patient notices. Often it will be biopsied because it looks like
some other kind of lesion and only then will its true nature be discovered.

▪ SAVE YOUR OWN LIFE

It is not an exaggeration to say that when it comes to melanoma, you
can save your own life. Regular skin exams by a dermatologist or other
physician or health care provider trained in skin exams, and skin self-

exams are two ways to diagnose any suspicious lesion at its earliest, most curable stage. Skin self-exams are also especially important because it has been shown that many abnormal skin lesions are often first discovered not by the doctor but by the patient.

SUN AND OTHER SOURCES OF ULTRAVIOLET RADIATION

When it comes to melanoma, the sun is a complicated risk factor. Some say that a single blistering sunburn in childhood increases your adult risk of melanoma several-fold. At the same time, dermatologists often diagnose melanoma in locations that never saw the sun.

Nonetheless, there is an environmental connection between sun exposure and melanoma and other skin cancers. Many questions remain unanswered. Exactly how much of a connection is there between sun exposure and melanoma? How much exposure increases the risk? How many years of exposure to sun increases your chances of getting melanoma? In what period of life (childhood, adulthood, old age) does exposure to the sun increase your risk by the greatest amount? We don't yet have the answers, but some patterns are emerging.

SAFE SUN: PRACTICING SKIN CANCER PREVENTION

- Apply a sunscreen thirty minutes before going out to allow the active compound to interact with your skin.
- Apply a broad-spectrum sunblock or sunscreen every two hours while outdoors.
- Wear a broad-brimmed hat. Although hats are disdained by golfers and tennis players alike, do try to find one hat that works for you (see Appendix 4 product guide).
- Wear sun protective clothing with a tight weave. The common T-shirt provides a sun protection factor of only 6. You don't have to wear a caftan, but you should be reasonably protected.
- Avoid the sun between 10 A.M. and 4 P.M. Take a siesta. Play some chess or cards in the shade.
- Be aware of the reflection of radiation off sand, water, and snow.
- *Protect* your children
- *Never* use a tanning bed.

▪ SUN, MELANOMA, AND YOU

Whether sun exposure turns out to be 50 percent of the cause of melanoma or 90 percent, we know at a minimum that it plays some important role in causing this deadly cancer. We also know that it is relatively easy to minimize our exposure to sun thereby reducing our risk of developing this disease. Reasonable and judicious sun avoidance combined with regular skin self-examination should permit each of us to lessen our risk of developing melanoma and dying from it.

There has been some debate recently in the media about whether the use of sunscreen creates a false sense of security, encouraging people to spend more time in the sun than is safe. The truth is, all scientific evidence suggests that anything you can do to minimize exposing your skin to the harmful effects of ultraviolet radiation will help prevent melanoma.

Sun protection and avoidance are the two most active steps we can take. A recent study of 1,300 women under sixty in the San Francisco Bay area evaluated whether sunscreen reduced the risk of cutaneous melanoma. Thirty percent of the women reported that they "almost always" used sunscreen products, 27 percent said they sometimes used sunscreens, and 43 percent said they never used sunscreens. After careful epidemiologic analysis, it became clear that women who used sunscreen sometimes or never had *twice the rate of melanoma* compared with those women who usually used sunscreens. While it is true that the number and type of moles that people have correlates better with melanoma risk than purely sun-related factors, exposure to sunlight cannot be ignored.

There are of course many things that one can do to minimize exposure to the carcinogenic agent we know as ultraviolet radiation. Sun-

CHOOSING YOUR SUNSCREEN

Sunblocks are physical agents, like zinc oxide or titanium dioxide, that actually reflect the sun's rays. They block UVA and UVB.

Sunscreens are chemical agents that absorb the ultraviolet radiation rather than reflect it. If choosing a chemical sunscreen, look for a product that provides both UVA and UVB protection. Use a product with SPF (sun protection factor) of 15 or higher.

screen is just one aspect of a total sun protection program (see box, page 242).

In addition to avoiding the sun when practical, the use of sunscreen, use of protective clothing, and a regular skin self-examination, special forms of surveillance are appropriate if you are at high risk for melanoma. You are in that category if you have had a melanoma before, have a history of melanoma in the family, have a history of atypical moles, are fair-skinned and/or have had excessive sun exposure. It should be noted that certain family syndromes have an especially high incidence of melanoma. Consult your dermatologist if you think you may fall into that category.

Even if you do not have the familial form of atypical moles, but have many atypical moles and are at risk for melanoma, photographic monitoring by your dermatologist can be helpful.

In one study of 18 patients followed for atypical moles, early diagnosis of curable melanoma was possible in 10 of the subjects as a direct result of changes that were detected in baseline surveillance photographs. In another study of 78 adults who had at least five atypical moles, 11 of 20 melanomas were detected solely because of changes that were evident when baseline photographs were compared with the changes detected in physical examinations.

Baseline dermatologic photography is now regarded as a critical aid in detecting melanoma in high-risk patients. Managed care has had a negative impact here, refusing to pay for these potentially lifesaving photographs. The American Academy of Dermatology and many dermatologists are currently attempting to obtain an official medical billing code that would permit reimbursement for photographs to monitor melanoma.

▪ EFFECTIVENESS OF SUN SCREENS

In protecting against skin cancer, not all sunscreens are created equal. Often people use a sunscreen with a high SPF rating, thinking this automatically protects them from all ultraviolet radiation. This is not the case, since only certain sunscreens offer broad-spectrum protection. The best sunscreens and sunblocks are those that state on the label that they protect against both UVA and UVB rays.

The best known sunblock is zinc oxide. This thick white cream, famous on the noses of well-tanned lifeguards, has evolved significantly over time. Now available in a range of colors and skin tones, it can be strikingly obvious as a fashion statement or less obvious by blending in when skin tones are selected.

Perhaps a more user-friendly sunblock is a chemical variation of zinc oxide called titanium dioxide. It is now used in a variety of high-quality products in which the sun-blocking compound is broken down into microscopic particles, so that each functions like a small mirror on the surface of the skin. Unlike its zinc cousin, titanium dioxide is virtually transparent as it reflects back the ultraviolet radiation.

Nowhere is the use of sun protection more important than in children. It is estimated that 85 percent of lifetime sun exposure is acquired by age eighteen. Chronic, repeated sun exposure leads, so we believe, to the genetic changes that cause skin cancer. Children spend a great deal of time outdoors and should be protected from the sun on a regular basis. Be sure to keep infants under the age of six months out of direct sunlight at all times. Sunscreen should be used only on children older than six months.

In addition to applying sunscreen approximately thirty minutes before going outside and reapplying after swimming or exercise, it is important to dress properly in the sun. If you look at pictures of midwestern farmers or railroad workers at the turn of the century, what strikes us today is that they were wearing long-sleeved shirts, long pants, and broad-brimmed hats even in summer. How these workers must have sweated while toiling! But one thing is for sure: I can guarantee few of them got skin cancer from overexposure to the sun. Nowadays, we frequently wear T-shirts and shorts in sunny weather. However, the typical T-shirt has a sun protection factor of only 6. Fortunately, it's now possible to buy lightweight clothes that, because of a tight weave, provide much more sun protection (see Appendix 4).

It is also important to stay out of the sun during the peak hours between 10 A.M. and 4 P.M. People who live close to the equator have known this for some time—their siestas are no accident. In addition, be cautious at high altitudes. For every 1,000 feet above sea-level, UVR increases 4 to 5 percent.

In recent years public agencies have provided additional information about ultraviolet radiation in our environment. Television weathercasts and newspapers provide us with the ultraviolet (UV) index. This new index is an estimate of the peak amount of ultraviolet radiation that will reach the earth's surface at noontime. Become familiar with the UV index and try to incorporate it into your sun-avoidance strategy.

▪ AFTER A MELANOMA DIAGNOSIS

After the doctor called with the biopsy results I was in a panic. I didn't know what the next step was. I thought I should get a second and third opinion.

—*Jane, graphic designer, 32*

Most melanomas are diagnosed in the earliest stage and treatment is straightforward. Once the diagnosis of melanoma has been made it is important to know its Breslow depth. The risk that you will develop serious problems with melanoma is directly related to how deep the melanoma is. Any melanoma that is up to 1 millimeter in depth has an excellent chance for cure. The cure rate following simple excision is in the range of 96 to 99 percent. Because it is not 100 percent, it is important to emphasize the need for regular monitoring and follow-up examination.

If the melanoma is just *in situ*, meaning it is not invasive and confined only to the epidermis, excision margins of 0.5 centimeters are sufficient. This is equivalent to about a fifth of an inch. The excision margin is the amount of extra, normal skin that is removed around the melanoma.

In order to determine how to treat a patient with melanoma and to make some predictions about prognosis, we categorize melanoma in stages.

When a melanoma is up to 1 millimeter in depth, excision with 1 centimeter margins down below the level of fat is all that is required. This procedure can be performed in the doctor's office under local anesthesia.

When the melanoma is between 1 and 4 millimeters thick it is classified as intermediate and may require margins of 2 centimeters when definitive treatment by excision is done. If the melanoma is more than 4 millimeters deep, the margin of safety around the melanoma should be 2–4 centimeters, if it is technically feasible. In some cases smaller margins may be acceptable.

It is extremely important to know that in the past decade doctors' attitude about the management of melanoma has changed in a meaningful way. Treatment of melanoma was based for many years on a single autopsy case performed at the beginning of the twentieth century. Back then autopsy of the patient revealed melanoma cells scattered throughout the surrounding skin, or about two inches away from the original cancer. Without much controversy or challenge, it was assumed that any melanoma, regardless of its stage, should be excised with *wide* margins of about two inches in order to get all the cancer out. Recent studies worldwide have suggested that under most circumstances wide excision of melanoma does not enhance survival or decrease the risk of recurrence of the cancer where it was removed.

Many physicians in practice today are not current on the latest management of melanoma. It is important to be sure that your physician is knowledgeable about current practices and understands that the amount of tissue that has to be removed is based on the thickness of the cancer as measured under the microscope. Of course, individual circumstances can vary, and there are certainly situations where it is necessary to be more aggressive than the thickness of the cancer alone would suggest.

▪ LYMPH NODES AND MELANOMA

Although we now better understand what the margins of excision for melanoma should be once it has been diagnosed by biopsy, new technology has raised questions about what to do next. Normally, once a melanoma has been diagnosed baseline chest X-ray and liver enzyme (LDH) readings (a simple blood test) are obtained so that the potential for spread of the melanoma throughout the body can be monitored. *If* melanoma is going to spread or metastasize it will usually go first to the lymph nodes and then to internal organs. The lung, liver, and brain are often affected eventually.

When melanoma is beyond more than 1 millimeter in depth, there is some controversy about whether the lymph nodes should be removed in an effort to halt the potential spread of the cancer. Usually physical examination by your physician helps evaluate whether there is any change in the lymph nodes. Feeling the nodes in the area that corresponds to the location of the melanoma will indicate whether they are enlarged or not. The most common lymph node areas are in the neck, armpit, and groin. A lymph node that is enlarged must be removed and studied.

If the lymph nodes are not enlarged, two approaches can be taken. One can wait and see, and through regular examinations the lymph nodes can be evaluated for evidence that melanoma has spread to them. Alternatively, the lymph nodes can be removed at the time of the original melanoma surgery and evaluated for the presence of cancer. Removal of lymph nodes is not without complications, so this procedure should not be performed without considering all the options.

▪ SENTINEL NODE BIOPSY

A new technique has been developed lately that may help us determine whether or not lymph node removal is more appropriate in melanoma management. Called *lymph node scintigraphy,* it involves injecting a radioactive substance at the site of the melanoma and tracking it with a scanner to help identify which lymph node group it drains to. Once that is identified, the cancer surgeon can remove what is called the sentinel node, or the first lymph node in the region to which that melanoma is draining. A biopsy of that lymph node during surgery using frozen sections permits a more precise analysis of whether the other lymph nodes should be removed. If no cancer is found, no further surgery is needed. The risk of complications from extensive lymph node surgery is thus avoided. However, if cancer cells are present in the sentinel node the rest of the lymph nodes can be removed, remaining firm in the knowledge that removal was necessary.

I must stress that sentinel node biopsy is not yet a standard part of practice. Although its logic is compelling, we are not sure whether this approach will in fact result in increased life expectancy from melanoma or allow us to identify metastatic melanoma earlier than we had been able to in the past. Therefore it is best if you discuss whether this new technique is appropriate with your dermatologist or surgical oncologist. At present, it is safe to say that such a procedure does give us more information about the melanoma and its extent.

It is important to note that if sentinel node biopsy is being considered, the excision of the melanoma must be done at the time the lymph nodes are mapped. It is not possible to have the definitive excision of the melanoma and the sentinel node biopsy done at different times.

▪ CHOOSING YOUR MELANOMA DOCTOR

When malignant melanoma is diagnosed early—or at least early enough—complete surgical excision of the cancer is the recommended course of treatment. Such an excision must include adequate removal of normal skin tissue around the site of the melanoma and also adequate depth of removal, including subcutaneous fat. The procedure can be performed by any physician trained in skin surgery who is knowledgeable about melanoma management.

Once a melanoma has grown thicker so that a wider margin is

WHAT IS MY PROGNOSIS?

Your prognosis, or survival rate from melanoma can depend on many factors. The most important information is how thick the melanoma is when it is removed. In general, the thicker the melanoma, the greater the risk that it will travel in the body and lead to death. This table gives only a very rough idea of how thickness corresponds to survival. Consult your doctor regarding your particular factors and remember that statistics apply to large groups of people, not to the patient as an individual.

Breslow Thickness	Survival Rate
Up to 1 mm	96%–99%
1.1–2 mm	94%
2.1–4 mm	78%
more than 4 mm	42%

required, reconstruction with a skin flap or graft may be necessary. This is generally done by a general surgeon, surgical oncologist, plastic surgeon, or dermatologic surgeon. The surgery itself is not necessarily the challenging part of management—it is deciding how much to remove, whether to check the lymph nodes, and how to manage the problem after the surgery.

To ensure your physician is skilled and knowledgeable about melanoma, you should ask several questions: What percentage of the doctor's practice is composed of melanoma patients? Does he or she have an association with a university-affiliated multidisciplinary melanoma panel? This type of group is usually not necessary for thin melanomas, but for more complicated cases, the input of several specialties is helpful. When a physician does have such an affiliation, you can be sure that you'll get the most up-to-date information, as well as the opportunity to join clinical trials that study new treatments for melanoma.

▪ PREGNANCY, ESTROGEN, AND MELANOMA

Recent studies have shown that pregnant patients do not do worse with early-stage melanoma than those who aren't pregnant. This concern has been raised because of the question about whether melanoma cells respond to the estrogen hormone.

As in any other situation involving skin cancer, continued skin self-examination is key to early detection, successful treatment, and cure. Since the size and shape of moles can change during pregnancy, the diagnosis of melanoma in a pregnant woman can be delayed. Because some change and increased irregularities are considered normal at this time, suspicious moles may be overlooked by patient and doctor alike.

Even though no link has been established between subsequent pregnancies and recurrence of melanoma, a waiting period between pregnancies is almost always recommended for a woman who has previously been treated for malignant melanoma.

The treatment for malignant melanoma discovered during pregnancy is the same as for melanomas diagnosed at any other time.

• RECURRENCE AND ADVANCED MELANOMA

When recurrence does develop—that is, when melanoma develops again at the site of the original cancer—it is often because of incomplete removal of the tumor the first time around. After removal of a recurrent melanoma, though, the overall five-year survival rate remains about 90 percent.

While early diagnosis is the best hope that the melanoma will not spread, the behavior of some cancers can often be hard to predict. If a melanoma is diagnosed with a thickness that poses a real risk that cancer cells will escape the skin and travel to other parts of the body, some have advocated removal of the draining lymph nodes. Currently there is no uniform view about the benefit of lymph node removal in melanoma. Sentinel node biopsy, as discussed above, may help clarify the debate in this area. At the present time it is best to discuss all options with your doctor.

As with all aspects of melanoma management there are many issues to consider. Once melanoma has metastasized the survival rate overall is about 20 to 30 percent. A whole range of treatment options exist, including vaccines, interferon, chemotherapy, and other approaches, but so far there is no magic bullet, no sure thing. Medical oncologists continue to research treatment for melanoma that has metastisized.

• ALTERNATIVE MEDICINE AND MELANOMA

The potential aggressiveness of melanoma leads some people to seek out alternative therapies, but I know of no alternative form of medicine that can cure melanoma. While the options available for melanoma once it has spread in the body may not be great, alternative therapies generally have shown no proven benefit.

Despite the lack of evidence that alternative treatments are effective in the fight against cancer, alternative cancer therapy is a multibillion-dollar business. Those who champion alternative treatments tend to be well-meaning people who genuinely believe that their treatments will be helpful.

If you are considering alternative therapy, it should be undertaken only in conjunction with traditional methods of treatment, including routine screening to measure the size of the cancer and whether it has spread. Discuss the risks and possible benefits of the alternative treatment with your oncologist and, if possible, proceed with his or her continued involvement.

One important question to ask your alternative medicine provider is whether there is any documented proof that the proposed treatment has been effective for other melanoma patients. What is the background and what are the credentials of the person who will be providing the treatment? Are there any attendant risks or side effects in undergoing this treatment? You should be wary of any self-published reports that advertise the value of the treatment. Instead try to find out whether the treatment has been described in any legitimate medical journals and whether it is monitored by any regulatory agencies.

• INVESTIGATIONAL THERAPIES

An important source of cutting-edge treatment for melanoma are clinical drug trials conducted at university medical centers throughout the country and at the National Cancer Institute. Unlike alternative therapies, these investigational therapies are carefully regulated and supervised. They are an important aspect of the treatment options available to melanoma patients. Usually, these trials evaluate whether a particular medication or technique is effective in curing melanoma or slowing its growth. If the study proves a success, the treatment is then made available for widespread use on a routine basis. There are dozens of clinical trials nationwide for melanoma. (See Appendix 6 for further information.)

Unfortunately, only 26 percent of Americans know that a new mole or changes in a mole are signs of melanoma. Continued education about the early signs of melanoma is critical. Read this book. Educate your family. Examine your family. See your dermatologist.

23 Basal Cell Cancer and Squamous Cell Cancer

*I had this thing on my nose for about a year. I
think it bled; then it healed up, so I figured it was
a pimple. Then it came back. Now there's always
a scab on it. I'm a golfer and I love tennis, so
maybe I got it there. I know what it is. How bad
do you think it's going to be?*

—Ken, orthopedic surgeon, 43

A young, attractive woman was referred to me by her
doctor, who had just diagnosed a basal cell cancer in
the corner of her eye, at the root of her nose. She was concerned about the diagnosis and frightened about her long-
term prospects.

"I don't understand it," she said, sitting anxiously on
the examining table. "I'm too young for this. My father
had many skin cancers, but he was so much older when
he got them."

Cheryl was a successful consultant in the banking
industry who had grown up in New Jersey. "We didn't know
a lot about sun protection then," she lamented. In our consultation, she told me about all those afternoons covered
with baby oil, and baking in the sun with an aluminum sun
reflector propped under her chin. "As soon as I heard the

word *cancer*," Cheryl said, "I knew it was bad news." In Cheryl's case, fortunately, that wasn't entirely true.

There are two principal kinds of non-melanoma skin cancers: basal cell cancer and squamous cell cancer. Basal cell can-

> ### EARLY SIGNS OF BASAL CELL SKIN CANCER
>
> - A "pimple" that heals but continues to recur. True pimples heal after a week or two.
> - A bleeding spot.
> - A new bump with a pearly surface.
> - An area that looks like a scar but there is no history of injury to the site.

cer is the most common cancer in the world. Squamous cell cancer is the second most prevalent skin cancer. Still, basal cell cancer outnumbers it four to one.

The good news is that each is easily treated and cured in most cases. In addition, neither one turns into melanoma—the one skin cancer that most people fear because it can metastasize and can be deadly. Nevertheless, if you have had many bouts with either basal cell or squamous cell cancer, you are at higher risk for melanoma and should examine your skin regularly for changes in existing spots or growths and for new growths.

Both squamous cell cancer of the skin and basal cell cancer arise from the skin's top layer, the epidermis. This layer, which is about twenty cells thick, or roughly the thickness of a sheet of paper, is our first barrier against all sorts of hostile environmental attacks, and as such is especially sub-ject to the harmful effects of ultraviolet radiation from the sun.

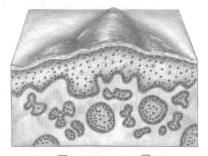

Basal cell cancer

▪ BASAL CELL CANCER

The primary cause of basal cell cancer is overexposure to the sun and those with fair complexions are especially susceptible. For the same reason, it occurs most often on sun-exposed areas of the body, which include the head and neck, the legs in women, and the trunk in men.

Because sun exposure is its main cause, the rates of basal cell cancer vary according to occupation (those who work outdoors are generally more at risk) and choice of recreational activities. The different styles of clothing that men and women wear, as well as changes in fashion, also have an impact on where on the body this cancer occurs.

The relation between the sun and multiple occurrences of basal cell cancer is vividly conveyed by an interesting pattern. In the days before most motor vehicles were air-conditioned, it was not uncommon for drivers to wind up with basal cell cancer on the left elbow and arm, and even on the left side of the face. We now believe that this was the result of drivers rolling their windows down all the way and comfortably resting their arm on the window frame of their cars or trucks. On long trips and over a lifetime of travel, the amount of sun exposure was indeed enormous, and the resulting skin cancer almost predictable.

Basal cell cancer is a cancer that has the least potential to spread in the bloodstream or metastasize. Worldwide there have been only about two hundred reported cases, in total, of basal cell cancer metastasizing, and those have usually been huge, neglected tumors. In part because it tends to be diagnosed early, basal cell cancer has a very high cure rate, if treated with the appropriate techniques,

The majority of basal cell cancers occur on the face. For this reason, the treatment that you select will have an impact on your appearance and on how you feel about yourself. In addition, this treatment choice must take into account first and foremost the cure rate.

▪ WHAT IT LOOKS LIKE

Under the microscope, in biopsy specimens stained with dyes to make the cancer cells visible, basal cell cancer appears relatively innocuous: purplish balls of cells organized symmetrically in a pattern that could be a design for interesting wallpaper. The microscopic tumor sits embedded in the normal epidermis and dermis. But this microscopic description does not tell the whole story. Just as cancer is a general term for a broad range of malignant growths, named for the organs from which they arise, and just as skin cancer itself has several different types, basal cell cancer has a variety of appearances and behaviors.

NODULAR BASAL CELL CANCER

The most common form of this condition is *nodular basal cell cancer*. It looks like a small bump and is often indistinguishable at first from a pimple or a colorless mole. The classic appearance of nodular basal cell cancer is that of a pearly surface, throughout which course small spider veins. The tumor, because it is very slow-growing, has often been present for some time before becoming a problem. Most frequently, people with this type of skin cancer first notice the growth when it begins to bleed. The site then heals completely for a month or two, only to erupt a month or two later and bleed again.

This illustrates one of the cardinal signs of skin cancer, recited in dermatologists' offices day in and day out: *Bleeding lesions require attention.* People often believe at first that the tumor is bleeding because it has been scratched or accidentally traumatized, but the real reason is that the very blood vessels that aid in the growth and development of the cancer cause a small amount of bleeding and oozing. In other words, this is part of the process of the cancer's formation.

MORPHEAFORM BASAL CELL CANCER

Another form of basal cell cancer is quite different from the typical nodular variety and harder to identify. *Morpheaform basal cell cancer,* also termed aggressive-growth basal cell cancer, is usually present for many years before it comes to the person's attention. Like the nodular variety, it does not have the potential to spread in the bloodstream, but it has a totally different appearance on the skin and under the microscope. It is often flat, firmer than the surrounding skin, and white or yellow. It has the texture and appearance of a scar, but if no history of trauma can be recalled, then it is important to have it evaluated. Its slow growth can be noticed over time, especially if photographs of the area from earlier occasions are available.

Morpheaform basal cell cancer is not widely known among primary care physicians, so it can be overlooked. This type of skin cancer tends to grow with deep roots under the surface of the skin and is often larger than it appears to the naked eye. Once diagnosed, it is easily treated and cured—the trick is to *make* the diagnosis. A firm diagnosis can be made only by a skin biopsy (see Appendix 1, guide to dermatologic procedures).

SUPERFICIAL MULTIFOCAL BASAL CELL CANCER

Superficial multifocal basal cell cancer tends to be shallow but broad. Although it doesn't have roots that extend deeply into the skin,

AN AFTERNOON AT THE BEACH: HOW A SKIN CANCER IS MADE

*In recent years, through research done by our collaborative skin cancer group at Yale, and by researchers around the world, we have developed a clearer idea of exactly how the sun causes skin cancer. Before we go to the beach to see what happens, let me introduce you to a cancer gene called **p53**:*

p53 is a tumor suppressor gene. It functions like the brake in a car, controlling cells that may go off wildly and divide, turning into cancer. This gene is present in the DNA of all our cells, including the epidermis. When the p53 gene is functioning normally, it produces a small molecule or protein that keeps the cell from becoming cancerous by killing abnormal or cancer-prone cells. For this reason, it is called a *tumor suppressor gene*. This braking or *suppressor* effect protects against the development of cancer. The p53 gene is a very important cancer gene because it is found in a whole range of cancers, including those of lung, breast, colon, and liver.

What Happens at the Beach

You have been playing volleyball but forgot to reapply your sunscreen after a dunk in the ocean. By the time you sit down for dinner, your forehead is tingling and the nape of your neck is on fire. You are sunburned. In fact, sunburn is a sign that skin cells have been injured by the ultraviolet radiation from the sun. As a result of this sun exposure, ultraviolet radiation has actually targeted specific molecules in the p53 gene for damage. When cells experience such a mutation from ultraviolet radiation and part of the DNA of the p53 gene is damaged, the stage is set for the cell not to die, as it should, but to continue to live and divide, passing on the abnormal DNA that was caused by the sun.

Fast Forward . . . the Following Summer

The cells that were mutated by the sun the previous summer have continued to divide abnormally, encouraged by more mutations from continued exposure to the sun. From a single epidermal cell that was mutated, a whole clone of cells have now grown that are at least precancerous and may even eventually turn into squamous cell cancer.

This understanding of how the sun causes cancer gene mutations in the skin is the strongest case for protecting ourselves against the harmful radiation from the sun.

TOUCH ME NOT?

Current popular ideas about cancer result, in part, from the studies medical ancients made of skin cancers and tumors on the surface of the body. From the time of Hippocrates through the period of medical enlightenment in the Renaissance, the concept prevailed that if one touched or manipulated a cancer, any cancer, one would only make it worse. This led to the commonly held belief, which persists to this day in some quarters, that manipulating a cancer will cause it to spread and that biopsying it to obtain a diagnosis is fraught with danger since you may introduce the cancer cells into the bloodstream. Neither is true. In fact, a biopsy is absolutely necessary for the accurate diagnosis of a cancer.

So pervasive was the perception that manipulation of cancer only made it worse, that the term *noli me tangere* (touch me not) was applied specifically to basal cell cancer since the Middle Ages. This phrase comes from the New Testament. Soon after Christ arose after the crucifixion, Mary Magdalene reached out to touch him, but he stopped her, saying "Touch me not, I am not yet arisen."

In reality, it was not the touching of the cancer that failed to remove it or exacerbated it, but rather the failure to remove the entire cancer. Some more enlightened minds during the Middle Ages understood that cancer of the skin had roots and that unless it was removed completely by its roots, a cure would not result. To this day, basal cell cancer that is not adequately treated may recur and be more aggressive the second time around.

it can sometimes be as large as a fifty-cent piece or more. It is not unusual to see people who develop one such skin cancer develop others in the same area. This may be due to the fact that radiation from the sun mutates several clones of cells and each develops into separate skin cancers.

Superficial multifocal basal cell cancer appears like a red, scaly patch. It has sometimes been mistaken for eczema or even psoriasis. If you have such a patch of skin, and it does not heal completely with topical corticosteroid, it should be biopsied to make sure it isn't this form of basal cell cancer.

RODENT ULCER

A fourth type of basal cell cancer is called the *rodent ulcer*. It earned that graphic moniker in eighteenth-century England, when neglected tumors would grow, outstrip their blood supply, and the center of the cancer would die. The resulting ulceration would fester and be especially unsightly. This type of basal cell cancer often develops after the growth has been neglected for some time. In general, basal cell cancer grows very slowly, so it takes many years for the cancer to develop to the point that it appears as a large nonhealing ulcer.

Before we move on to squamous cell cancer, let me stress that basal cell cancer almost never metastasizes. It is considered a malignancy because it will continue to grow unabated and destroy the tissues around it, but in fact it has no practical potential to spread in the bloodstream. Although this ability to metastasize is a fearsome feature of malignant tumors in general, it's usually not true of basal cell cancer.

▪ SQUAMOUS CELL CANCER

Squamous cell cancer is another common skin cancer that is thought to result most often from sun exposure. It arises from plate-like cells in the epidermis. Unlike basal cell cancer, squamous cell cancer can metastasize to the lymph nodes and even to internal organs.

The risk of metastasis is low as long as the cancer is treated early. Once the cancer has metastasized, treatment options are fewer and, if surgical excision does not get all the cancer, other choices are limited. In general, though, even if the squamous cell cancer has spread, up to 50 percent of cases can be cured.

Another way squamous cell cancer can cause trouble is when it grows along nerves. This occurs in fewer than 1 percent of cases, but it is very serious when it does happen. Once a squamous cell cancer of the face or scalp has spread to the nerves of the skin, it can track along the nerves and even gain access to the brain.

As with basal cell cancer, some squamous cell cancers are more aggressive than others. They may grow rapidly and invade deeply, so they must be treated with respect. Squamous cell cancers occur more frequently in men than in women, by a 4-to-1 ratio.

Squamous cell cancer usually appears as a crusty, scaly, warty bump. It may range in size from pea-sized to chestnut-sized and is usually raised.

Although squamous cell cancers grow slowly, the sooner you see your doctor and the cancer is diagnosed and treated, the less complicated the surgery to remove it will be and the faster you will make a complete recovery.

The treatment for squamous cell cancer varies according to the size and location of the lesion. The surgical options are much the same as those for basal cell cancer. While the next section focuses on treating basal cell cancer, almost everything applies equally to squamous cell cancer.

▪ TREATING NON-MELANOMA SKIN CANCERS

If you have reason to believe that you have a basal cell cancer or a squamous cell cancer, first stay calm. Whether you have a growth that is nonhealing or one that looks just like the basal cell cancers I have described, reassure yourself by recalling that basal cell cancer does not spread in the bloodstream and is easily treated in the doctor's office. A variety of treatments are available, all of which yield a far less noticeable scar than you might fear—as long as the cancer is treated *early*. The most effective step you can take now is to make an appointment with a dermatologist you know, or one to whom your primary care physician refers you. He or she will evaluate the area you are concerned about and, if suspicious that there may be a basal cell cancer, will likely perform a small biopsy. This very brief procedure (it takes no more than a minute or two) will confirm or rule out the diagnosis.

Once a diagnosis of basal cell cancer has been made there may be several options for treatment. These include excision, scraping and burning, and Mohs micrographic surgery. At this point, however, you may wonder whether it's necessary to do anything. In fact, some of my patients ask, "If basal cell cancer does not spread in the bloodstream, why should I bother treating it?" The answer is clear and simple: *Basal cell cancer is a cancer.* Cancer cells divide abnormally and in an uncontrolled fashion, all at the expense of normal tissue. Basal cell cancers can be very destructive and, if they are not treated early, they will have to be managed sooner or later down the road. Squamous cell cancer can, in a low percentage of cases, metastasize.

The best treatment approach depends on the type of cancer, its location, your age, and whether the cancer is recurrent or not. Most of the treatment options are surgical and have varying cure rates. There are several new nonsurgical treatments currently under investigation, but they have either not yet been proven effective or have not been approved by the FDA.

Whenever basal cell cancer recurs, the risk of its being much larger than the original one is great because of the growth of the cancer cells within the scar bundles remaining from the previous surgery. It is important, therefore, to consult with your physician and determine what technique will provide the highest possible cure rate.

SURGICAL EXCISION

In surgical excision, which is really a simple form of plastic surgery, the skin cancer and the area around it are numbed with a local anesthetic such as lidocaine. The doctor then makes an incision through the full three layers of the skin around the obvious area of the skin cancer. The size of the margin must be estimated and there is a risk that the physician may take too little tissue and not get all the cancer, or take too much, resulting in a bigger scar than necessary. Skilled dermatologists can often estimate quite well.

> ### DOES BASAL CELL CANCER TURN INTO MELANOMA?
>
> Basal cell cancer and squamous cell cancer do not turn into melanoma. They are not even birds of a feather. However, people who get many non-melanoma skin cancers are at increased risk of getting melanoma.

The specimen, roughly the shape of a football, is removed and the edges of the wound are pulled together using plastic surgery techniques. Two layers of stitches are used: a bottom layer that consists of an absorbable material, which is usually synthetic, and a top layer that uses nylon or other synthetic nondissolving stitches. The superficial top stitches are removed in approximately five to seven days depending on the location. The deeper set provide the wound support; these stitches usually dissolve in about four weeks, by which time the wound has begun to heal on its own. Once the stitches are removed, small tapes may be placed over the wound and remain in place for three to five additional days. It is important to note that there are many variations on the procedure just described and your doctor will select the technique he or she thinks is best for you.

You should expect that with time the surgical scar will improve. In the early months, however, there may be redness, especially if you are fair-skinned, as well as bumpiness related to slow absorption of the dissolving stitches. If the surgery was on the face, you must be very patient, since facial wounds take approximately nine to twelve months to look their best. I know that waiting so long can be difficult, but it's only at the end of this period that the optimum result can be expected—try not to rush to judgment about the cosmetic appearance of a surgical wound. The benefits of surgical excision include an improved cosmetic result, compared with scraping and burning. The cure rate with this technique is in the 90 percent range for a first-time basal cell cancer. If, after the specimen has been removed and has been evaluated by a dermatopathologist, it turns out that residual cancer cells are present at the margin, meaning that it has not been completely removed, further treatment is often necessary (see "Mohs Micrographic Surgery," page 262).

SCRAPING AND BURNING

For basal cell cancers that are superficial and confined to the top layer of the skin, a simple treatment is available that has an 80 to 90 percent cure rate. Scraping and burning, also known as *electrodessication and curettage*, is a quick and easy technique for removing a skin cancer. It should be used only for superficial basal cell cancer and small nodular basal cell cancer on the arms, legs, and trunk. It will usually leave an innocuous round pale scar.

The disadvantage of this technique is that no tissue is available afterward to evaluate whether the cancer has been completely removed. If the cancer should recur, treatment using the Mohs micrographic surgery technique is the preferred approach.

In the scraping and burning procedure, after the skin cancer and the area around it is anesthetized, a sharp curette, or scoop, is used to aggressively scrape the area and a small margin around the skin cancer. (The cells of the cancer lack the microscopic hinges that connect one cell to the other. Normal skin, which possesses these connections, does not scrape away, whereas the soft and mushy skin affected by basal cell cancer will yield to the curette.) The more aggressively one curettes and burns the area, the greater the risk of an unsightly scar. So, through experience, an individual physician can identify whether a tumor requires multiple treatments or simply a single scraping and burning.

After the scraping, an electric needle is used to cauterize the base and edges of the skin cancer site. Some people believe the needle is a laser, but lasers play no major role in the management of skin cancer.

Scraping and burning is not appropriate for morpheaform basal cell carcinomas, recurrent basal cell carcinomas, or large, nodular basal cell carcinomas.

MOHS MICROGRAPHIC SURGERY

The most thorough method for treating basal cell cancer and squamous cell cancer is a technique called *Mohs micrographic surgery*. This office-based procedure, once not widely available because only a limited number of individuals had been trained to perform it, is now available at every major university center and in many communities throughout the United States, Canada, and Europe.

Named after Frederick Mohs, a general surgeon at the University of Wisconsin, the technique is based on the notion that normal pathology specimens, cut like a bread loaf, evaluate only about 3 percent of the total surface area of the margins of the cancer. By contrast, the Mohs technique allows evaluation of the complete surface area. This is important because many basal cell cancers grow with fingerlike projections or roots, and the random sampling of the specimens used by conventional pathology may not permit a thorough assessment of residual cancer. In addition, the Mohs technique requires that the dermatologist, *who must be specially trained*, not only excises the cancer from the patient but maps it out with special colored inks for purposes of orientation, and then evaluates the microscopic cancer. That one physician controls all three aspects of the process, I believe, is an important factor in the very high cure rate. Indeed, Mohs surgery has the highest cure rate of any of the methods mentioned, approaching 98 to 99 percent in most cases.

Because of the mapping technique, the complete cancer and only a minimal amount of normal tissue is removed, so Mohs micrographic surgery is a tissue-sparing method. Therefore it has the best cosmetic outcome, since there is often no need for the large plastic surgery reconstruction that would normally be done with traditional surgical excision. Often, simpler plastic reconstruction can be done at the same time that the Mohs micrographic surgery is performed. Moreover, because the cancer can often be removed in a very thin layer, the wound may, in some cases, be allowed to heal on its own, which can yield a better cosmetic result than plastic reconstruction. In cases where the cancer is large, Mohs micrographic surgery provides the assurance of the highest cure rate while permitting optimal reconstruction.

Under local anesthesia, the cancer is excised from the patient in a disk-

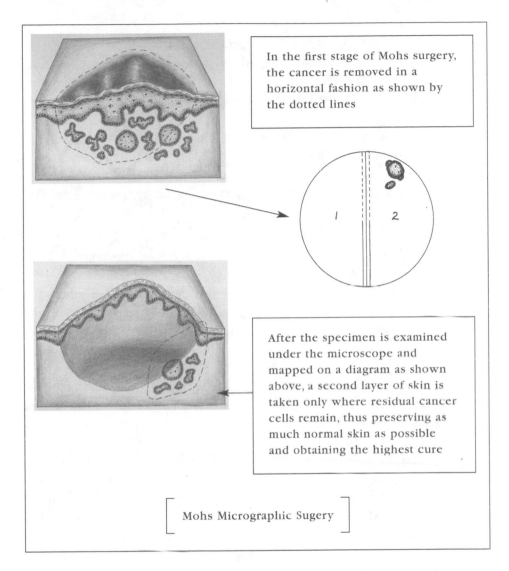

In the first stage of Mohs surgery, the cancer is removed in a horizontal fashion as shown by the dotted lines

After the specimen is examined under the microscope and mapped on a diagram as shown above, a second layer of skin is taken only where residual cancer cells remain, thus preserving as much normal skin as possible and obtaining the highest cure

Mohs Micrographic Sugery

like shape (see box above). The specimen is divided into pieces and carefully mapped with different colors. The tissue pieces are then processed and studied under the microscope in such a way that it allows the complete peripheral surface and undersurface to be viewed at once. This enables the Mohs surgeon to determine whether there is any cancer at the undersurface of the specimen as well as at the periphery, an advance that is extremely important. If residual cancer is present, an additional specimen is removed, but only at the specific site designated by the map.

Once all the cancer has been removed through Mohs surgery, if a shal-

---

SKIN CANCERS THAT CAN BENEFIT FROM MOHS MICROGRAPHIC SURGERY

Basal cell cancer or squamous cell cancer that is

- located near the eye, ears, lips, or in the central face.
- the morpheaform subtype, that is, the doctor cannot easily tell the margins of the cancer.
- greater than one centimeter.
- in a location where tissue preservation is important and the best cosmetic result is desired.
- recurrent.

---

low wound results it can be allowed to heal naturally, without additional surgery. The wound will generally heal within three to four weeks, but may remain red for some time after that. Makeup can be applied, but one should not expect the best cosmetic result to occur until nine to twelve months have passed.

More often than not, the type of skin cancer that requires Mohs micrographic surgery will, upon its removal, need reconstruction of the wound area. The majority of Mohs surgeons in this country are specially trained in plastic reconstruction of facial wounds.

If your plastic surgeon or other reconstructive surgeon does not mention Mohs surgery as an option and describes a very complex reconstructive process, stop and question whether a simpler approach might not be acceptable. It is extremely important to have open lines of communication with your physician.

Because of the high cure rate, the logic of the procedure, and the opportunity to get the best cosmetic outcome, Mohs surgery is the method of choice for any recurrent skin cancer, any large skin cancer, and certainly any facial cancer where the best cosmetic result is desired.

RADIATION

Radiation therapy is a widely used treatment for the management of many cancers, and is best used only for very specific situations when it comes to skin cancer. Technologically, radiation therapy has improved enormously in the past two decades and the latest generation of X-ray devices permit the delivery of finely tuned and specific doses. In this pain-less technique the tumor is identified and radiation is applied in a series of short daily treatments which usually span four- to six-weeks.

Radiation has some disadvantages, however. No tumor is excised, so the margins of excision cannot be identified. As a result, and to compensate, a radiation field, identified on the patient prior to treatment, may include a wide area of obviously normal skin, thus irradiating tissue unnecessarily.

In addition, if the radiation therapist is not that familiar with the particular type of cancer, such as a morpheaform basal cell cancer, and does not understand that its roots may extend beyond what is obvious, undertreatment may result, with recurrence of the cancer later on. Another disadvantage of radiation therapy is that it is delivered in small, fractional doses over a long period of time to get the best cosmetic results. For elderly patients, it is not often feasible to make the daily trips for treatment.

The principal advantage of radiation therapy is that when it is per-formed correctly on the properly selected cancer, it can yield a good cos-metic result. It should be noted that although no incision is made radiation therapy may still leave a scar. Radiation therapy is especially helpful for basal cell cancer and squamous cell cancer that is inoperable, or as an adjunct treatment after removal of a high risk cancer.

CHEMOTHERAPY

Chemotherapy has little role in the management of basal cell cancer and squamous cell cancer of the skin. However, for decades a form of top-ical chemotherapy has been used for precancers such as actinic keratoses and can be effective when used properly.

While the diagnosis of cancer is upsetting and the diagnosis of a cancer that occurs on your face may be of even greater concern than if it occurs elsewhere, it is important to remember that techniques are available that can result in the highest cure rate possible and the best cosmetic result. It is important to help your physician help you understand how the different options would best apply.

▪ A HAPPY ENDING

After extensive discussion about the various ways to treat her skin can-cer, Cheryl elected to undergo the Mohs technique. She arrived at the office for the procedure and, after the site was identified, my nurse anesthetized the cancer and the skin around it with lidocaine solution. Although that stung briefly Cheryl was amazed that she felt none of the rest of the surgery. I took the first layer of tissue, or *Mohs stage,* and after processing was able to study it under the microscope. I offered Cheryl a peek under the microscope and she was relieved to see just a small collection of cancer cells in the area that mapped out toward the eye. She returned to the procedure room, and with the area already numb, I removed a sliver of tissue smaller than the white of your nail. After studying this piece, it was clear no more cancer remained.

Cheryl was delighted that the cancer was completely removed and we turned our attention to the reconstruction. The option of skin graft, linear closure, where the edges of the wound are simply pulled together and sewn, and a skin flap in which a piece of adjacent tissue is elevated and transposed into the wound to fill it were discussed in detail. She asked about allowing the penny-sized wound to heal on its own. Because of its location I was concerned that it would pull on the corner of her eye and perhaps distort the tear duct, so we elected to perform a small skin flap. This surgery took only twenty minutes, and soon after, Cheryl, wearing a large pressure bandage, went home with her husband. When I called her at night to see how she was doing, she explained that she was a bit tired and a bit tearful but amazed that she had so little pain. I reminded her that she would probably get a black eye in a few days, but that after the stitches were removed, she would feel much better about the healing and the prospects for minimal scarring on her face.

WHEN IS MOHS MICROGRAPHIC SURGERY THE BEST ROUTE?

The high cure rates and tissue-sparing benefits of this technique are well suited to facial surgery where it is best to minimize the chance of recurrence and optimize the cosmetic result. An important benefit of Mohs surgery is that because a very thin layer of tissue is first taken, if clear of cancer cells, the shallow wound may be allowed to heal naturally and look better than if a skin graft or skin flap is placed. If plastic surgery is required, it can be performed at the time of cancer removal.

Cheryl's sutures were removed in five days and when I saw her for follow-up six weeks later, she was pleased that the scar had already begun to fade. She carried a bottle of sunscreen with SPF 15 and asked if it was the correct one to use. I told her that it was, and the hat she had taken to wearing in bright sun, with its wide brim, was likely to help as well. "I don't let the children outdoors without their sunscreen, either," she said, highlighting the strongest action step she could take to prevent skin cancer in the next generation.

COMMON SKIN PROBLEMS V

24 Common Skin Conditions

*Jimmy scratches all day. When he's under stress,
it gets worse and then the scratched skin gets
infected. I feel so bad for him. It's hard to see your
child suffer like this.*

*—Leanne, 38, mother of an 8-year-old
with severe eczema*

The bad news about common skin conditions is that they are just that—common. The good news is that the majority of problems you and your skin may face over a lifetime are treatable and can be fixed. In some cases, the skin ailment is chronic, waxing and waning in severity, so knowing how to handle it on an ongoing basis will make you a comfortable partner with your condition. In other cases, the problem is acute and once it's over, it's done with (some of these acute problems are covered in "Skin Emergencies," Appendix 3).

▪ XEROSIS

Dry skin, what doctors call *xerosis* (pronounced zir-OH-sis), is both common and annoying. It is caused in part when the skin cannot retain water. Although young

FIXING CRACKED FINGERTIPS: KRAZY WHAT?

Cracked fingertips can be a big problem for people with dry skin. When deep, painful fissures occur, try to apply Aquaphor or some other thick ointment. If this fails or objects start to slip from your grasp, I advise patients to apply a thin layer of cyanoacrylate (one brand is Krazy Glue). This forms a water-protective coating that sheds in time when your top layer of epidermal cells sloughs off naturally. Be very careful when using this glue, since it is not officially recommended for this use and can stick your fingers together. BE CAREFUL!

people can develop xerosis, as the skin ages its water-retaining abilities wane, so dry skin especially becomes a problem of older individuals. Dry skin is often exacerbated by a cold, dry climate, the use of forced-air heating, and excessive washing of the skin without appropriate moisturization.

The main complaint of people with dry skin is itching. The skin appears rough, cracked, and scaly. The natural markings of the skin become pronounced. Look at the back of your hand under a magnifying glass and you will see many fine crisscrossing lines surrounding the hair follicles. These are the so-called natural skin markings. In severe cases of xerosis, there may be horizontal superficial cracks or fissures, which have been likened to the appearance of a cracked, dry riverbed.

In all cases of xerosis, prevention is the key. Simple steps such as decreasing the frequency of washing, using gentle and non-irritating soap, and frequently applying moisturizers are recommended.

For most mild cases of xerosis treatment with bland emollients such as Eucerin cream is effective. Thicker creams and ointments are the best moisturizers to use and these should always be applied after any type of hand washing or bathing. In more severe cases of xerosis—those in which fine cracking or superficial fissuring is present—a week of topical corticosteroid may often be necessary to reverse the changes. Heavy-duty moisturizers such as Lac-Hydrin, which contains lactic acid, can be helpful—although it stings a bit at first on irritated skin.

▪ ITCHING

Itching, also known as pruritus, is perhaps the most common symptom of all skin diseases. You feel an unpleasant sensation that elicits a compelling desire to scratch. There are many potential causes of itching in the skin. Just a few of the physical stimulants that can trigger it are vibrations, chemical irritants, certain drugs, various underlying internal diseases, dry skin, aging of the skin, and various forms of eczema. Stress and other psychological factors can also play a role in itching.

Because dryness of the skin is one of the most common reasons for a person to experience itching, the initial treatment of pruritus should always include rehydration of the skin, with frequent application of an effective moisturizer. If you have tried this general treatment and the itching persists, or if there are obvious signs on the skin suggesting another problem, see your dermatologist.

Treatment of pruritus includes identifying the underlying cause and some general symptomatic relief measures. Avoid extremes in temperature at home and at work. Also avoid very hot showers and overly warm clothing. Hot environments, hot showers, and the like usually make the itching worse. Generous application of an effective moisturizer frequently throughout the day can often help. There are also several over-the-counter itch preparations that provide excellent relief; one such product is Sarna lotion, which contains menthol and phenol. In severe cases, a physician may prescribe oral antihistamines, such as Benadryl or Zyrtec, to provide additional relief. Avoid topical lotions that contain diphenhydramine, the active ingredient in Benadryl, because it may worsen the situation by causing an allergic reaction of the skin.

In rare situations, persistent unexplained itching may be a sign of serious internal disease. If you've had unremitting itching, consult your doctor.

▪ DERMATITIS

A word that simply means inflammation of the skin, dermatitis is often used synonymously with eczema. Both words are broad general terms that need to be further qualified by the type of dermatitis and its location. Regardless of the type three stages are often recognized: acute, subacute, and chronic. Each of these represents a stage in the evolution of the inflammatory process that underlies dermatitis.

Acute eczematous inflammation is an intense redness of the skin with tiny little blisters. Severe itching is often present. In the subacute stage, there may be redness, scaling, and overlying cracking or fissuring of the skin. Itching is also a common symptom at this stage, as are pain, stinging, and burning. In the chronic stage of eczematous inflammation, there is thickening of the skin with accentuation of the normal skin lines, in addition to cracking, fissuring, and evidence of scratching. Dermatologists can usually tell you've been scratching by the long scratch lines where your fingernails wandered in search of relief.

Let's take a look at the main types of dermatitis or eczema.

▪ ASTEATOTIC ECZEMA

Asteatotic eczema, which is also known as eczema craquelé or dry skin eczema, is actually a severe form of xerosis. It arises after excess drying of the skin and is most common in elderly people and during the dry winter months. The inflammation process can be seen on almost any skin surface area, but by far occurs mostly on the lower legs. In addition to rough and scaly skin, there are often thin, red raised patches with cracks (now you know where "craquelé" comes from), which can bleed. Pain rather than itching is associated with these patches. Further scratching of the skin or applying agents that further dry out the skin (for instance, calamine or alcohol-based lotions) will invariably worsen the condition.

When asteatotic eczema is mild to moderately severe, it can be treated simply with bland lubrication such as Vaseline or Aquaphor and a low-potency topical steroid ointment such as hydrocortisone ointment 1% twice daily. In its more severe form, you may need to resort to open wet

---

CHICKEN SOUP FOR YOUR SKIN

An excellent way to soothe and heal dry or otherwise irritated skin is to apply open wet dressings. Follow these instructions:

1. Soak a cotton pillowcase or handkerchief in tepid tap water.
2. Wring it out so it is still damp.
3. Apply to the affected area and leave in place for 10 to 15 minutes.
4. Apply lubricant after removing.
5. Repeat several times a day as needed.

dressings (see box, page 274), followed by the application of a moderate-strength topical steroid ointment.

Once the condition subsides, prevention is key. As with all types of xerosis, you should pay particular attention to avoiding activities and substances that excessively dry out the skin, such as frequent bathing, harsh soap, and lack of lubrication. Once the problem has been reined in, concentrate on daily lubrication of the skin with an over-the-counter thick moisturizing cream or ointment.

▪ ATOPIC DERMATITIS

Atopic dermatitis is a chronic eczematous condition that frequently flares into an acute stage. It usually begins early in life and waxes and wanes. At various stages throughout life, the disease may behave differently. Infants and very young children often have outbreaks on the face and either patchy or generalized eczema of the body. In adolescents and those adults still affected—the condition often abates in adulthood—the eczema is generally localized in a symmetric fashion in such areas as where the arms bend and the back of the knees. The hands may also be involved.

Several factors are thought to play a role in this disorder: genetic susceptibility (it often runs in families); a personal or family history of atopy, meaning the presence of hay fever, very dry skin, asthma, or eczema; alterations in the immune system; and, possibly, allergies to such airborne substances as house dust, mites, or mold.

An outbreak of atopic dermatitis usually starts with redness and severe itching. Scratching leaves the skin dry, scaly, and thickened. This scratching causes more itching, creating more scratching—this is a textbook example of the "itch-scratch cycle" made famous in television commercials. There can also be a superficial infection that results from breaking the protective barrier of the skin; this is characterized by a honey-colored crust overlying the eczematous areas. As the injured area heals, areas of lightened or darkened skin may linger, although they gradually improve with time.

Other features associated with atopic dermatitis may include keratosis pilaris (tiny rough red bumps on the upper arms), darkening of the skin around the eyes, an increased number of lines on the palms, and marked sensitivity to irritants such as wool, clothing, fabric softeners, and cold dry weather.

Several factors are known to worsen atopic dermatitis and trigger acute exacerbations. If you understand these aggravating stimuli and try to control them, you'll have a better record of keeping this disorder in check. Anything that increases dryness or aggravates the sensation of itching, stimulating the desire to scratch, can trigger an outbreak. Avoid extremes of and changes in temperature, activities that cause profound sweating, decreased humidity, excessive washing of the skin, and contact with topical irritants such as harsh soap and detergents or irritating chemicals. As with any chronic condition, stress can be an aggravating stimulus. Avoiding stressful situations is easier said than done, but if you can manage your life in a way that reduces stress, your skin will love you. Certain foods may also provoke an acute flare-up of atopic dermatitis.

When topical treatments such as moisturizers, open wet dressings, and corticosteroid creams and ointments fail, depending on how severe the problem is, oral prednisone or an injection of corticosteroid may be used to end the need to scratch and give your skin a chance to recover. Antibiotics may even be used if there is also superficial infection of the skin, such as impetigo.

Spend time trying to understand which specific factors trigger your atopic dermatitis, and try to come up with ways to avoid them or minimize their presence in your life. Adjust your environment to become more agreeable. This may include maintaining a cool stable temperature in the home, avoiding overdressing and situations of excessive sweating, humidifying the house, and minimizing airborne allergens and dust. Relaxation techniques such as meditation work well for some people.

▪ NUMMULAR DERMATITIS

Nummular dermatitis is a common and often chronic condition that usually occurs in middle-aged and older adults. Its coin-shaped red lesions are often quite itchy, starting as small marks with tiny blisters and expanding and coalescing into larger patches. There is often crusting over the center of these lesions and evidence of superficial infection. The usual locations are the back of the hand, the forearms and calves, the flanks, and the hips.

It is not clear what causes nummular dermatitis, but in most other kinds of eczema, these lesions are more common during the winter months.

As with all types of dermatitis, it's a good idea to use a gentle soap, avoid frequent washing, and keep your skin well lubricated. During an outbreak of nummular dermatitis, the acute, subacute, and chronic stages may all be present at once, so a combination of treatments may be used. Treatment options include a strong topical corticosteroid, oral antibiotics, open wet dressings, and anti-itch medications such as oral antihistamines.

CONTACT DERMATITIS: WHEN YOUR SKIN TOUCHES SOMETHING IT SHOULDN'T

Dermatitis that is caused by allergy to certain compounds is one of the most frequent skin problems. It occurs when cells in your skin react to chemicals or compounds to which they have become sensitized in the past. Through a very complex mechanism, your immune system remembers that it does not like a particular "allergen," and, in response, mounts a full-blown defense against it. Cells march to the area of contact and pour out chemicals that cause severe itching, blistering, and even breakdown of the skin. Once the itching and blistering have resolved, hyperpigmentation, or discoloration of the skin, may last for some time.

Allergic dermatitis due to poison ivy or similar plants is usually obvious. Avoiding the plant is the best defense. When you have developed a reaction to another compound, such as nickel, nail polish, perfume, or latex, but it is not clear what you are actually allergic to, patch testing by your dermatologist will help identify the culprit. In this procedure tiny amounts of dozens of chemicals are placed on your back and, a few days later, are studied for a reaction.

The best way to deal with an acute allergic contact dermatitis like poison ivy, sumac, or oak is:

1. Wash the area with soap and water.
2. Wash your clothes to remove the resin.
3. Apply a topical corticosteroid cream.
4. Use a moisturizer.
5. Take an antihistamine pill for itch.
6. Do open wet dressings (see page 274).
7. In severe cases, where swelling is uncomfortable and itching severe, your doctor may prescribe several days of an oral corticosteroid called prednisone.

▪ HAND DERMATITIS

An eczematous inflammation of the hands, which may be uncomfortable and can interfere with work, is usually caused by irritant contact dermatitis or allergic contact dermatitis. It is no surprise that people in certain occupations, such as cleaners, hairdressers, nurses, and others who wash their hands frequently or come in contact with chemicals and other irritants, are more prone to develop hand dermatitis.

The symptoms are similar to those of other dermatitis conditions. A detailed history by your dermatologist can help sort out exposure to irritants or substances that may cause an allergic contact dermatitis. You may be asked to keep a diary for a week or two in order to reveal a pattern that zeroes in on the offending agent or situation.

If an allergic contact dermatitis of the hands is indeed suspected, your physician will most likely order a series of patch tests to try to identify the causative agent. Your condition will improve if you can eliminate exposure to the chemical that is causing the reaction. However, other conditions can be mistaken for hand dermatitis, so your doctor should also check for fungal infection and psoriasis.

In severe cases of hand dermatitis, which do not respond to topical treatments such as liberal use of moisturizers and topical corticosteroid creams, ultraviolet phototherapy can sometimes be helpful. This is a treatment prescribed and monitored by dermatologists in which a light booth is used to deliver carefully controlled ultraviolet radiation to skin.

▪ DYSHIDROTIC ECZEMA

Dyshidrotic eczema is a reaction that develops on the hands and feet. The exact cause of this condition, which is characterized by tiny itchy blisters, is not known, but stress seems to play a role.

Dyshidrotic eczema seems to go through several stages, beginning first with moderate to severe itching with subsequent eruption of numerous fine blisters on the palms, the soles, and the sides of the fingers and toes. The tiny blisters slowly resolve in several weeks, followed by peeling of the palms and soles.

Treatment is similar to that for other forms of eczema. Identifying and eliminating stressful circumstances in your life may also be helpful.

▪ STASIS DERMATITIS

Stasis dermatitis occurs most often on the lower legs in patients with bad venous circulation. Venous insufficiency, another term to describe the circulation problem, simply means that the blood flow from these far reaches of your body back to the heart is impaired. Signs of venous insufficiency may include swelling of the lower legs and varicose veins. The eczematous eruption, however, does not develop in all patients with venous insufficiency, and the reason for its presence in certain individuals is not clear.

Acute inflammatory stasis dermatitis shows up as a very itchy isolated red patch on the lower leg. There often is weeping of fluid, crusting, and at times tiny blisters. In severe cases, a more generalized itchy eruption can occur on various other parts of the body. This is called an *id* reaction.

In the chronic form of stasis dermatitis, a brawny, reddish brown discoloration of the lower calves develops. As the problem gets worse, a reddish brown lesion with some bluish tint is seen on the lower inside calf. Scarring ensues and this area often becomes firm with overlying skin thickening. The skin may have a bumpy cobblestone appearance. It is at this stage that one is at risk for leg ulceration. Because the skin is often quite tight and scarred, the slightest trauma can break down the skin, resulting in ulcer formation. Such ulcers are sometimes quite hard to heal, but the use of new artificial skin is promising. Chronic stasis dermatitis is best treated with topical corticosteroids and daily compression with prescription compression stockings; the latter is critical for healing and to prevent further acute inflammatory attacks.

▪ SEBORRHEIC DERMATITIS

Seborrheic dermatitis is a common chronic condition that arises in oily areas of the head—specifically the scalp, the scalp line, the eyebrows, around the nostrils and mouth—and on the chest. Less frequently the armpits, the groin, and the buttocks are involved. The cause is not known, but a yeast called pityrosporum ovale is probably a player.

In infants and children, seborrheic dermatitis appears first as cradle cap and later as dandruff in the scalp. The typical appearance in adults is that of redness throughout the scalp and scalp line. In addition, scaling over the eyebrows, nose, beard region, and chest can be seen.

When a moderate to severe amount of fine dry white scaling—commonly known as dandruff—is seen throughout the scalp (or on your navy blue suit), some people interpret it as dry skin and cut back on washing. That's not a good idea—by decreasing the frequency of hair washing, more scale accumulates, which may cause further inflammation throughout the scalp. Treatment therefore includes more frequent hair washing (daily or every other day) with an anti-dandruff shampoo that contains selenium sulfide or zinc. Regardless of which one you choose, the shampoo should be lathered up generously throughout the scalp and left on for five minutes before rinsing off. A non-greasy topical corticosteroid solution may also be prescribed to apply throughout the scalp twice a day to combat the itching.

For treatment of the red scaly areas on the face or chest, a low-potency topical corticosteroid cream and an anti-yeast cream (Nizoral) to combat pityrosporum ovale should help.

Since seborrheic dermatitis tends to be a chronic recurring process, maintenance therapy with anti-dandruff shampoo and the other treatments mentioned may be necessary.

▪ PSORIASIS

Psoriasis is a relatively common inherited disease of the skin which is characterized by overproliferation of the skin layers. While it often bears the brunt of Madison Avenue glibness ("the heartbreak of psoriasis"), it can indeed be a difficult problem for those who have it. It affects approximately 1 to 3 percent of the population. The exact cause of psoriasis is not fully understood, but major advances in the study of this skin condition have taken place in the last several years and it is becoming clearer that inherited abnormalities in the immune function of the skin definitely play a role.

Psoriasis has favorite locations where it likes to set up house, including the scalp, elbows, knees, and buttocks. A typical patch of psoriasis can be a circle, an oval, or even an irregular shape; it is red (often brick red) with overlying thick, silvery scales. When the scale is peeled off, one can usually see tiny areas of bleeding, like pinpoints. On the buttocks, the armpits, or the groin, psoriasis often appears as a red smooth lesion without much scale. Patches of chronic psoriasis tend to remain fixed in their one position for months.

Guttate psoriasis is a common form of the condition that often erupts following a streptococcal sore throat or a viral infection of the upper respiratory tract. It is a generalized eruption of many pinpoint to 1 centimeter pink-red papules with overlying scale.

Certain types of arthritis may coincide with the skin lesions of psoriasis. Factors known to provoke or exacerbate psoriasis are trauma to the skin, infection such as strep throat, certain medications, low calcium levels, and stress. Psoriasis may also be more prevalent in the HIV-positive population (though of course having psoriasis does not mean you have AIDS).

Psoriasis is treated with topical creams, oral medication, and ultraviolet light therapy. The exact treatment depends largely on the type of psoriasis and the extent of cutaneous involvement. For limited psoriasis, your dermatologist will probably prescribe a topical therapy such as corticosteroids, a topical vitamin D compound called calcipotriene (Dovonex), tar preparations, a topical vitamin A derivative called tazarotene gel, or anthralin. Should these topical therapies not work or if the extent of the psoriasis is significant, your dermatologist may recommend an oral medication such as methotrexate, acitretin (a derivative of vitamin A), or cyclosporine (a medication that affects the immune system). Ultraviolet light therapy may be suggested in tandem with oral psoralen, a compound, which when taken by mouth and absorbed, interacts with the ultraviolet light to reduce psoriasis patches.

Various specific treatments are also available when psoriasis has broken out on your scalp, including medicated shampoos containing tar or salicylic acid, baby oil to put in your hair at night to loosen up the scale, or topical corticosteroid solutions. Psoriasis tends to be a chronic condition—although it often responds to therapy, it nevertheless frequently recurs. By rotating several of the treatments that have been outlined, your dermatologist can help you achieve the best control of this skin condition.

▪ PITYRIASIS ROSEA

Pityriasis rosea is a common skin condition that is usually seen in young adults. The exact cause of this eruption is not known. Typically, its first symptom is an isolated 1- to 3-inch, round-to-oval pink lesion with a tiny central collar of scale. This isolated first patch, called the herald patch, can arise anywhere but is most commonly seen on the chest or upper arms and legs.

Several days or weeks after the onset of the herald patch, similar but smaller lesions erupt over the entire trunk, arms, and legs, sometimes in the pattern of a Christmas tree. (Typically, pityriasis rosea does not involve the face). Most of these lesions do not cause any discomfort, but sometimes there is a mild itching sensation.

This skin disease usually runs its course over a period of four to twelve weeks. No specific treatment is necessary, but in cases with severe itching, your dermatologist may recommend a topical corticosteroid or ultraviolet therapy.

▪ Dermatosis Papulosa Nigra

Dermatosis papulosa nigra is an entirely benign condition that many black people experience. Multiple brown or black bumps, each no bigger than a peppercorn or millet seed develop most often on the face and neck. Under the microscope they look very much like seborrheic keratoses, the growths I call "barnacles of life." The easiest way to treat this condition is to gently scrape the papules off. Some physicians like to gently burn or freeze them, but I prefer a technique that simply scrapes the bumps off at the level of the epidermis—this minimizes hyperpigmentation, or worse, white spots.

▪ Common Pigmentation Problems

VITILIGO

Vitiligo is a relatively common disorder of pigment loss with great social impact. People with the condition develop white patches on their skin where the pigment-producing melanocytes have been destroyed. Because of the resemblance of vitiligo to some forms of leprosy, in certain parts of the world it is confused with the ancient infectious disease. In those situations, the social stigma historically associated with leprosy is wrongly attached to patients with vitiligo.

Vitiligo is thought to be an autoimmune disease. Somehow the body sets up a process whereby the immune system destroys the melanocytes. In fact, because of the autoimmune nature of the disease, it is sometimes seen in the skin of people with other diseases in which the immune system attacks the body's own cells, such as thyroid disease, pernicious anemia, and collagen-vascular diseases.

Vitiligo, which occurs in all populations but is more noticeable in people of color, usually starts suddenly with white patches on the skin. It develops most commonly on the hands, feet, genitalia, and face. It also appears on the cheeks, around the eyes and near the mouth. Vitiligo may occur in one spot or one segment of the skin, such as on an arm or leg, or it can be generalized, appearing over the whole body.

Vitiligo usually appears first in childhood. Itching can be an early symptom—it's probably a sign that the body's immune cells are slugging it out with the melanocytes. Because of the emotional toll this condition carries, it is especially frustrating to physicians that we cannot easily predict or control its course.

Treatment has generally been unsatisfying and consists of the use of topical corticosteroids. Since tanning in the sun can stimulate pigment production, this is one of the few areas where dermatologists, under carefully regulated circumstances, make use of ultraviolet radiation combined with an agent called psoralen. Melanocytes can repopulate the vitiligo patch from pigment cells that survive in the hair follicles and from the adjacent normal skin.

Many people, frustrated by their condition, have tried tattooing, surgical treatments, and cosmetic covers. Because none of these approaches is predictably successful, some people with vitiligo seek the help that comes from attending support groups. When there is a 50 percent or greater pigment loss over the whole body, depigmentation may be recommended in order to make the skin a uniform color. This is an irreversible step: if the person doesn't like the result, there will be no means of changing back to the original pigmentation. A topical medicine called monobenzone is used daily modifying the treatment frequency as the pigment fades.

Surgical solutions to vitiligo have been tried and consist of grafting normally pigmented skin into the depigmented area. Punch grafts of normal skin have been used but result in a confettilike appearance of pigmentation. Recently, I published a technique that I invented for the treatment of vitiligo that has proved simple, quick, easy to perform in the doctor's office, and does not appear to result in the irregular pigmentation. I call it the Flip-Top Pigment Procedure and an example of the results are shown in the "Color Atlas of Your Skin."

HYPERPIGMENTATION AND HYPOPIGMENTATION

In people of color, the effects of trauma to the skin may become more obvious than in more lightly pigmented individuals. Common causes of post-inflammatory hyperpigmentation are acne, lacerations, eczema, and even a special type of reaction to medication called *fixed drug eruption*. It can develop in response to ampicillin, tetracycline, sulfa, or other medications. In this case a circular patch of jet black discoloration can develop in dark-skinned people and persist for months, getting worse with each subsequent exposure to the medication. It is harmless, but until the cause is known, and then avoided, it will not resolve.

After skin injury, whether from an abrasion, rash, or other disruption of the skin surface, post-inflammatory hyperpigmentation can develop. When the trauma occurs in the epidermis, there is an increase in the transfer of melanin molecules to the surrounding epidermal cells. When the dermis is also injured, pigment-containing scavenger cells, or melanophages, set up house in the dermis for a long time, resulting in discoloration of the skin that can last for years.

There is no perfect treatment for post-inflammatory hyperpigmentation. It will get better with time so patience is essential, but topical corticosteroid cream can help in some cases. Minimizing sun exposure is also important. In my experience, laser treatment does not work, and may in fact worsen the situation.

Hypopigmentation can occur for the same reasons as hyperpigmentation and similarly requires patience and time for improvement. Because hypopigmentation just represents a decrease, rather than complete absence of pigmentation, recovery can be expected as the pigment cells from adjacent areas step up to the bat.

In order to determine the nature of your skin pigment problem your dermatologist will likely examine you under a Wood's light—a black light that helps determine the extent and depth of pigmentary change.

▪ DID MEDICINE CAUSE MY RASH?

Three out of every thousand prescriptions in this country result in some sort of allergic reaction. Although all medications come with an extremely long list of potential side effects, it is important to identify a true allergic reaction to medication, because taking the same medication again can result in further problems. Similarly, if you do not actually have an allergy to a medication but merely couldn't tolerate it in the doses given, you need to keep that in mind should you need that medication in the future.

It is helpful to distinguish between the latter situation and a true allergy to a drug. Fewer than 10 percent of adverse drug reactions are due to a true allergy to the medication. In an allergy the body's immune system responds to a foreign chemical, typically a protein, and such reaction will happen every time the person takes the drug.

The most common types of drug reactions, however, are not allergies, but intolerances. For instance, if erythromycin is taken on an empty stomach, it might cause nausea or vomiting. That is not an allergy, however, it is an adverse reaction to the drug. Likewise, many women who take antibiotics find that they result in a yeast infection. This is also not an allergy, but an adverse event due to a change in the bacteria that normally grow in your gastrointestinal tract.

When a drug causes a reaction on the skin, it often will involve wide areas of the skin. There will also be a correlation between when the drug was taken and when the rash started.

About half of all drug reactions on the skin are called exanthems. An exanthem is the splotchy type of flat red rash with clear areas. It may cover most of the trunk, legs, and even face, but does not usually involve the palms and soles. This kind of rash will typically begin within ten days of starting a new medication, and some people develop a fever as well. The most common drugs causing this type of reaction are antibiotics: ampicillin, amoxicillin, trimethoprim/sulfamethoxazole (Septra, Bactrim, Co-Trimoxazole). The rash will typically go away on its own within one to two weeks of stopping the medication. Scaling and peeling may follow after the red rash fades.

Hives are also common, constituting about one-fourth of all drug reactions. When you get hives from drugs, it usually happens within thirty-six hours after starting the medication. An individual spot of hives will last fewer than twenty-four hours. Again antibiotics are the most common culprits, and 1 in 50 people taking amoxicillin and 1 in 100 people taking either ampicillin or cefaclor will end up with hives. Upon discontinuing these medications, the eruptions should cease within one to two weeks, if not much sooner.

The sun can also cause a number of drug-related reactions. When a medicine is absorbed by your body, it is distributed throughout the various tissues, including the skin. When the skin is exposed to ultraviolet light from the sun or even a tanning booth, certain itchy types of rashes can occur in uncovered areas. Drugs that commonly cause these type of eruptions include sulfa drugs (including some water pills and diabetes pills), nonsteroidal anti-inflammatory drugs (such as piroxicam), members of the tetracycline family, and griseofulvin, a common antifungal medication. Drug rashes occur in children, and, like those in adults, usually resolve promptly. Very rarely more serious rashes develop in children and adults in response to medication and require medical attention.

If you develop a drug rash while taking more than one medication, it may be necessary to use the process of elimination to determine which medication is causing the rash. This should be done only in close consultation with the doctor prescribing the medications. The watchword is to be patient, but your dermatologist, internist, or family doctor will likely be able to get to the bottom of your drug rash.

▪ BIRTHMARKS

Birthmarks, which doctors call hemangiomas, are benign tumors of blood vessels that appear on the newborn or soon after birth. Some birthmarks disappear on their own during childhood. The term birthmark is also used for other skin lesions present at birth, but I have found that most people mean hemangioma when they use the term. Before we take a look at some of the most common types of birthmarks and treatment options, let's clear up some myths about their cause.

Birthmarks don't have anything to do with what Mom ate during pregnancy, bad thoughts she might have had, or problems with delivery. These growths sometimes seem to be stimulated by estrogens, which is why many resolve over time following birth, as the estrogen levels in the child change or as those estrogen receptors present on the birthmark itself change.

STRAWBERRY HEMANGIOMAS

A common type of birthmark, the strawberry hemangioma, occurs in children, developing shortly after birth. A strawberry hemangioma typically starts as a small red bump and grows rapidly over two to three months. Then its growth stops and a process called involution, when a hemangioma shrinks in size, begins. In most cases it leaves little evidence that it was ever there.

Strawberry hemangiomas are red or purple on the surface and are raised above the surface of the skin. Sometimes the mass or lump under the skin can be sizable. If it is near the neck or mouth it can interfere with head movement and eating; near the eye, it can interfere with eyesight and thus affect the infant's proper development of vision; near the nose, breathing can be affected. Any hemangioma near the mouth, in the mouth, or near the nose is of special concern. Though it is rare, this can herald the development of a similar growth in the throat so any child suspected of having this problem should be evaluated by a pediatric ear, nose, and throat specialist.

Parents are obviously concerned about the appearance of these lesions on their children, which can make management of strawberry hemangiomas a bit controversial. On the one hand, a conservative approach is called for. We know that the majority of hemangiomas of this sort go away on their own. Ten percent go away by age one and 90 percent will have vanished by age ten.

But what about those that don't go away or resolve too slowly? Most parents and doctors would like the hemangioma to be gone by age four or five, the time when the child is about to start school and make new friends.

Many doctors are resistant to excising, or completely removing, these growths, whether with traditional or laser surgery, because they can be large and the resulting permanent scar may cause more cosmetic problem than the original birthmark. In addition, incomplete excision of the hemangioma can result in recurrence within scar tissue, which can become more problematic. Most important, a hemangioma should not be excised during the rapid growth phase.

If the hemangioma is in a vital location, treatment with corticosteroids—by mouth for a defined period such as a month or two, or even by direct injection by a skilled physician—can slow or even reverse growth. In rare cases where life is at risk, interferon, a naturally occurring chemical that affects the immune system, can be used as well.

Whether to excise or not is a decision that should be made in consultation with experts who treat hemangiomas as a routine part of their practice. Dermatologists, plastic surgeons, and ear, nose, and throat surgeons may all have expertise in this area and should consult closely with the child's pediatrician. My advice is to be conservative when feasible; when function is compromised, as when the birthmark is close to the eyes, nose, or mouth, of course be aggressive. When the situation falls in between, consider excision if the plastic surgeon believes the resulting permanent scar will be superior to that which would result from natural resolution.

EROSIONS

A common problem that does occur with hemangiomas is that during the involution phase the surface skin may break down, causing a depressed area or erosion. This can be painful for the child. Proper wound care can help speed healing and eliminate the pain. Follow your doctor's instructions carefully; this will probably involve using an antibiotic cream such as Bactroban and keeping the area covered with a nonstick dressing such as Telfa. In more advanced cases, a special dressing called Vigilon, which is a soothing gelatinlike material, can help a great deal (keep it refrigerated between uses so it will have a cooling effect as well). Never use alcohol or peroxide, which sting terribly and are not helpful; instead, tap water and gentle soap will do the trick. A topical anesthetic cream such as ELA-Max may help control some of the pain that the child feels.

PORT WINE STAINS

Port wine stains, another common birthmark, are flat red or purple discolorations of the skin that is visible at birth. Some port wine stains can be associated with a condition called Sturge-Weber syndrome; your pediatrician will know whether this possibility should be further investigated, depending on the size and location.

When lasers first became available to treat these tumors, there was much excitement about their potential to remove the entire hemangioma. We now know that there are birthmarks of this type that can get 50 to 80 percent improvement, but complete eradication with current technology is not always possible.

Each treatment course must be tailored to the child. For example, with a very young child, parents must discuss the use of general anesthesia with the dermatologist and pediatrician. Although this approach does allow the dermatologist to be more complete in treating the birthmark than office treatments done with topical anesthetic, there are minimal risks associated with anesthetizing a young child that must be taken into consideration. New lasers that cool the skin make it much easier to treat large areas on children in the office setting.

By the time a person reaches adulthood, port wine stains have often evolved from the original pink or red childhood mark to a purplish birthmark. When lasers were first introduced, we thought that only pale birthmarks responded to the treatment but, happily, this has not proven to be true. Medical insurance does not normally cover treatment for such birthmarks because it is considered cosmetic.

Whatever approach you take with laser, remember that it is a gentle, prolonged approach that slowly eliminates the growth under the surface of the skin (see chapter 13).

STORK BITES

Stork bites on the back of the neck are a form of port wine stain that do not resolve on their own but are not an issue for most people. You don't see them every day and hair covers them. Similar lesions over the eyes, so-called angel's kiss, tend to resolve on their own.

FUNGUS OR CANCER:
THE STORY OF LYMPHOMA OF THE SKIN

A group of skin rashes that look something like early psoriasis or mild eczema may actually be precursors to outright lymphoma, a form of cancer of the white blood cells. This serious condition is important to know about because it may occur in areas that are not sun-exposed, and may be mistaken for eczema or psoriasis. It can also develop as early as the teen years. In general if such a rash does not go away with topical corticosteroid medication, it should be biopsied by your dermatologist.

The disease can pass through several stages, including a flat or patch stage, a stage with large, raised scaly areas, and a tumor stage in which nodules are present on the skin. In a small number of people, the rashes progress to involve the bloodstream and the lymph nodes.

The key player in what is called *cutaneous T-cell lymphoma* (CTCL) is the T-cell type of white blood cell (the same type of cell that becomes infected with HIV). When these special T-cells in the skin start growing out of control, they can cause several different types of skin lesions.

In its earliest stages, CTCL can be treated with topical therapies including super-potent steroids or topical nitrogen mustard. Photochemotherapy, or the use of an oral photosensitizing drug along with ultraviolet A light (PUVA), is also a helpful therapy for such patients.

Dr. Richard Edelson, chairman of dermatology at Yale since 1985, pioneered the use of a clever therapy called *photopheresis.* In this treatment, the patients ingest the same photosensitizing drug that would be used in PUVA. The patients then have their blood filtered, as though on dialysis, and about 10 percent of their white blood cells are removed. These white blood cells are then exposed to the same ultraviolet A light that is used in PUVA therapy for psoriasis. Finally, these cells are then injected back into the patients. In some patients, this therapy can result in improvement of the more severe forms of the disease.

An indication of how quickly science progresses is the fact that even this procedure, relatively new by conventional standards, is giving way to more specific ways of manipulating the abnormal T-cells that are at the root of the condition.

Jack, a busy salesman, came to see me because he had developed an enlarging circle of redness and tenderness on his hand. He didn't recall injuring the area but was concerned that it was not going away. When I examined him, I found the classic picture of an infection: redness, warmth, a raised surface and pain. I did a culture and then started him on antibiotics right away. When I got the results of the culture the next day, I found out that the antibiotic I had prescribed was active against the bacteria and he got better within a couple days.

Skin infections come in all shapes, sizes, and locations. Many are trivial and will get better without any special attention. A tiny few can be lethal. Most fall in between these two extremes.

Infections capture our imagination in some special way because they are one area of medicine where cause and effect is clear and never in doubt. For example, shingles is caused by the herpes zoster virus, impetigo is caused by the staph bacterium, and yeast infection is caused by the candida species. In short, infections are diseases that result from the presence of germs.

Few things in medicine are so clear-cut. Kill the bug, get better.

Not so long ago, infections were a challenge to treat. The Scottish scientist Sir Alexander Fleming noted in 1928 that a blue mold growing in his laboratory released a compound that inhibited the growth of bacteria colonies. His famous discovery about the antibiotic effects of penicillium mold changed the course of the world forever: no more would so many people die from infections like pneumonia; no longer would injured soldiers perish from battlefield infection; no longer would new mothers be at risk for death from infection.

When Fleming discovered penicillin, the greatest revolution in the history of modern medicine began: we had identified the enemy for a century—with small microbes of all shapes and sizes darting frenetically on the microscope slide. Now we finally had a weapon to subjugate them.

Combating infection is a major part of any dermatologist's practice. Dermatologists are in fact infectious disease specialists of the skin. The skin is our major barrier to the outside world, and that world is teeming with forms of life we can't see or feel. Early on, much of the field of dermatology actually included the study and treatment of syphilis and related venereal diseases. In the 1980s, dermatologists played a key role in identifying and describing the dreadful new disease that shattered the immune system of young gay men and others, leading in many cases to the growth of the purplish skin tumors of Kaposi's sarcoma.

When a dermatologist talks about a skin infection, he or she is referring to any skin problem where germs of one sort or another have set up shop and are disrupting the normal state of affairs. Skin infections can be caused by viruses, the smallest of germs (so small that they really just consist of a patch of DNA), bacteria (included among the top ten are staph and strep), and even larger germs called fungi. Because the skin is our first defense against the outside world, it is subject to infection on a daily basis and must therefore have built-in defenses against those life-forms we would rather not share our body with.

Some of us seem to suffer from every imaginable skin infection; others bounce through life unscathed. While we may not have a choice as to which microscopic demons we encounter in our daily rounds, the more knowledge we have about that lump, bump, rash, or blister, the more effectively we will be able to send it packing.

In general, infections are equal-opportunity destroyers: they don't differentiate between rich and poor, the famous and the unknown, women and men, blacks, Native Americans, Caucasians, and other races. There is a correlation between risk and poor living conditions and lifestyle, but in general, germs seem to follow the policy of catch as catch can. And most are pretty good at it.

Infections have been with us since recorded time began. Ancient people were most familiar with those that showed on the skin. If you have a moment, pick up your family Bible and turn to the Book of Leviticus 14:1–32. The lengths to which the ancient Hebrews went to shun those with leprosy is sadly evocative of our own early response to AIDS.

Despite the valiant efforts of early physicians and scientists, the understanding of disease, derived largely from what could be observed, was limited. But that did not prevent infectious disease, rampant in the form of epidemics, from playing a role in history second only to war when it came to shaping our destiny.

Bubonic plague, a condition with obvious skin symptoms, helped shape the course of European history as no other influence had in its time. Caused by a bacterium spread by rats or fleas, it manifested with lumps—enlarged lymph nodes, really—beneath the skin. These lumps were called buboes. In the middle of the fourteenth century, the plague killed a third of the European population at a time when the total world population was a fraction of what it is today. The plague wrought tidal changes in politics, wealth, power, and control.

Lest you think the bubonic plague is gone forever, be aware that a smattering of cases continue to be reported to the Centers for Disease Control (CDC) in Atlanta. This federal agency is charged with monitoring all reportable and communicable (infectious) diseases that could represent a public health threat. Whether it is in identifying a new disease by noting geographic clustering and common dermatologic findings (as with Lyme disease) or being alert to unusual infections in a population that shouldn't be getting rashes and fevers (in the early days of HIV), the CDC staff, assisted by researchers at universities and state health boards, plays a critical role in protecting us against both known infections and those that have yet to rear their ugly, threatening head. New strains of germs burst on the scene with an unsettling regularity: the two just cited and Legionella pneumonia (also known as Legionnaire's disease) are three examples.

If Darwin was right, we can expect the development of new infections to continue as long as there are hosts for the germs to thrive on. Here you will read about common skin infections— whether they are serious or not, how to identify them, and what to do about them. Of course, there are many more infectious conditions of the skin than those listed here, so consider these the hit parade.

▪ BACTERIAL INFECTIONS

*So Satan smote Job with sore boils from the sole of his foot even
into his crown. And he took him a potsherd to scrape himself
therewith as he sat among the ashes.*

—*Book of Job, 2:7–8*

Bacterial infections were popular tools of punishment in the Bible.
Throughout time, the amazing diversity of bacteria has made a special
impact on skin.

Bacteria are self-sufficient single-cell organisms. Unlike amoeba, they
aren't very mobile, so they must eat and do everything else where they sit.
Small enough that millions could dance on the head of a pin, most are far from angelic. However, it is true that our skin is host to a wide range of good germs, which actually help our skin to stay healthy on a regular basis. Some live deep

> ### SELF-SHIELD PROTECTION
>
> The skin plays an active role in killing surface
> bacteria. Amazingly, about 20 percent of people
> carry some skin bacteria that produce antibi-
> otics that can inhibit other germs. In general,
> though, infection occurs when unfriendly bac-
> teria gain a foothold in your body.

down in hair follicles, others live on the scalp or in sweat glands, causing
characteristic body odor.

Perhaps the first cruel fact of life is that although we are born sterile,
as we pass through the birth canal we are immediately baptized with bacteria. Within the first twenty-four hours of birth, there will be more than
6,000 bacteria *per square centimeter* in our tiny armpits alone. As Grandma and Grandpa and Aunt Felicity pass us around, they colonize us with
those bacteria that will help keep our skin in balance over our lifetime.

Good bacteria are just that: good. It is the evil bacteria that most concern us here. There are various types of these tiny organisms and they
cause many forms of bacterial infections. Unlike viral infections, bacterial
infections are often responsive to treatment with a course of antibiotics.
On rare occasions, the bug, somewhat smarter than we are, outmaneuvers
us and develops resistance to antibiotics. But more about this later.

▪ IMPETIGO

Impetigo (pronounced im-pe-TIE-go) is a highly contagious infection that is limited to the skin. It occurs most often on exposed areas of the skin, including the arms and legs, face, and scalp. It may also occur at the site of injury, such as an insect bite or cut. It occurs spontaneously, most often in children. When it develops in adults, it's almost always a complication related to a more serious skin condition, such as severe eczema.

Impetigo starts with minuscule blisters. Imagine a cluster of translucent bubbles, each no larger than a pencil point. In fact, all you really can do is imagine them, because it is unlikely you will ever see them. By the time impetigo is a big enough problem to be noticed, the blisters have ruptured and the localized infection begins to color the skin. Thus what you'll probably see first are crusty, honey-colored scabs. The area may itch or burn. A halo of redness may surround the area as well, the result of the increased blood flow the body is bringing there in an attempt to contain the infection and fight it with its own defense mechanisms, such as activated white blood cells.

TREATMENT

If a child has impetigo, he or she should be encouraged not to scratch the blisters or scabs because these lesions are filled with bacteria. All the admonitions in the world notwithstanding, people and pets will scratch. Since some scratching is almost inevitable and impetigo can spread rapidly, you should contact your child's pediatrician. The doctor will probably prescribe a ten-day course of treatment with an antibiotic such as erythromycin or dicloxacillin, or treatment with a topical antibiotic ointment, such as Bactroban.

In the meantime you can begin washing the skin with an antibacterial soap, such as Lever 2000, a few times a day and restrict any sharing of towels, washcloths, or clothing. Don't wash excessively.

PREVENTION

While there is no sure way to prevent impetigo from recurring, regular hand washing at home, school, and/or day care can minimize the chances of transmission. If your child has had a case of impetigo before, an antibacterial soap should be used. Don't get obsessive about hand washing, though.

Excessive washing can deplete the skin of important oils, which are part of its natural protection against infection. (Lady Macbeth probably had very clean hands but exceptionally dry skin.)

▪ CELLULITIS

Cellulitis (pronounced sell-u-LIE-tis) is a highly visible infection of the skin that is generally more serious than impetigo. The bacteria cause inflammation of the loose connective tissue of the skin, so what you see is an enlarging patch, or plaque, of red, hot, tender skin. From the time it is diagnosed its progress can be monitored—that is, response to treatment can be measured by marking the advancing red edge of the infection with a black pen and determining how far it has moved in a 24-hour period. If treatment is successful the red area will begin to shrink, not expand.

Cellulitis is usually preceded by some sort of injury—naturally occurring, such as an ulcer, or an accidental puncture or cut. People with diabetes or who are immune-suppressed are at special risk for getting cellulitis.

Cellulitis is usually caused by the streptococcus bacteria, also called strep. It occurs mostly on the legs, although any part of the body can be affected. Unlike other bacterial skin infections, you might actually get a fever, feel fatigued, get chills, and develop enlarged lymph nodes. Erysipelas

---

HOW DOES MY DOCTOR KNOW
WHAT INFECTION I HAVE?

The most important principle in medical practice is: make the correct diagnosis. When it comes to infections this is done by doing a skin culture of the affected site. A sterile swab is passed over the area and put into a tube with "culture or transport medium"—a solution intended to keep the germs alive. Once in the laboratory, the swab is plated on petri dishes that contain different nutrients. After a period of time, the bacteria grow and form identifiable colonies. By testing which compounds destroy the colonies or limit their growth, sensitivity to particular antibiotics can be determined as well. In many cases, though, it may not be possible to do a culture and antibiotics are started based on what the doctor believes is the true germ at fault.

is an extreme form of strep cellulitis that usually occurs on the face and is potentially fatal. Diabetics are prone to infection with strep as well as pseudomonas, a bacterium that produces a characteristic green color.

If cellulitis is suspected, see a doctor at once. The site should be cultured if possible and antibiotics begun immediately pending final test results. Depending on your general health and the nature of the cellulitis, intravenous antibiotics may be required.

▪ BOILS

Boils are most notable historically because they were one of the ten plagues visited upon Pharaoh (in the Book of Exodus) in order to motivate the ancient Egyptians to liberate their enslaved workers. Then, as now, boils, or inflammatory infections of the hair follicle unit, were considered a major pain, especially if they occurred on the thick skin of the neck, in which case they were considered a pain in the neck.

WHAT IT IS

A boil starts in a hair follicle. Also know as a furuncle, a boil is a bacterial skin abscess and begins as a small, firm nodule. An abscess is a small (or even large) pocket of pus. Many people today don't realize that this material is actually a good thing—the ancients were so enamored of this sign of battle against infection that they called it "laudable pus."

In the case of a boil, the nodule becomes inflamed, red, and warm and increases in size. It sits in the dermis and as it enlarges it emerges like a red dome over the surface of the skin. Boils at this stage feel tense. Some of us might even describe the appearance of an inflamed boil as "angry." They can be especially tender, probably due to the stretching of skin nerve fibers by the expanding growth.

Not much has changed since the time of Hippocrates. Boils are classic examples of infection. Before microscopes and stethoscopes, doctors relied on obvious signs of infection, which were *rubor* (redness), *tumor* (mass), *calor* (warmth), and *dolor* (pain). The inflammation and expansion of the boil, typical of any internal or external infection, are a result of the effort of the body to fight, seal off, or otherwise contain infection. Thus the contents of the boil actually are an immunologic stew. The pus consists of white blood cells, fibrin, proteins, and other materials the body produces or eliminates in the course of fighting infection. In any infection that produces pus, a way must be found for it to escape. Warm compresses sometimes help, but it is not unusual to require simple draining.

Boils may appear anywhere on the body where there is hair, which means practically everywhere. However, they are most common on the buttocks, under the arms, on the back, and on the scalp.

A carbuncle is a boil that sits deeper in the skin. It can be extremely painful. Although anyone can develop boils or carbuncles, some people are more prone to get them. When a person has multiple boils or recurrent boils, the condition is referred to as furunculosis. People with AIDS and other immune-deficiency diseases are at special risk for boils, as are people with long-term or poorly controlled diabetes.

WHAT IT LOOKS LIKE

Boils vary in size. They are swollen and red, and usually shaped a bit like a cone. It's not a stretch to think of a boil as a small volcano, given the heat it sometimes generates. Boils are hot and tender to the touch. As the infection progresses, the boil may become extremely painful as it changes into a more deeply seated carbuncle. When a boil nears the point of rupturing a yellowish white "point" appears in the center of the abscess.

WARM COMPRESSES THE MODERN WAY

Warm compresses are helpful in many skin problems. Try this method.

1. Soak a washcloth in tap water and wring it out.
2. Place in a plastic sandwich bag but don't seal it.
3. Place in your microwave for fifteen to thirty seconds.
4. *Make sure the pack is not too hot.*
5. Apply the washcloth in the bag to affected area for five minutes at a time.
6. Repeat process, paying close attention to make sure pack is not too hot.
7. *Caution*: If you are diabetic or have circulatory problems, consult your doctor before using warm compresses.

RESISTANCE TO ANTIBIOTICS

Antibiotics should always be used cautiously. There is much legitimate concern about their excessive use leading to antibiotic resistance of bacteria. However, in a particular situation the risk of ongoing infection must be balanced against the risk of antibiotic resistance. By varying antibiotics among different types and not staying on one particular agent for too long, risk of resistance can be minimized and a chronic problem with furunculosis or any other skin infection can be controlled.

TREATMENT

Don't pick, pop, or scratch a boil—you'll only cause yourself more pain and discomfort. Warm compresses applied several times daily can help speed the natural process of the lesion rupturing and the subsequent healing. All you need do is soak a washcloth in warm water, wring it out, and apply it to the boil until it cools. Alternatively, see the method described on page 297.

If the boil persists for more than ten days, if it is particularly painful, or if redness develops around the area, call your doctor. He or she will want to examine it and may decide to use a small scalpel to lance the hard, swollen lump in order to aid drainage and healing. An antibiotic, either oral or topical, may also be prescribed. If you suffer from furunculosis, a daily prophylactic dose of an antibiotic for a period of a few months under the supervision of your doctor will be helpful.

PREVENTION

Whether you get boils and carbuncles or not is largely a function of your genetic makeup (what isn't?). Occasionally, circumstances arise where you can take some preventive steps. If you have diabetes, tight control—that means keeping blood glucose levels within the normal range, with as little day-to-day variation as possible—will help control outbreaks of boils.

Be tuned in to your body. At the first sign a boil is developing, treat it with compresses and/or antibiotic ointment to try to prevent its further growth into a deeper carbuncle.

▪ VIRAL INFECTIONS

Viruses are infectious particles many times smaller than bacteria. If millions of bacteria could dance on the head of a pin, millions of viruses could party on the back of a bacterium. New viruses continue to pop up, causing disease and havoc throughout the world. But they serve a useful purpose as well.

In the annals of medicine, a very special viral skin infection played a most important role. Everything we do today to immunize our children against infectious diseases is based on the ingenious and courageous observation two hundred years ago made by an English country doctor, Edward Jenner. His ability to observe was probably Jenner's greatest genius. Most important, he could, as we would say today, think out of the box.

It was Jenner's attention to the countryfolk of Gloucestershire that led to his special experiments. He observed that dairymaids often contracted cowpox, a disease of cattle; this seemed to confer protection against getting smallpox, a common cause of death in eighteenth-century England. Jenner reasoned that perhaps he could protect humans against lethal smallpox by inoculating them with the much less dangerous cowpox. Although he had no idea that a virus caused the problem or that the two diseases were caused by members of the same viral family, he assumed they were somehow related based on the dermatologic similarity of the conditions.

In 1796, Jenner inoculated an eight-year-old boy named James Phipps with some material taken from the pustule of Sarah Nelmes, an infected dairymaid. Although the boy developed a fever, he recovered without incident. Almost two months later, Jenner inoculated the boy with smallpox material, which failed to take. By 1799, over 5,000 people were vaccinated and the vaccine's value was so widely recognized that Napoleon had his whole army inoculated against the smallpox virus.

Immunization against viral infections, begun with the pioneering work of Jenner, has limited our risk of infection greatly. Several dermatologic infections, however, are caused by viruses for which immunization is not yet possible because of the plethora of subtypes. Venereal warts, common warts, and herpes simplex are just some examples.

▪ COLD SORES

Cold sores are one of the most irritating, painful, and common of all skin infections. Even though they are rarely serious, they can cause tremendous irritation both physically and emotionally. At one point little could be done for cold sores, but the advent of antiviral therapy has made it possible for people who develop them frequently (say several times a year) to use prophylactic treatment (as I shall describe below).

WHAT IT IS

Cold sores are caused by the herpes simplex virus, also known as herpes simplex type I. This is a cousin to herpes simplex type II, which is the cause of genital herpes. Once contracted, herpes virus type I stays in your skin. It lies dormant in the nerve root cells, but can cause recurrences of fever blisters intermittently throughout your lifetime. Recurrences may be triggered by stress, sunburn, menstruation, excessive fatigue, or another infection, such as a cold. Trauma from facial surgery is a special risk. If you have a history of this problem and will be having facial surgery (even something as trivial as a biopsy) you should advise your doctor.

Cold sores are highly contagious and are spread most easily by kissing. So, alas, while recuperating from your fever blisters you should refrain from kissing others and having any other direct bodily contact that involves the infected area. As mentioned, the herpes virus type that affects the mouth is different than the type that causes genital herpes infections.

WHAT IT LOOKS LIKE

Cold sores usually appear on or around the lips. They may also appear on the cheeks, chin, or nose, but rarely on other parts of the body. The good news is that certain symptoms foretell the onset of a cold sore; this gives

SKIN IS AN IMMUNE ORGAN

Cold sores frequently break out after exposure to sunlight. Research over several decades has shown that the skin acts as an immunologic organ. It is thought that ultraviolet radiation from the sun destroys or alters important immunologic cells in your skin, thus permitting a reactivation of cold sores.

If you get outbreaks after sun exposure, try wearing a good sunscreen and use prescription antiviral medication.

you a fighting chance of controlling it. Because the virus lives in the nerves, burning, stinging, itching, or some other sensation will usually be felt before the rash breaks out. Antiviral medication should be used at the first sign of a symptom (it is of less benefit once the blisters have developed).

The common cold sore consists of a cluster of tiny blisters. The cluster itself is generally small, ranging from about the size of a pencil eraser to a penny. Since fever blisters generally appear on the face, they are easily identified. Unfortunately, they are also noticed by others, which causes a certain degree of embarrassment. Not only do they do nothing to enhance our appearance, but others may confuse the cold sores with the herpes II virus, which causes genital herpes.

TREATMENT

Cold sores are treated with an antiviral medication (generally Denavir, Famvir, or Valtrex), which slows down the replication of the virus at the site of infection. Denavir can be applied topically when cold sore symptoms are first experienced and has been shown to reduce healing time. Valtrex and Famvir must be taken by mouth. Currently there is no medication that can completely eradicate the herpes simplex virus from the body.

At home, you may apply ice to the affected area to relieve the itching and burning. You may also want to apply an over-the-counter antibiotic ointment during the healing process to avoid further bacterial outbreaks on top of the viral infection. Eroded skin is more prone to bacterial infection. When the blisters become crusty, apply a warm, moist cloth to the area to soften the scabs and avoid bleeding. And, of course, *do not pick*. Bad outbreaks can result in scarring, but with proper care this usually does not happen.

PREVENTION

You can't easily prevent cold sores, but there are measures you can take to limit their recurrence. If you know your cold sore outbreaks are stress related, try to reduce the stress in your life. (Easier said than done.) If they are related to exposure to the sun, wear a hat whenever you go out in the sun and use the highest SPF sunscreen you can find. You might even want to use flesh-colored zinc oxide on the affected lip area.

The antiviral medications mentioned above can speed the healing of your fever blisters. Since the average cold sore sufferer has only two to three outbreaks per year, taking oral medication all year as a preventative may be excessive. Alternatively, if you begin to take the medication, topical or otherwise, at the first sign of an outbreak, you'll at least decrease healing time and perhaps the severity.

Some old soldiers in the cold sore wars insist that taking folic acid regularly minimizes the frequency of cold sores. In addition, those all too familiar with this viral nuisance swear by L-lysine, a dietary supplement. It must be noted that there are no clinical studies that have verified the efficacy of these preventive measures, though many cold sore sufferers swear by them. Better to swear by science and use a medication we know affects the activity of the virus.

▪ SHINGLES

Shingles are also called herpes zoster. Both shingles and chicken pox are caused by the varicella-zoster virus, and anyone who's had chicken pox may develop shingles. The most important thing to know about shingles is that the real difficulty can begin after the rash has healed. Postherpetic neuralgia, a special type of pain that persists after the infection and rash are gone, can cause untold misery. Thankfully, some new medications are beginning to show promise in controlling this bad side effect.

WHAT IT IS

Once you've had the chicken pox, the varicella-zoster virus will lie dormant in a nerve root in the spine, poised to flare at some unknowable and unpredictable time in the future.

A case of shingles is accompanied by an obvious red rash that contains small blisters that may rupture. The first sign that a case of shingles is on the way involves a painful burning sensation that seems to wrap around one area of the body, generally an arm or a leg or one side of the face or body.

Because the virus lives in the nerve root, its distribution is along the lines of the nerves that supply a particular distribution of your skin.

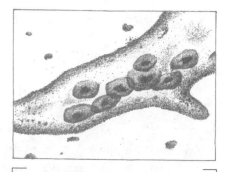

A diagnosis of herpes is made from cells scraped from the blister and examined under the microscope.

SHINGLES AND PAIN

One elderly patient came to see me after he had a protracted course of shingles over his forehead and eye area. His pain was unbearable. We tried a whole range of medications and finally referred him to our pain management clinic. It is hard to know for sure, but if he had been put on antiviral medication right away, perhaps with a steroid as additional therapy, his degree of pain would have been less.

There is one nerve root on each side of the body and it supplies branches of nerves that circle the body to the midpoint. For this reason the rash will stop sharply on the midline. In fact, the word *zoster* means girdle, reflecting the way the rash distributes itself.

Multiple blisters appear within the reddened area. These blisters may range in size from a quarter to the size of your palm. Shingles around the eye occurs more frequently in the elderly and can be very painful. The pain can be a continuous burning or shooting spasms.

TREATMENT

Early diagnosis will ensure the most successful treatment of shingles. This means starting therapy within forty-eight to seventy-two hours of the first tingling sensations and the appearance of the red rash. As soon as you have the first inkling of a case of shingles, call your doctor. He or she will prescribe an antiviral medication (such as Valtrex or Famvir) to prevent progression of the eruption and decrease the postherpetic pain syndrome. To be effective, the drug must be started within seventy-two hours of the onset of the shingles symptoms. Some believe that the use of steroids, taken orally in the form of prednisone or injected into the site of pain, will mitigate postherpetic neuralgia.

PREVENTION

Until recently there was no way to prevent shingles, but the new varicella vaccine available to prevent chicken pox may also help protect you from getting a case. Unfortunately, for those of us who have already had chicken pox, this is not of much benefit—but be sure that your children

---

POSTHERPETIC NEURALGIA

Early aggressive treatment of shingles can reduce the chances of pain afterward, especially important in patients over sixty who are at special risk for this complication.

- Start antiviral medication within seventy-two hours of getting the rash. This reduces the risk of pain by up to 50 percent.
- Use corticosteroids—they will decrease the acute pain even though they probably won't decrease the chronic pain afterward.
- In some older patients, amitriptyline (Elavil) used for three months, as soon as shingles starts, can reduce the persistent pain. Similar drugs are helpful if you can't tolerate Elavil.
- Neurontin (gabapentin) with or without Elavil can help with the pain as well.
- Topical anesthetics such as lidocaine cream (ELA-Max) can be applied to the painful area and might decrease discomfort.

---

and grandchildren get immunized. Pediatricians consider the vaccine safe and effective.

▪ WARTS

As old as witches and toads, warts are among the most common skin infections in the world. They are caused by one of seventy-five different types of the human papilloma virus, or HPV. Each of these versions of HPV causes a different kind of wart, depending on where on the body it occurs.

HPV is medically important because several forms of the virus that cause warts can lead to cancer. Chief among these are the genital HPV types, which can cause cervical cancer. Nonetheless, rest assured that the majority of warts that we encounter in daily life are mundane and noncancerous.

Warts can be unsightly, and if they appear on the soles, as plantar warts, they may also be painful. However unsightly, warts are rarely a serious condition. Though not dangerous, warts can and often do recur despite treatment. Eventually, though, most warts resolve on their own.

WHAT IT IS

Medically speaking, a wart is a verruca. A verruca is not a famous fashion model or a great, exotic new dance, but a benign skin lesion that is raised and rough to the touch. They generally appear on the hands and feet. The wart virus is contagious and can be spread by direct or indirect contact (the latter means that yes, you can catch HPV at the gym or in the shower). The virus is transmitted more easily if you have a cut or a scratch on the skin. The types that occur most frequently are *common warts* (obviously) and *plantar* (foot) *warts*. Common warts occur most frequently on the hands. When they develop in and around the nails, they are

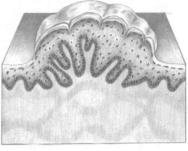

Common wart

extremely difficult to treat and may, if present for many years, evolve into squamous cell cancer (see chapter 23). While warts mainly plague children and young adults, they can occur at any age. They are very common and problematic in kidney and heart transplant patients, because these individuals are immune-suppressed.

Because a wart is in fact a tumor (an abnormal growth of excess cells), it requires an extra supply of nutrients. These nutrients are brought to the growing wart by blood vessels that the wart itself generates. If you examine a wart closely you can see small, clotted blood vessels on the surface.

KIDS AND WARTS

Warts can be a problem for children. They tend to be unsightly and often occur on their hands, where they are especially noticeable. Even though most warts will resolve completely on their own—once the body's immune system finally recognizes that the virus is an unwanted visitor—dealing with unsightly growths remains a concern. Try a cautious and conservative approach; use topical over-the-counter remedies first. If these don't work, some prescription remedies may help. Finally, if those don't work, freezing or burning the wart off can be effective.

THE PROFESSOR AND THE COUNTRY GIRL

Some time ago, early in my practice, I was vacationing in the wonderful town of Amalfi on the Italian coast. The manager of my hotel discovered I was a dermatologist and asked if I would be willing to see a patient (the closest dermatologist was in Naples, many miles away). I agreed and was ushered into a dimly lit hotel ballroom. There, lined up against a back wall were eight elderly ladies, all dressed in black, and a beautiful girl of seven or eight. I was introduced in a long flowery speech in Italian, as if I were the surgeon general of the United States. Be that as it may, the little girl showed me her hands on which she had multiple clusters of common warts. I studied her carefully, intent on not missing anything (I didn't have malpractice insurance to practice in Italy, let alone a license). Finally, I completed my exam and announced to the concerned relatives that this was not cancer and that it would all go away on its own. They were delighted to hear this but were clearly skeptical. I finished my vacation, happy to have been of help.

About four months later, I received a call at my office in New Haven. The hotel manager had come to America on business and sought me out. He told me that about two weeks after I left the girl's warts all disappeared. I apparently had won the relatives' confidence. Who knows what they believe now about the American doctor who cured the little girl just by talking to her!

Their appearance, as little black dots, almost certainly confirms that the growth is a wart and not some other lesion.

When a plantar wart "blossoms" on a weight-bearing part of your foot—the heel or ball of the foot—it will flatten as you walk on it and can become very painful. A plantar wart can be confused with a corn, except that corns do not have those telltale pinpoints that identify it as an HPV infection.

WHAT IT LOOKS LIKE

Warts are rough, hard bumps. They are usually pea-sized or smaller, though a wart the size of a dime is not uncommon. They may be white, pinkish, or tan in color, depending partly on the pigmentation of your skin.

WARNING!

If you have a wart that occurs around the fingernail (a periungual wart) and *it has been present for more than ten years*, it should be biopsied. It could be squamous cell cancer. The cancer is confined to the top layer of the skin and has no risk of traveling in the body, but it *is* cancer and should be treated. The best method of treatment is Mohs surgery (see chapter 23).

Often, warts can cluster to give the appearance of a much larger area of affected skin.

TREATMENT

Warts may be treated at home with an over-the-counter patch or liquid that contains salicylic acid. But keep in mind that warts do not necessarily have to be treated—unless, of course, they are causing pain and discomfort. Common warts are neither cancerous nor precancerous. And given enough time, a wart will likely "miraculously" disappear over time and without any treatment (usually within one to two years). Thus, if you are a patient person, you may do best simply to watch and wait.

If patience is not your greatest asset, your doctor can remove a common wart by freezing it with liquid nitrogen. This is an office procedure that requires no anesthetic and little recovery time. Expect the site to hurt while the procedure is being done and to throb a bit after. Although people rarely need any painkillers, when treating the fingertips Tylenol may be helpful.

Other means of removing a common wart include laser vaporization and the surgical procedure curettage and electrodessication (scraping and burning). In both cases there can be permanent scarring, so one must consider that risk when treating a condition known to disappear on its own.

It should be emphasized that none of these procedures can guarantee that a wart will not recur in the same spot months—even years—after removal. This happens because the wart virus lives in the apparently normal skin as much as one-third of an inch away from the wart itself.

Treatment options for plantar warts are the same, as are the chances of recurrence.

MY FAVORITE TREATMENT

Because I like to eschew aggressive treatments for conditions that usually vanish of their own accord, I've adapted a technique that has been used by dermatologists for a long time. For years we have advocated taping warts to make them go away. Unfortunately many people use porous cloth tape or duct tape. I have found that if you apply waterproof plastic tape and keep it in place over the wart twenty-four hours a day for two weeks, you can see a 50 percent decrease in the size of the wart. Since the area is waterproofed, this treatment will not hamper a child's activity. It will have the added benefit of concealing the unsightly warts, which the child is likely to be self-conscious about.

The process can be repeated for another two-week period, until the wart, which is swollen from moisture, simply undergoes cellular death and disappears. Since the tape is likely to fall off during the two-week period, simply replace it.

PREVENTION

There is no way yet to prevent warts; indeed, most of us who have ever had a wart have no idea when or where we contracted it. To minimize the chance of getting warts, however, you can try to avoid "wart friendly" environments, such as the gym, though sticking with your exercise plan is definitely worth the risk of a wart or two.

▪ GENITAL WARTS

Here is one key fact you should know about genital warts. In a study of 97 people who had intercourse with partners known to have genital warts, 64 percent developed such lesions themselves within nine months.

Genital warts are contagious. Perianal warts can accompany genital warts through local spread. Genital warts in children are sometimes an indication of sexual abuse and should be carefully investigated—however, bear in mind that warts of the nongenital subtype can occur in genital areas in children through diaper changing and other normal handling by individuals with common warts.

CATCHING WARTS

- *Plantar warts* can be caught in a swimming pool or on the floor of the shower room (water-softened skin is more susceptible to wart virus infection).
- *Common warts* may spread around fingers through nail biting; shaving may spread warts over beard area.
- *Genital warts* are most common at sites of highest friction.

Genital warts should not be viewed with the same laissez-faire attitude as other warts. They can be associated with other genital infections, so a thorough examination and follow-up is required. Regular Pap smears and gynecologic exams are essential for women documented to have human papilloma virus (HPV) since it is a risk factor for cervical cancer.

WHAT IT IS

Genital warts are one of the most common sexually transmitted infections. One estimate suggests that about 30 percent of sexually active adults have the virus. Genital warts are transmitted by skin contact with an infected person, usually during sexual activity. Once transmitted, the virus multiplies in the skin cells, forming small bumps on the labia, vagina, penis, or in the anal region. Because these bumps are usually painless and flesh-colored they often go unnoticed. In addition to increasing the risk of cervical cancer, in rare cases HPV can increase the risk for penile or anal/rectal cancers.

TREATMENT

Although genital warts can be identified fairly accurately by their appearance, your doctor may perform a biopsy in order to be certain of the diagnosis. Sometimes, if the extent of the warts is not obvious because they are subtle and fade into the surrounding skin, a test called aceto-whitening can be done. By soaking the area in a weak solution of vinegar for a few minutes, subtle warts can be identified.

Because of the risks presented by genital warts, they should be treated. Topical therapies include a compound called Aldara (imiquimod) and

TO LASER OR NOT?

When skin lasers became popular more than a decade ago, there were claims that this new method would be ideal for treating warts. Along with many other doctors, I treated thousands of lesions believing that this new technique would minimize scarring and be more comfortable for patients. Our experience did not bear this out. The carbon dioxide laser that we used causes a burn. Wound care was critical and some discomfort was inevitable. Patients did get scars and warts recurred. The reason for this is that warts are caused by a virus that is detectable more than 1 centimeter away from the obvious growth. For this reason, we treat what we can see but we don't kid ourselves into thinking that the virus—and thus the risk for new growths—has been eliminated. To laser or not? Ask your doctor for the least painful, most effective option he or she has.

Condylox (podophyllin), which is painted on the warts by the patient. Scraping and burning or freezing are also options, and laser treatment may be helpful in resistant cases.

In situations where all these approaches fail, or where the warts are too widespread, there is evidence that interferon injection can help. Interferon, a compound manufactured naturally by the body, is now used as an immune modifier. The side effects of interferon include a mild flulike syndrome, but it can be controlled by taking Tylenol prior to injection.

PREVENTION

Although condoms are by no means fail-safe, they can help prevent the spread of genital warts. Since condoms do not cover all areas that may be affected by genital warts, if you have an outbreak of HPV, the best thing to do is to tell your partner and abstain from sex during the course of treatment. In addition, all women with genital warts and all women whose partners have genital warts must be monitored closely by their gynecologists with routine Pap smears to make sure there is no evidence of cervical cancer.

▪ FUNGAL INFECTIONS

Fungal infections are no picnic, particularly because they love to feast on the top layers of your skin. These infections can be very uncomfortable and in many cases keep coming back like a bad penny. The good news is that they are rarely dangerous and often can be treated at home, without even a visit to the doctor.

A picnic is a good metaphor to understand superficial fungal infections of the skin. Fungal skin infections can be broken down into three different groups based on what they eat: proteins, carbohydrates, or lipids (fats). The group of fungus infections that go by the name *tinea* are germs that eat keratin, the protein that makes up nails, hair, and the dead top layer of skin. Yeast infections caused by candida occur in moist areas, especially in people with high blood sugar (people with diabetes or those on oral steroids such as prednisone), because yeast eats glucose, our natural blood sugar (a carbohydrate). Another type of superficial yeast infection known as *pityriasis versicolor* (formally known as tinea versicolor) completes the fungal menu by subsisting on fats from our sebaceous (oil) glands. This infection is usually first seen in the teenage years, when the oil glands that accompany the hair follicles blossom.

▪ ATHLETE'S FOOT

Athlete's foot is officially called *tinea pedis*. *Tinea* is derived from a Latin term referring to insect larva (as though hearing about pus wasn't enough for you!). Old concepts seep into the language of skin and remain long after science should have eliminated them. In this case, these infections were once thought to be spread by insects.

Athlete's foot is a fungal infection that can be either very bothersome or hardly annoying at all. It occurs between the toes or on the soles where you might see a scaly, pink rash. If the toenails get infected, they can become thick, yellow, and brittle. Occasionally, if the space between the toes gets worse, a bacterial infection can also result.

WHAT IT IS

The athlete's foot fungus is often acquired in public showers (though you can contract it in a private shower), since it likes to grow in warm, moist environments. As athletes tend to use communal showers, they have a special predilection for contracting it. In one study comparing the kind of shower use to the rate of infection, 9 percent of day school students, 22 percent of boarding school students (who share showers), and 90 percent of miners (who share industrial showers) had tinea pedis.

Believe it or not, athlete's foot has a favorite set of toes—it occurs most frequently between the fourth and fifth toes. This happens because these toes tend to press closely against each other, providing a location of maximum moisture and warmth. Athlete's foot may, however, cover the sides or the soles of the feet.

Athlete's foot occurs most often in young men (again, it's not being an athlete that is the risk factor; it's the use of communal showers or pools, as well as sweating and wearing shoes that don't "breathe"). About 80 percent of men in industrialized nations will develop athlete's foot at some point. In some respects, tinea pedis is a penalty for wearing shoes. In cultures in which sandals or no shoes are worn, tinea pedis is rare.

WHAT IT LOOKS LIKE

Many first-timers, unfamiliar with athlete's foot, initially mistake the fungus for dry and flaky skin. Flaky skin between any of your toes or on the sides or soles should in fact make you suspicious that the fungus may be lurking and warrants at least a call to your doctor. Scaling and cracking of the skin in these areas are definite signs of athlete's foot. In more extensive cases even small blisters might form.

TREATMENT

A number of over-the-counter products are effective. These include creams, sprays, and powders that contain the antifungal ingredients clotrimazole, miconazole, and more recently terbinafine, which is arguably the most effective topical antifungal cream available with or without a prescription. When you use one of these products, you should use it daily, continuing for at least a week after the condition has disappeared in order to avoid the chance of recurrence.

If the condition does not clear up with the use of an over-the-counter treatment over a two- to four-week period, you should make an appointment to have your doctor examine your feet to check for other skin conditions, such as psoriasis, eczema, or an allergic reaction. Additionally, if a case of athlete's foot has been treated incorrectly or not treated at all, it may become complicated by a secondary bacterial infection; this may required the addition of an antibiotic. For fungal nail infection, known as onychomycosis, there is now oral medication that is proven effective but it requires a prescription.

PREVENTION

There is no way to ensure 100 percent protection against athlete's foot. It's an infection, and people do get infections. Nevertheless, there are plenty of precautions you can take.

Because athlete's foot is so highly contagious, your first line of prevention is to wear sandals when you shower or use a pool in a public place. Also, never share a towel with anyone.

In addition, dry your feet carefully after every shower or swim, and change your socks if they are wet. Depending on how prone you are to the infection and/or how obsessive you are about unsightly skin infections, you may also want to wash your feet thoroughly with an antibacterial soap once or twice daily. (Remember to dry them carefully.)

▪ RINGWORM

Ringworm is officially referred to as *tinea corporis* (tinea of the body), *tinea cruris* (tinea of groin), and *tinea capitis* (tinea of the scalp). Though commonly referred to as ringworm, you'll be glad to know worms play no part in this fungal infection.

WHAT IT IS

Ringworm is a contagious fungal infection that may appear anywhere on the body, though it is most often seen on the arms, legs, back, and chest. The fungus that causes ringworm is usually transmitted by human contact or by contact with animals, especially young cats and dogs. Ringworm patches spread to about two to three inches in diameter and may appear in clusters on one part of the body. This fungal infection occurs most often in children.

WHAT IT LOOKS LIKE

The ringworm fungal infection got its common name because it appears as a ring-shaped lesion. The lesions have a slightly elevated border. When they appear on the scalp, they infect the hairs and produce redness, flaking, and often hair loss. And anywhere they appear—they *itch*.

What makes self-diagnosis of this infection difficult is that the fungus may easily be confused with eczema, psoriasis, or other common skin problems.

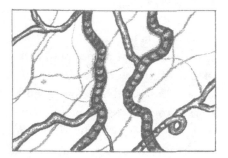

TREATMENT

Unless ringworm appears on the scalp, it can easily be treated with over-the-counter antifungal medications, just like athlete's foot and other minor fungal infections. However, just as self-diagnosis is difficult, so self-treatment may easily fail. If

A scraping of fungal rash as seen under the microscope confirms the diagnosis.

the lesions and redness on your skin persist, see your doctor for a professional look. Your dermatologist will probably take a scraping of the fungus to confirm the diagnosis. Correct medication can then be prescribed.

PREVENTION

It's hard to prevent ringworm because there are so many ways it may be transmitted. Sharing combs, brushes, or towels, standing on a bath mat after an infected person has done so, and wearing someone else's hat or gloves are all ways the fungus that causes ringworm can be transmitted. The fact that children share everything, from hats to napping mats, is a major reason ringworm is so common among the younger set. You can do your best to keep individual wardrobes and personal possessions separate, clean, and disinfected, but into many a family's life some ringworm does enter.

▪ JOCK ITCH

Jock itch is also called *tinea cruris* (ringworm of the groin), and anyone who has had it knows how it got its nonscientific name. It itches (and burns) and can be a painfully unpleasant experience.

WHAT IT IS

Jock itch is a common fungal infection occurring in the groin area. Although it is more prevalent in men, a small number of women suffer from it. As with almost all fungal infections, this one loves the excessive heat and moisture trapped in the groin area by tight underwear or athletic gear, where the fungi multiply very quickly. For this reason, jock itch occurs mostly in warmer weather.

WHAT IT LOOKS LIKE

Jock itch appears as a scaly rash in the groin region and sometimes on the inner thighs. It rarely affects the scrotum. Because it itches, burns, and is uncomfortable, this fungal infection is fairly easy to identify.

TREATMENT

Over-the-counter antifungal creams and powders usually eliminate jock itch within two weeks. If such self-treatment isn't effective, call your doctor. As with other fungi, jock itch can be confused with more serious skin conditions, and a skin scraping may be necessary to confirm the diagnosis.

PREVENTION

Easy ways to prevent jock itch include wearing loose underwear and outer clothing in warm weather, changing underwear often in warm weather, changing athletic clothing immediately after exercising, washing towels frequently, and not sharing towels.

Check your feet to see whether you have athlete's foot or toenail fungus—these are common sources for recurrent jock itch infections. If you think you have tinea on your feet or nails, put your socks on first, in order to prevent picking up unwanted hitchhikers as you put on your underwear.

You may also want to wash your groin area with an antibacterial soap (such as Phisohex) during the warm weather. Dry the area carefully after washing.

▪ PARONYCHIA

Paronychia, a painful infection around the fingernails, can be caused by yeast or bacteria. In this common condition there is an acute swelling of the tissues around the nail, mainly just before the nail fold. The swelling, which can be tender and painful, is caused by separation of the nail plate from the tissue underneath it and from the infection. Usually nail separation is due to trauma and infection is facilitated by excess moisturizing of the fingers from constant exposure to water.

Paronychia occurs most often in bartenders, waitresses, nurses, and others who wet their hands frequently in the course of work. The moist grooves of the nail become invaded by bacteria and yeast.

In the case of yeast the most common cause is *candida albicans,* whereas staphylococcus and streptococcus are the bacterial causes. If there is a green tinge to the area it is likely that *pseudomonas aeruginosa,* yet another bacterium, is the culprit.

The best treatment for bacterial paronychia is incision and drainage when the condition is acute, followed by antibiotics. Keeping the fingertips dry is essential.

▪ PERLECHE

Perleche (pronounced purr-LESH) is a yeast infection that occurs in the corners of the mouth. Most often it occurs where the folds of the mouth get deeper with aging—saliva and moisture pool in the area during sleep. Candida albicans, a common yeast that can cause vaginal infections as well as yeast infections around the fingernails, sets up house in that environment because it likes it.

People who have little fissures or cracks in the corners of their mouth can get perleche as well. (A common cause of the fissuring may be ill-fitting dentures.) Children who lick their lips, drool, or suck their thumbs may also develop perleche.

A standard treatment is a topical anti-yeast cream such as ketoconazole. If the person has diabetes, the condition may persist until the diabetes is brought under control. An alternative solution might be to try to improve the fissuring in the corners of the mouth by adjusting dentures or even by surgically tightening the skin in the area or by injecting Zyplast collagen to fill out the area.

In resistant cases, where bacteria may be growing as well, a combination of anti-yeast and antibacterial cream may be effective.

▪ PARASITES

Although many bacteria that live on our skin are friendly and helpful, the same cannot be said for larger microbes known as parasites. Just the term *parasite* can send shivers down the spine—at this moment you might even feel like throwing this book down and running to the shower. Take a deep breath. This book is parasite-free. Reading about these tiny trouble-makers will only help should they come knocking some day. The distinguishing thing about parasites, microbial and otherwise, is that they are "takers" rather than "givers." Like an ungrateful relative, they live off you without returning anything of benefit. To extend the analogy, they do so in a very irritating way.

▪ LICE

Mention lice to any parent of young children and you'll get responses that vary in intensity from moans and groans, through expressions of horror, to cries of "Stay away from me and my child." Lice do not discriminate. They show up in public schools, homeless shelters, and the most proper and pristine boarding schools (well, maybe not so pristine after all!). Only a privileged few of us who have raised children have managed to avoid at least one or two bouts with head lice.

WHAT IT IS

Lice are parasites that thrive on the blood of their hosts. (If you're feeling queasy, think of them as tenacious mosquitoes, and this discussion may become easier.) They are tiny—so small that finding them is like locating the proverbial needle in a haystack. Lice are wingless insects, black mites that look as if they might fly but never will. That's why they stick to your body, whether your scalp, eyebrows and eyelashes, or groin.

This is not the worst of it, though. Lice eggs, or nits (guess where the word *nitpicker* came from), are equally horrible culprits and more subversive. They are smaller than the head of a pin and can be mistaken, even by an experienced observer, for ordinary dandruff. Nits are the terrorists of the parasite set and they're what may keep a lice problem chronic. If someone in your family has lice, you must search for nits assiduously and treat your whole house and your car as a potential nit-infested area.

TREATMENT

Treatment of head lice must eradicate both the lice and their nits. Permethrin Crème Rinse or lindane (Kwell) shampoo must be massaged into the scalp for four or five minutes, rinsed out, and dried. Any remaining nits must be individually removed with special combs and tweezers. The wash should be repeated in one week. (Keep in mind that pregnant women should not use lindane.)

Combs and brushes should be washed or replaced. Family members should be treated. Sometimes a sulfa antibiotic may be used because it kills the bacteria in the guts of the adult lice, and without these bacteria, the lice die.

Pubic lice can be treated with lindane or permethrin cream, lotion, or shampoo. The area should be retreated after ten days. Sexual partners should be simultaneously treated, regardless. If these lice are on the eyelashes, petroleum jelly should be applied thickly each morning and evening for eight days. After this, remove remaining nits mechanically. Clothing should be machine-washed and dried.

Body lice, also known as vagabond's disease, is the most easily treated. That's because body lice do not live on the skin, but in the seams of clothing. Simply laundering the clothing and taking a bath usually solves this problem.

PREVENTION

If someone in your family or one of your friends has head lice, don't share combs and brushes, and use a shampoo treatment yourself.

▪ MITES AND SCABIES

Mites do not make right. Worse, they can cause a painful infestation called scabies.

WHAT IT IS

Scabies, from the Latin verb that means "to scratch," is an infestation caused by a microscopic mite. The female mite (*Sarcoptes scabiei*) burrows into the skin and causes an allergic response. Once firmly embedded, the mite happily lays its eggs, enjoying the warmth you provide.

Once those eggs have been laid, it takes about a week to ten days before the allergic response to the mites occurs. This is when severe itching usually begins. The rash scabies causes often progresses from tiny red bumps to larger and scattered lesions that are scaly and crusty.

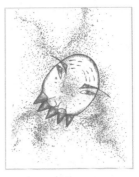

Scabies mite

WHAT IT LOOKS LIKE

The first sign of scabies is usually a bunch of small scaly bumps that are often ignored. When the itching starts, there can be no ignoring these bumps. Once scratched, the bumps scale, crust over, and often turn red.

Burrows also indicate scabies; they occur most frequently in the web spaces between the fingers, on the inner wrists, on the penis, scrotum, nipples, and on the ankles. Burrows are very thin raised lines, less than one-quarter inch in length, with a telltale black dot at one end. To confirm that you have scabies, your dermatologist will typically look for burrows and place a drop of mineral oil at the end of it. He or she will then lightly scrape the surrounding skin onto a glass microscope slide, which will be examined for the mite or its telltale signs.

TREATMENT

Scabies should be treated immediately, and you ought to enlist your doctor's help. Prescription drugs such as lindane lotion (Kwell) or permethrin cream (Elimite) work well against scabies. Every member of your household should use the prescription to avoid passing the infestation back and forth. Apply the medication at night from the neck down (include the head when treating children). Then wash it off in the shower the next morning. Ivermectin, an oral medication, is available for less difficult cases.

PREVENTION

No matter how good your hygiene, if you come in contact with a person who already has scabies or touch their clothing, towels, or washcloths, you can contract the infestation. Scabies are a problem in group homes and nursing homes, so in these settings be alert to the possibility if you walk into a common room and notice everyone is scratching.

▪ TICK BITES

Many types of ticks bite humans, but it is the deer tick we fear the most. The deer tick has achieved celebrity status because it is the carrier of Lyme disease—an easy disease to contract and a hard disease to cure. Another dangerous disease that can be carried by another type of tick is Rocky Mountain spotted fever.

WHAT IT IS

Ticks live in the woods, in the grass, on bushes, and on animals. Although the bite of a tick may seem innocuous, some ticks are more dangerous to humans than others. You might not even feel the bite, but ticks may carry toxins, viruses, or bacteria that cause infection and illness.

WHAT IT LOOKS LIKE

Lyme disease: The deer tick causes Lyme disease, which got its name from a town in Connecticut where the disease was first described by Yale infectious disease experts in the 1970s. You may assume that anywhere deer are or have been, there may be deer ticks. The rash associated with Lyme disease is bright, red and resembles a bull's eye—the central area is clear with a dot in the middle and a circle of red surrounds it. However, Lyme disease is not always associated with a rash, and even when a rash occurs, it doesn't have to be this classic one.

Rocky Mountain spotted fever: Once you have been bitten by a tick carrying Rocky Mountain spotted fever, you will notice a rash that starts on the soles and palms that consists of small, purple or red spots. It will then spread to other parts of your body.

TREATMENT

If a rash resembling those described above begins to develop, it is imperative that you see a doctor. If you suspect that the rash you have may be the result of a bite from a tick infected with Rocky Mountain spotted fever, and you can't reach your doctor, go to an emergency room. Immediate attention may save your life. If dealt with promptly with a seven- to ten-day course of antibiotics, Rocky Mountain spotted fever is not dangerous.

If your case is particularly severe, intravenous administration of antibiotics may be necessary. Rocky Mountain spotted fever is particularly dangerous for the elderly.

Lyme disease exposure may also come to your attention because after some time outdoors you notice a tick clinging tightly to your skin. At first glance, it might look like a tiny mole. In the Northeast, it is not unusual for people to come to their doctor's office with the culprit neatly wrapped in tissue paper for purposes of identification. One tick that is often offered up is the wood tick, a relatively benign creature but a parasite nonetheless.

If your doctor confirms a diagnosis of Lyme disease, you will be treated with a course of antibiotics (usually ten days), such as doxycycline, amoxicillin, tetracycline, or cefuroxime (Ceftin). If the disease is discovered in its later stages, you may have to take antibiotics for a prolonged period.

One of the alarming aspects of Lyme disease is that it can cause so many different symptoms, including neurologic changes, cardiac malfunction, arthritis, and fatigue. There are blood tests available to confirm whether you have Lyme disease, but no test is foolproof and interpretation is dependent on the expertise of your doctor.

The advent of a Lyme disease vaccine promises hope of preventing Lyme disease in those people especially at risk. However, multiple inoculations are required, the protection is not permanent, and the benefit is not fully known at this time. Like so many advances in medicine, this innovation is sure to be refined and improved over time.

PREVENTION

Whenever you are in a wooded or grassy area, wear long pants, long sleeves, shoes, and high socks so that no areas of skin are exposed. When gardening, always wear gloves. This is especially important if you live in an area known to harbor the deer tick.

THE RIGHT WAY TO REMOVE A TICK

Although Mom or Dad may have told you to remove a tick by lighting a match behind it, this will only aggravate the problem because the tick will respond by burrowing into the skin more deeply. The tick secretes a substance that hardens to form a super-glue hold between its mouth and your skin.

The best way to remove a tick is to take a pair of tweezers, grab the tick as close to the skin as possible, and pull back. If ticks are removed within twenty-four hours of contact, it is very unlikely that you will get Lyme disease, even if the tick was a carrier.

▪ SEXUALLY TRANSMITTED DISEASES

The number of cases of sexually transmitted diseases (STD) or infections is increasing at an alarming rate all over the world. In the United States alone, there are 20 million new cases of STDs diagnosed every year. Almost every sexually transmitted infection is accompanied by symptoms that affect your skin—this is one more very important reason to value your skin as the source of important clues to the status of your overall health.

Persistent itching or burning sensation in the genital area should send you to your doctor. Itching in the pelvic area is often a symptom, in women, of *candida albicans* infection. This yeast infection is usually associated with oral antibiotic use, poorly managed diabetes, and pregnancy. While *candida vaginitis* is less frequently sexually transmitted, it still can be; however it is transmitted, it needs to be treated. Men can also get candida infection of the penis, so-called *candida balanitis*, and transmit it during intercourse.

Itching may be caused by pubic lice (or crabs) and scabies. As discussed earlier in this chapter, both infections may be transmitted through infested towels, washcloths, bedding, or shared clothing, but they may also be sexually transmitted.

Painful urination is often the first symptom of a sexually transmitted infection in men, but women suffering from an STD may also experience painful urination. While this symptom may be associated with a bladder infection from another cause, it can be caused by STDs such as gonorrhea or chlamydia. The pain is caused when the infection enters the urethra, the tube that leads from the bladder.

Both gonorrhea and chlamydia (the fastest growing sexually transmitted infection in the United States) are treated with antibiotics and cause no permanent damage if attended to promptly. If neglected, however, either disease may affect fertility. If untreated, chlamydia may lead to other complications, such as pelvic inflammatory disease (PID).

Genital sores are frequently a symptom of an STD. Genital sores are most commonly a symptom of genital herpes, syphilis, or chancroid (a highly infectious disease caused by a spore-producing bacterium.)

SYPHILIS

The one general statement that can be said about syphilis, once in the purview of dermatology, is that it is decreasing in incidence. The reason syphilis had long been the focus of dermatology is that in its different stages it shows classic skin signs. Some of the skin sores that patients with syphilis get are infectious to touch. For this reason, doctors must know what syphilis looks like on the skin or in the genital area and take appropriate precautions.

GENITAL HERPES

Genital herpes is caused by the herpes simplex II virus. After initial contraction of the infection, the virus resides in the skin and can be reactivated. The classic sore is preceded by a tingling or pain in many cases. While the herpes infection is active it is contagious and sexual contact should be strictly avoided. Antiviral medications such as Famvir and Valtrex are available to decrease the healing time. In people prone to many outbreaks of genital herpes, preventive doses of this type of medication may be prescribed.

BITES, STINGS, AND OTHER NASTY THINGS, OR HOW TO DEAL WITH BITES WHEN YOU CAN'T BITE BACK

CREATURES WITH WINGS

Most stings from flying bugs hurt for a while and become a memory, having conditioned us to stay away from the hive or nest, which is exactly what the aversive conditioning of the bug was intended to achieve. However, I wouldn't be including this section in this book if bee, wasp, and hornet stings weren't also potentially deadly. In fact, more than half the deaths caused by bites from venomous animals are attributable to bee and wasp stings.

All the venomous stinging insects are from the Hymenoptera order. The specific insects are honeybees, hornets, fire ants, paper wasps, and yellow jackets. Any sting from one of these insects is venomous, but only the honeybee leaves its venomous stinger behind. A honeybee stinger should be removed immediately. Avoid using a tweezers when removing the stinger, because this may cause more venom to be released. Instead, use a flat edge of a credit card or table knife and, pressing it against the skin, swipe it across the sting area. This method minimizes the chances that more venom will be released.

After a sting or multiple stings, the victim may experience an immediate or delayed reaction. In all cases, after someone has been stung, you should monitor the person's breathing closely. (Allergic reactions to stings often include swelling, followed by blockage of the airways.)

Local reactions to stings include itching, swelling, and reddening of the area, as well as pain. These reactions usually subside in a few hours—unless the person experiences an allergic, or anaphylactic, reaction. Anaphylactic reactions usually occur within the first half hour after a sting has occurred. The sooner such a reaction occurs, the more severe it will be. An anaphylactic reaction involves internal swelling and breathing problems and is caused by a hypersensitivity to an antigen—in this case, venom. In such cases, call 911 immediately. While waiting for help to arrive, remove all restrictive clothing and jewelry, monitor the person's breathing and circulation, and be prepared to administer cardiopulmonary resuscitation (CPR). A severely allergic person should carry an emergency medical kit. The kit should include a syringe, a tourniquet, epinephrine (EpiPen), and an oral antihistamine. Family members of a severely allergic person should be skilled in CPR.

If the reaction to a sting is only local, the area should be washed with soap and water. Additionally, all restrictive clothing and jewelry should be removed. A baking soda paste, made with baking soda and water, may relieve the itching, or you may want to use an over-the-counter ointment or cream containing hydrocortisone. An ice pack can also relieve pain. Should a sting occur in the mouth, sucking on an ice cube or a drink of cold water will help to relieve pain and swelling. Even in a nonallergic person, a sting in the mouth or throat or on the tongue may cause enough swelling to block the airways. Thus, you should monitor the breathing of any person who has been stung there.

OCEAN CREATURES

Marine animal stings can be very dangerous, both because there are many lethally venomous marine animals and the chances of drowning increase dramatically due to disabling cramps and shock from the venom.

The most common marine animal stings are jellyfish stings. These stings range in seriousness, depending on the type of jellyfish. The venom from a poisonous jellyfish retains its potency even after the tentacles that carry it have been severed and after the jellyfish is dead.

Probably the most infamous of the venomous marine invertebrates is the Portuguese man-of-war. It is a bluish, bladderlike float, or jellyfish, with long stinging tentacles found mainly in tropical waters. Stingrays are similarly dangerous.

In all cases of marine animal stings, attend to the victim immediately. If the victim is having a severe reaction or if he or she has been stung many times, get emergency assistance at once.

IS IT A HUMAN BITE OR LESS DANGEROUS KIND OF ANIMAL?

Any emergency room doctor will attest that bites by humans are much more common than you think. I'm not talking about toddlers and older kids who don't play well with others—in these cases, grown-up is not synonymous with adult.

Bites by humans actually have a lot in common with those of other animals. The mouths of all animals contain a multitude of bacteria and sometimes viruses. Thus if the bite breaks the skin, an infection may develop. The only difference here is that a bite by a dog, or other nonhuman animal may carry the risk of rabies in addition to other diseases.

If a fellow *Homo sapiens* or dog bites you, check first to ascertain if the bite has broken the skin. If it hasn't done so, wash the area thoroughly with water and an antibacterial soap to avoid infection. Next apply a cold compress or ice pack to avoid contusions or bruising. When an animal bite has broken the skin, you must see your doctor. Make sure you tell the doctor whether the animal, human or otherwise, was a stranger to you.

▪ CREEPY CREEPING CREATURES

BEDBUGS

A flat wingless insect, the bedbug is darkish brown and lives on furniture and floors. It is found most often in beds, hence the name. These nasty little things do come out at night to bite humans, so the old nighttime blessing "Don't let the bedbugs bite" is no joke.

If you are bitten by a bedbug, you'll notice itching in the area soon after the bite. A lesion then develops, usually with a hemorrhagic mark in the center. Since the bedbug sucks blood from several sites, a small cluster of lesions may occur. The bite or bites will then redden and perhaps blister, particularly in children. The lesion usually subsides in a matter of hours. The bites may appear anywhere the body touches the bed. These bites are generally harmless, unless they become infected.

Bedbugs may be eradicated by using an insecticide. Use an insect bomb but also wash all clothes and sheets and dry them on HOT.

SPIDERS

Spider bites are usually not dangerous. However, two species of spiders are responsible for most of the serious spider bites in the United States: the widow spider—most notoriously, the black widow—and the brown recluse or band spinning spider.

Brown recluse spider: It is as antisocial as its name implies. The brown recluse spider lives in dark, warm areas like attics or sheds. It has markings on its back that resemble a fiddle. Originally found mostly in the midwestern United States, it is not so antisocial that it has limited its travel—it can be a problem in the eastern United States as well. Within twelve to twenty-four hours after the bite, there is a dull, aching pain. In the next twenty-four hours, a blue-gray blister that contains blood forms. Over the next three days the skin around it gets red, hard, and swollen.

It takes about five months for complete healing. Antivenin that will neutralize the brown recluse spider venom is under development. If you think you have been bitten by the brown recluse, get medical attention immediately.

Black widow spider: You will know the black widow by her look. She has a large crimson shape like an hourglass on her belly. Her bite causes swelling, redness, and limb pain within twenty minutes. During the high-risk hour that follows the bite, abdominal cramps, cardiac changes, and kidney shutdown can occur. Emergency treatment with a widely available antivenin, as well as other medications, is needed.

SCORPIONS

There are over six hundred species of scorpions worldwide and they are of special concern in arid parts of the world such as the southwestern United States, the Middle East, India, and Mexico. The business end of the scorpion is the tail, which contains a stinger that inflicts the wound. Although the venom of scorpions varies from species to species, the poison belongs to a broad class of chemicals known as neurotoxins. The scorpion venom can cause internal problems as well as local injury in the skin itself.

In general scorpions sting when they feel threatened, and most injuries occur on the arms or legs, head or neck. At first there is a sharp burning pain at the sting location, which may be followed by numbness of the surrounding skin. Swelling can also occur. The internal symptoms include convulsions, coma, irritability, and cardiac abnormalities. Treatment of the sting consists of elevation of the area, application of ice packs, and antihistamines to control the inflammation. Antivenin is available, but its usefulness is not definite. In the case of internal symptoms, get help immediately.

SNAKES

Some reptile bites can be harmless, except for the pain they cause, while others can be lethal. Although there are many kinds of snakes that can bite, fortunately, there are only four poisonous types found in the United States. Copperheads, rattlesnakes, and water moccasins (also known as cottonmouths) are all pit vipers. The coral snake is the sole non-viper in this dangerous group.

If you believe you or someone you are with has been bitten by a poisonous snake call 911 or the emergency number in your area. Do not wait for the medical team to arrive to begin treatment.

Before telling you what might be effective, let me first dispel two myths about snake bites. First, trying to suck out poisonous venom with your mouth will *not* help the victim and could hurt you. Never use suction on a poisonous snakebite unless instructed to do so by an emergency dispatcher. Second, cutting into the bite with a knife—the way they do in old westerns—will not help the victim and may actually hurt the victim even more by adding the risk of infection to an already traumatic situation.

When a person is bitten by a poisonous snake, the most frequent cause of death is shock. Here is what you can do to avoid shock in the victim:

1. Have the person lie down. Snakebites nearly always occur on an arm or leg. Make sure the bitten extremity is *lower than heart level*.

2. Remove all clothing and jewelry that may be restrictive.

3. Whenever possible, bandage the area above the bite tightly, tourniquet-style, to slow blood flow and the spread of the venom through the bloodstream. If bandages are not available, use duct tape, masking tape, a necktie, or whatever is available. Be creative—anything is better than nothing, *as long as the material is not wire*. The bandage should restrict circulation but should not cut it off. If the skin is very pale below the bandage, you'll know immediately that the bandage is too tight.

4. Keep a close watch on the person's breathing and circulation. Also check the pulse until help arrives.

Most medical texts also advise trying to identify and kill the snake without endangering yourself, as well as administering emergency first aid.

In cases of snakebites by nonvenomous snakes, follow the same procedure as you would for any other animal bite.

*I keep breaking out and drugstore medications
don't help. Now I'm getting scars and I hate the
way my face looks.*

—Janine, 18, college student

Advances in medicine in the past two decades have dramatically changed the nature of adolescence. Effective topical and oral medication can now control the effects of raging hormones that result in acne. There are even options for adult acne sufferers.

Acne is such a part of growing up that when you think about the most noticeable bodily change in the teenage years, it is acne. I think the way we commonly dismiss this as a trivial problem may have something to do with our own discomfort and unease through those difficult years. In fact, acne is a very serious problem. Having a condition that affects self-image while your self-image is being shaped is a bit like your mother drinking too much wine or smoking while she was pregnant with you: the issue isn't the drinking per se, it's that the behavior occurs at a time when it can have profound effects beyond those intended. And so it is with acne, a common medical concern but like none other I have seen in younger patients.

Acne really consists of two problems: the acute symptoms of discomfort with cystic acne and the appearance of active lesions; and second, the long-term permanent effect of facial scarring that can result when acne is not properly controlled.

During puberty, 100 percent of boys and 90 percent of girls will have some acne lesions. There are in fact many types of acne—as many as fourteen different kinds, affecting newborns to the elderly. So if you're one of the lucky few who hasn't had acne by the time you graduate from high school, it's no guarantee you won't run into trouble.

In the last decade, about five million visits were made to dermatologists annually for acne problems, and this doesn't include all the visits to family doctors who often are the first line of treatment for this common and unsettling condition.

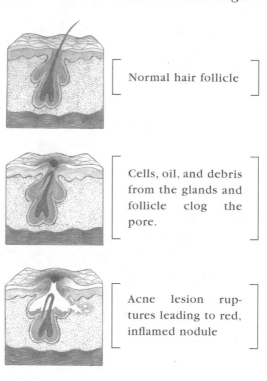

Normal hair follicle

Cells, oil, and debris from the glands and follicle clog the pore.

Acne lesion ruptures leading to red, inflamed nodule

I have a special interest in early successful management of acne because in my practice I am often asked to help people with post-acne scarring, which is one of the more difficult challenges in dermatology. As with everything in life, it is far better to fix a small problem than wait for it to become overwhelming. Nowadays there are so many effective treatments for acne, from topical agents to oral medications such as Accutane, that I honestly believe that any teenager who does not pick at his or her face should not have scarring of any significant degree. In this way, acne scarring should be considered preventable. The trick is to diagnose the condition early, jump on it with the whole range of treatment options, and stay on top of the problem until the body chemistry has changed and the hair follicle oil glands, no longer pumped up and frenetic, slide into a more comfortable and less antagonistic relationship with their host.

Acne vulgaris is the most common type of acne (*vulgaris* in fact means "common"), which plagues the vast majority of teenagers. Acne vulgaris has several different subtypes, so sufferers may experience some or all of the following lesions: *comedonal* (pronounced koh-me-DOAN-ul), papular, pustular, or cystic.

Any form of acne, whether in a teenager, adult, or child, can range from mild to severe. People like Janine are subject to acne vulgaris (95 percent of people will have at least one outbreak of it) in their teen years but adults are also at risk for at least one outbreak in their lifetime. Adult types of acne include perioral dermatitis and acne rosacea, These can make people as upset as any teenager in the throes of acne vulgaris.

▪ ACNE VULGARIS

Acne vulgaris is a natural consequence of what makes men as we know them. That's because one of the key factors that lead to acne vulgaris is increased sebum production, a direct result of increases in the male hormone—in both men and women—during puberty.

Abnormal blockage of the hair follicle opening may be the causative factor that is acne's smoking gun. This blockage is thought to result from an increased amount of "sticky" keratin due to hormonal changes and the increase in sebum production. These keratin cells accumulate in the hair follicle canal directly above the opening of the oil gland duct, resulting in a plug formation known as a *microcomedone*. This microcomedone then enlarges just beneath the surface of the skin in the pore itself. Later it becomes visible as a *closed comedone*, or whitehead, which is a firm white papule. If, however, the pore dilates, an *open comedone*, or blackhead, will

---

ACNE MYTHS

All of the following ARE NOT TRUE:

- *Chocolate and greasy foods cause acne.* Oil in your follicles helps cause acne, not tasty food in your tummy.
- *Sun helps acne get better.* There is no proof of this.
- *Not washing your face causes acne.* Acne is not caused by dirt.
- *Masturbation causes acne.* Truly a myth.

CONCEALING

Concealing stubborn lesions is OK, but follow these rules:

- Use as little concealer as possible.
- Make sure the product is labeled non-comedogenic (won't cause pimples).
- Remove it when you no longer need it.
- Try to use a concealer that has an active ingredient, like salicylic acid or sulfa.

occur. Further enlargement of the open comedone can cause the pore to enlarge further, resulting in the large pores often seen in patients with acne. Although these open and closed comedones, blackheads, and whiteheads themselves are not inflammatory, they set the stage for inflammatory lesions that may occur.

Another important cause of acne is a bacterium known as *Propionibacterium acnes* (often referred to simply as *P. acnes*). This tiny germ normally lives happily in the oil gland yet plays a significant role by producing substances that contribute to the inflammation of acne. As this bacterium incites inflammation in the follicle, the wall of the hair follicle becomes thinner and eventually may rupture. When this happens, you get yet another manifestation of acne: the red, hot bump, or papule. Once it actually ruptures, a bit like a volcano in turmoil, a much larger inflammatory red papule or pustule may develop, a lesion that can be exquisitely tender.

But acne is not exclusively an "inside" job. Oil-based makeup and hair gels, hormonal changes that occur in the premenstrual period, and pregnancy can make things worse, as can frequent manipulation of skin lesions. In fact, one of the commandments of dermatology is: *Do not pick*. Picking your face can make acne lesions worse and, of greater concern, can lead to discoloration and even scarring.

▪ TREATING ACNE VULGARIS

I mentioned earlier that acne vulgaris is eminently treatable, and treated it should be. Remember, untreated acne may leave scars that will last a lifetime. The cost of treating acne, whether you have insurance or not, should not be an impediment to therapy. An entire year of topical therapy for mild to moderate acne may cost as little as $30 to about $200.

UH-OH! I HAVE A RED-HOT PIMPLE THAT WON'T GO AWAY AND I HAVE A RED-HOT DATE

For large acne cysts that get inflamed, injection with a steroid solution can provide rapid relief. Often, the cyst will begin to subside within twelve hours. While this treatment should not be used routinely, it is a reliable emergency approach that dermatologists frequently use.

Occasionally, once the cyst has calmed down, excision may be the only way to ensure that it does not rear its ugly head again.

If you have more severe acne and require Accutane, treatment is more expensive—including medication costs, blood tests, and doctor visits, it can run about $2,000 for a twenty-week course. On the other hand, if it works, the nice thing about Accutane is you may never need treatment again.

In treating acne, an extensive history is taken to determine how you wash your face and what substances you have been putting on it, since several of these can irritate your skin and worsen the acne. Next, an exam of your skin will result in an inventory of the type of acne lesions you have. That will help in rating the severity and developing a treatment plan. In general, in this area of dermatology, we do not use an elephant gun to kill a flea. However, if you fall into a more severe category with the larger papules, nodules, and cysts, the most aggressive appropriate therapy should be undertaken.

Basic management steps include washing with gentle soaps or nonsoap cleansers such as Cetaphil and decreasing the frequency of moisturization. Remember, one of the causes of acne is the oil your own glands produce. Why import extra oil to the scene of the potential disaster? It's okay to use moisturizers, but they must be specifically designed for people with acne. Such products will often say "non-comedogenic" (won't cause pimples) or "oil-free" on their labels.

Several topical agents can correct the abnormal accumulation of keratin in hair follicles; this decreases the amount of follicular plugging, thus getting at one of the causes of acne. Such compounds include Retin-A (tretinoin, a form of vitamin A that has been chemically altered); Differin (adapalene gel); and benzoyl peroxide, which comes in many formulations and a range of brands. Benzoyl peroxide, in low concentration, is available over-the-counter while Retin-A and Differin require a prescription. Ben-

IF WE KNEW THEN WHAT WE KNOW NOW

While we believe that the treatments being used for acne today are safe and will stand the test of time, when medicine was not as sophisticated, technology we did not fully understand was used to treat this frustrating and widespread disease.

More than fifty years ago, X-ray was used to treat acne. It was thought it would dry up the oil glands. It was even used to remove facial hair. And it worked. Fast-forward to today and guess what? Patients who received radiation to the face for these purposes now have an increased incidence of skin cancer. Everything in medicine is a trade-off, but today we do not consider skin cancer a reasonable risk in the treatment of acne.

zoyl peroxide kills the bacteria of acne better than any topical or oral antibiotic, and because it kills *P. acnes* by producing oxygen (*P. acnes* cannot live with oxygen), the bacteria never develops resistance to it. Benzoyl peroxide is the cheapest, most effective over-the-counter acne remedy.

Salicylic acid can be used alone or along with a sulfur product. Salicylic acid works as an anti-inflammatory agent and is an excellent first-line choice for mild acne. It is the active ingredient in many over-the-counter drying agents.

For treating severe acne a cousin of Retin-A, isotretinoin, known as Accutane, is extremely effective. Isotretinoin helps to markedly diminish sebum production, normalize the growth pattern in the follicle, and also may work to diminish the activity of *P. acnes*.

A warning about Accutane: isotretinoin can cause birth defects. Unfortunately, many of the people who would benefit most from Accutane are women of child-bearing age, so special precautions are needed when using this drug. Other side effects of Accutane, which must be thoroughly explained to you by your doctor and weighed against the drug's benefits include changes in night vision, hair loss, headaches, dry eyes, dry mouth with cracked lips, dried nasal lining that could lead to nose bleeds, and even calcification of the Achilles tendon and other musculoskeletal problems. Accutane can increase blood lipids, so it's very important that these be monitored throughout therapy. The side effects clear up when the standard twenty-week course of treatment is completed.

Oral antibiotics are a good approach to managing acne because they

---

ACNE RULES

- **Don't pick.** If you find that you are tempted to pick your lesions, go find something else to do with your hands. Peel an apple, knit, play the drums.
- **Do not overwash.** Wash your face once a day with a gentle nonsoap cleanser. Do not use abrasives: sandpaper is for wood and the bottom of birdcages.
- **Do not put a lot of stuff on your face.** Avoid oils, creams, and other agents that are oily and can plug up follicles.
- **Take your medication as prescribed.**
- **DON'T PICK.**

---

seem to strike at *P. acnes*, the bacterial instigator of the problem. Tetracycline, the old standby, is inexpensive and works well, but some patients develop sun sensitivity. Minocycline, a once-a-day medication (which makes it easier to remember to take), can be very effective, but does have rare side effects such as discoloring the skin and dizziness. If you will benefit from minocycline, most dermatologists consider these side effects well within the reasonable risk-benefit ratio.

Tetracycline and minocycline also possess anti-inflammatory properties apart from killing bacteria, which may play a role in calming down inflamed acne lesions. Whatever your treatment plan, none of the medications will work if they stay in your medicine cabinet. Managing acne is a daily task. Your body makes new acne lesions daily, so it makes sense to fight it daily with total compliance with the prescribed plan. And remember: Don't pick!!!

Once acne lesions clear they may leave behind either scars or a dark or light patch on the skin. The scarring that results from acne can often be bothersome and permanent, so it is best to get your acne under control while the getting is good. (For a discussion of how dermatologists treat scarring, see chapter 18.) The dark and lighter discoloration in the skin is a result of the skin's reaction to the inflammation of the acne lesions. This discoloration often does fade, but it may take many months to do so. It does not indicate that the acne is still active. Very often, after the acute acne flare settles down, redness may persist for many months, depending on your skin type. If you are fair, redness would not be surprising; if you are more darkly complected hyperpigmentation may result.

SPECIAL CONSIDERATIONS IN PEOPLE OF COLOR

There is a significantly lower incidence of inflammatory acne in blacks than in whites. However, when it does occur, it can have a range of unwanted manifestations that can last a lifetime, and from a cosmetic point of view, post-inflammatory hyperpigmentation is an important issue.

Pomade acne is a variety of acne that is often seen in darker-skinned individuals. It results from the oils, greases, and waxes used in hairstyling that address the unique features of black hair. Some of these agents clog up hair follicles, stimulating the production of acne lesions. Because they clog up hair follicles, these compounds are called comedogenic. Acne lesions usually develop in the immediate area of the hairline. The acne can spread anywhere on the face if the grease, wax, or oils come in contact with facial skin.

To correct the problem, refrain from using such oily products as much as possible. Given the hair "issues" you may be facing, it's unreasonable to suggest giving up your favorite products altogether. One compromise would be to use nongreasy pomades. For example, agents that contain glycerin or silicon oils may be less acne-causing. Apply hair grease every other day, if possible, and pursue a regimen for acne prescribed by your dermatologist. Washing with an acne cleanser that contains salicylic acid may be helpful as well. But don't overdo or you'll simply irritate the skin and cause yourself more skin problems.

ACNE ROSACEA

Acne *rosacea* (pronounced row-ZAY-shah) is an acnelike eruption seen most often in fair-skinned individuals of northern European extraction. Although it may look like typical acne, it lacks one of the classic features of acne—the comedone. You may have acne rosacea if you have redness of the forehead, cheeks, and nose; a mild swelling of the face; papules and pustules; and dilated blood vessels, also known as telangiectasias. People with rosacea often have a history of flushing or blushing easily.

Some patients with rosacea have the redness, papules, and pustules; some have only redness and telangiectasias; and still others have a combination of all of these features. The condition is chronic, with periods of exacerbation and remissions. In its extreme form, it gets deep into the many oily follicles of the nose and the inflammation can result in thickening of the end of the nose. This condition is known as rhinophyma. In roughly half of all patients with acne rosacea the eye can be affected, with such symptoms as conjunctivitis, soreness, decreased tear production, and redness and scaling of the eyelids.

The exact cause of acne rosacea is a mystery, but it is known that certain factors can exacerbate it by dilating facial blood vessels. Among the things that can make rosacea worse are alcohol ingestion, sun exposure, and warm drinks. It is also felt that a mite named *Demodex folliculorum*, which lives in the hair follicles, may be in on the act; in some individuals with acne rosacea, the concentration of such mites is significantly increased.

Treatment of acne rosacea must be customized to the person. For very mild cases, Metrocream or Noritate, brands of topical metronidazole cream has been shown to be effective. For moderate to severe cases, an oral antibiotic such as tetracycline or minocycline might be required. These medications are used for many months to keep the problem, once tamed, under control. Combinations of oral antibiotics and topicals are also very popular. Another topical agent is sulfacetamide and there are several commercially available preparations with this antibiotic in tinted form to minimize the redness. For the most severe cases, isotretinoin is sometimes prescribed.

> ### MONEY CAN'T BUY HAPPINESS
>
> J. P. Morgan, the famous banker and richest man of his day, suffered terribly from a form of acne rosacea called rhinophyma. Morgan was so devastated by his appearance that he curtailed his social life on account of it.

To take care of the redness and telangiectasias, once the acne rosacea is under control, laser surgery can be quite effective and results in a high degree of patient satisfaction. Although there is no proof that laser does anything other than remove the broken blood vessel, or has an effect on the flushing that comes with rosacea, in some patients I have noticed a decreased need for topical medication after several laser treatments. (It could just be coincidence.)

For treatment of rhinophyma, resculpting the nose with the carbon dioxide laser, or even the less sophisticated but equally effective wire loop cautery, can result in remarkable improvement.

Rosacea of the eyelids responds nicely to oral antibiotics, but before that is even tried, wiping the eyelid edges daily with Johnson's Baby Shampoo applied with a Q-tip can clear up the mildest cases.

▪ PERIORAL DERMATITIS

Perioral dermatitis, another acnelike eruption with a distinct pattern, occurs mainly in young women. It is by far one of the most frustrating forms of acne, because it occurs not long after a person thinks she was through with acne forever. Just when she thinks she's out of the woods, whammo! The follicles, like the Terminator, are back for more. But don't despair—good therapy abounds.

Perioral dermatitis distinctively occurs most often around the mouth, the nostrils, and sometimes the outside corners of the eyes. In these areas there is a background of redness, sometimes scaling, and studding with tiny pinpoint pustules.

The exact cause of this eruption is not known. It has been postulated in the past that the frequent use of moisturizing creams in these areas can significantly worsen the condition. Although the application of a mild topical corticosteroids has been shown to improve perioral dermatitis, stronger steroid creams may worsen it.

Treatment includes a several-week course of anti-inflammatory oral antibiotics such as tetracycline or erythromycin. Use of moisturizing creams or any topical corticosteroids in the affected areas should also be discontinued. Once the eruption has cleared, the dosage of the antibiotics can often be lowered and then stopped. For resistant cases, however, long-term oral antibiotics are sometimes needed.

▪ FOLLICULITIS

Folliculitis—a very common condition— is an inflammation of the hair follicles that can result from an infection, chemical irritation, or mechanical irritation. The inflammation in the hair follicle may be either close to the surface of the skin or deeper down within the hair follicle.

A superficial folliculitis often manifests on the skin as a tiny pustule with a rim of redness. Such a lesion heals without scarring, although it may leave behind an area of hyper- or hypopigmentation. A deeper folliculitis can show up as a larger red nodule under the skin that can be tender and swollen; it may eventually form a pustule and will leave scarring as it clears up.

Infectious folliculitis can be caused by bacteria such as *Staphylococcus aureus,* yeast such as candida or *Pityrosporum ovale,* or mites such as *Demodex folliculorum.* One can also develop a bacterial *Pseudomonal* folliculitis on the trunk after spending time in a hot tub that has not been properly sanitized. (Be wary of getting in hot tubs with lots of froth—the froth is produced by dead skin protein, upon which such bacteria feast!)

Folliculitis from chemical irritation can develop on skin that has been covered with plastic dressings or casts, or after the application of topical ointments such as petroleum jelly. Also, cooks exposed to a lot of cooking grease tend to develop folliculitis.

Frictional and mechanical injury to the skin can also result in folliculitis, commonly seen in athletes who accumulate sweat under heavy pads and other sports equipment. Another type of mechanical folliculitis is *pseudofolliculitis barbae.* This results from a foreign-body reaction to one's own hair and is most commonly seen in people with hair that curls back and digs into the skin after shaving. For this reason, it is most commonly seen on the beard and neck area; the scalp, armpits, pubic areas, and legs are other areas often affected.

To treat folliculitis the doctor must first determine the underlying cause. Cases of infectious folliculitis can be treated with oral antibiotics in combination with topical antibiotics. Yeast and candidal folliculitis are most often treated with topical anti-yeast agents and, if more extensive, an oral anti-yeast medication. Fungal folliculitis is likewise treated with antifungal topical agents in limited cases and oral antifungal agents in more extensive ones. Folliculitis caused by mites such as *Demodex* can be treated with topical anti-mite preparations. For folliculitis that is induced by chemical irritants, withdrawal of the agent usually results in the lesions clearing up. Lastly, folliculitis caused by mechanical trauma is best treated by eliminating the direct cause. In the particular situation of pseudofolliculitis barbae, for instance, it is best not to shave the hair so closely to the skin; special razors and shaving creams are available to help with this problem.

WHEN BAD THINGS COME IN THREE: FOLLICULAR OCCLUSION TRIAD

A problem more common in darker-skinned individuals than others is the follicular occlusion triad. This consists of *hidradenitis suppurativa, acne conglobata,* and *dissecting cellulitis* of the scalp. These three conditions all have in common blockage of the hair follicle unit followed by inflammation of the apocrine glands. These small glands are found in the area of hair follicles responsible for secreting pheromones in most mammals (however, their role in humans is not entirely clear). Hidradenitis suppurativa can be a severely debilitating condition, resulting in drainage, scarring, and discomfort. Acne conglobata, which occurs on the face, buttocks, and back, can result in scarring and nonhealing tracts or channels in the skin. Dissecting cellulitis of the scalp consists of large inflammatory nodules, and nonhealing areas that can result in hair loss and permanent scarring. In all these conditions, the first line of therapy is to use tetracycline or minocycline, two common antibiotics.

Many doctors recommend a course of Accutane (isotretinoin), but unfortunately the drug is not as effective in this problem as it is against common acne. Surgical removal of the affected skin is sometimes attempted but is not always successful.

▪ ACNE KELOIDALIS NUCHAE

Acne keloidalis nuchae, a chronic, progressive, and scarring condition seen in black men, presents a real challenge to dermatologists. It's very frustrating to the patients, since treatment is difficult, and even surgical intervention is no guarantee of a cure. Acne keloidalis usually affects men starting in their twenties. Symptoms include small, pea-sized bumps on the back of the head that, when infected, can get much larger and tender. A common result of this inflammatory reaction is scarring with hair loss in the diseased area. The cause of this condition is not known, and although testosterone levels were elevated significantly among patients with acne keloidalis in one study the meaning of this finding is not known.

With respect to treatment, it is best to be conservative at first. While some men are fond of the shaved-head look, hair should be allowed to grow long in the affected area. Mechanical irritation caused by clothing, such as a tight collar, should be minimized. Antibiotics, either topical such as clindamycin or erythromycin or oral, such as Keflex—can be a mainstay of treatment. Benzoyl peroxide should be avoided, because, although it is an excellent medication for controlling follicular inflammation, it may bleach the hair. Hair oils and greasy skin products should be avoided at all times. Occasionally, a course of Accutane can be helpful.

Once the infection has been brought under control, the scars, the "keloid" part of keloidalis, may be managed with an injection of Kenalog corticosteroid (see "Keloids" in chapter 24, "Common Skin Conditions").

If the keloids continue to grow and steroid injections are not helpful, sur-gical therapy is the next step.

If no significant improvement of lesions is obtained after half a dozen injections, excision using any surgical technique that your physician is comfortable with makes the most sense. It is important that the excision be done down through the full layer of skin into the fat and that the wound be allowed to heal naturally—although some doctors obtain good results by suturing the wounds.

At Yale, we use a regimen of radiation therapy which is supposed to inhibit the activity of the fibroblasts, or scar-producing cells, that become active during the healing phase after surgery. Superficial radiation treat-ments are applied to the wound area itself after the keloid has been excised. Radiation therapists believe that such radiation in young patients is not an especially great concern, given the limited treatment period of three days and the relatively low dose of radiation used.

Although laser has been touted as a magical approach to managing this problem, in my experience it provides no additional benefit over the other treatments described.

Most of the practice of medicine involves old-fashioned detective work. Indeed, doctors and detectives have always had a special relationship (Arthur Conan Doyle, author of the Sherlock Holmes series, was a physician). In attempting to understand a medical problem, doctors rely on a host of clues: laboratory tests, the history of the problem as related by you, the patient, and the physical exam.

In this tricky and challenging clue-finding effort, our skin proves very valuable. In addition to being our largest sensory organ and, by some standards, our largest organ overall, skin functions as a window to our overall health. While some of the changes in the skin as a result of health problems occur further down the road than we would like, others can be a bit like an early warning system, advising your doctor to order a blood test or an MRI scan to see what is going on inside.

In this chapter I discuss some of the more common skin signs in health and disease. However, please do not try to self-diagnose. If you notice a skin sign that is similar to something you think you have, contact your doctor. Don't panic; don't fuss; just make the appointment. The truth is, most times the skin sign you see will prove to be transient and unrelated to any serious internal problem.

Here is a brief rundown of some skin signs and what they can indicate about internal health problems.

- *A persistent rash across the nose and cheeks* can be a sign of lupus erythematosus. This red rash resembles a butterfly in shape and may be accompanied by raised reddish rashes elsewhere on the body and increased sensitivity to the sun.
- *Cracked skin or bleeding at the nipple* may indicate a form of breast cancer. Other cancers may manifest themselves on the skin as hard nodules.
- *Yellowing of the skin, or jaundice,* may be a sign of hepatitis due to liver disease.
- *Thickened skin,* usually on the backs of the hands and around the neck, can develop in people who have had diabetes for a number of years.
- *Excessively dry skin and dry, brittle hair* may be signs of an underactive thyroid or hypothyroidism.
- *Painful blisters inside the mouth and on the palms and soles* may indicate hand, foot, and mouth disease. This infection is caused by a virus that affects children most frequently. The firm blisters may also be accompanied by red spots or a low fever.
- *A bluish discoloration of the skin,* accompanied by numbness, burning, or tenderness of the fingers and toes, may be a sign of a rare disease of the blood vessels called thromboangiitis obliterans, or Buerger's disease. Most common in smokers, it can cause skin ulcers and, if not treated, even the loss of fingers or toes.

For details on some of these skin signs and the conditions they represent, read on.

▪ CANCER AND THE SKIN

Certain internal cancers cause changes in the skin. In these cases, the evidence of disease on the skin will appear after or at the same time that the internal cancer begins to grow.

Studies have shown that the most common cancers to appear on the skin before they are discovered internally are those of the lung, ovary, and kidney. Additionally, studies suggest that somewhere between 1 and 4 per-

DO DOCTORS GET SICK?

In 1862, the French physician Armand Trousseau drew attention to the association of superficial migratory thrombophlebitis and internal cancer. Characterized by the development of blood clots in the veins just beneath the skin surface, this condition was a sign of cancer of the stomach. What is interesting and tragic about *Trousseau's syndrome* is that Dr. Trousseau himself died of gastric cancer, manifesting his own syndrome at death.

cent of internal cancers will spread to the skin. The cancers most likely to do this include those of the breast, stomach, lung, uterus, kidney, ovary, colon, and urinary bladder. When these malignant tumors travel to the skin they should not be mistaken for skin cancer, which is a different condition altogether. Unfortunately, by the time any of these internal cancers spread to the skin, the cancer must be considered widespread.

When an internal cancer causes signs on the skin, those signs will wax and wane as the internal cancer waxes and wanes. Multiple hard, nontender nodules can form on the skin as metastases.

▪ LIVER DISEASE AND THE SKIN

One of the most common skin signs of internal disease in the digestive system is jaundice, derived from *jaune*, the French word for yellow. Jaundice results from the buildup of bilirubin in the skin. It occurs in newborns and disappears with simple treatment or no treatment at all. The body normally forms a substance called bilirubin from the breakdown of hemoglobin in red blood cells that have become old and need to be recycled. Typically, people with jaundice have a yellow discoloration in areas where there is a high content of elastic tissue. The first place that jaundice occurs is the whites of the eyes, followed by the skin of the face, the roof of the mouth, and the abdominal wall.

Jaundice can be seen best in bright daylight. Some cases of jaundice may exhibit a different color than yellow, depending on where the buildup of bilirubin or its breakdown products have occurred within the body. A greenish hue can be seen in jaundice if the liver has processed the bilirubin and cannot get it out of the bile duct and into the intestines. This occurs most often when there is a cancer blocking the exit of the bile duct into your intestines.

While jaundice is one sign that can be seen in patients with acute or chronic liver disease, there are, of course, many more signs associated with chronic liver disease. All these skin signs, including jaundice, are signs of advanced liver disease.

Itching is common if there is a problem anywhere in the system that produces bile. For instance, there can be a malfunction with the liver processing bilirubin or a blockage of the duct out of the gallbladder that releases bile into the intestines. Either of these can result in intense itching that leads to uncontrollable scratching. This irresistible scratching can lead to skin abrasions from fingernails, resulting in an increased blotchy discoloration and a thickening of the skin.

Some people with cirrhosis of the liver develop red palms and bruise very easily; this happens when factors necessary for blood clotting are no longer being produced in the liver in adequate amounts. Some people lose large amounts of their body hair and men with chronic liver disease develop increased estrogen (the female hormones); this can lead to enlargement of the breast, shrinking of the testicles, and loss of hair in the armpits or trunk.

Finally, swelling of the ankles is sometimes due to advanced liver disease.

▪ KIDNEY DISEASE AND THE SKIN

People with kidney disease experience many changes in their skin. In one large study of patients with failure of the kidneys, 70 percent demonstrated changes in skin color. Forty percent of the subjects had a yellowish tinge to their skin, while 30 percent had an increased tan or brown color to their palms or soles. Again, 70 percent of those studied had fungal infections of their fingernails, toenails, or the bottom of their feet.

About two thirds of kidney-failure patients also have changes in their nails. The most common change is called "half and half" nails, in which the half of the nail closer to the cuticle is white while the other half is normal or pink. This is thought to be due to increased fluid underneath the nail itself.

Almost all people with kidney failure have very dry skin; two-thirds of them experience severe itching. In some cases, this itching gets even worse with dialysis. Although the cause of this itching is unknown, it can get better with artificial ultraviolet light treatment.

▪ DIABETES AND THE SKIN

The most common fungal skin infection in people with diabetes is candidiasis. When not enough insulin is present, the amount of sugar in the blood increases. The sugar in the blood serves as food for the yeast known as candida. The most common sign of candidiasis is bright red areas that may have adherent white tissue surrounded by small pimples. These splotches are found in or near mucosal areas, such as the groin, on the tongue, and inside the mouth. People also get these infections in areas of skin folds, such as underneath the breast, or between folds of fat skin, between the fingers, at the base of the fingernails, or even in the nails themselves. Anyone with frequent skin infections such as these should be screened for diabetes.

In addition, approximately one-third of diabetics get thin, scarred dark bumps on the shins that often develop in tandem with thick yellow skin. This condition is called diabetic dermopathy.

A rare skin disease associated with diabetes is *necrobiosis lipoidica*. In this disease, round yellow and brown or orange smooth lesions are seen on the shins. In advanced cases, they may form ulcers. While 90 percent of patients with necrobiosis lipoidica have some problem with their sugar metabolism, only three out of every thousand patients with diabetes have this condition.

Adults who develop diabetes normally produce enough insulin but have cells that don't respond to the insulin they make. Those with this insulin resistance may get a condition called *acanthosis nigricans*. Folds of velvety skin, especially in the armpits, neck creases, and the backs of the fingers, develop over time. The skin looks dirty, but this is only because the excess skin possesses increased melanin compared with what is normally present.

Diabetics also develop bacterial infections, including folliculitis (see p. 338), or skin abscesses due especially to staphylococcal bacteria develop. Diabetic patients are also prone to get infections of their ear canals with a bacterium known as pseudomonas.

▪ THYROID DISEASE AND THE SKIN

The thyroid gland, which sits in the front of the neck just below the Adam's apple, produces a hormone that regulates the overall energy metabolism of the body. When low amounts of thyroid hormone are produced, fatigue, weight gain, and temperature changes can occur. In mild cases of hypothyroidism (*low* hormone), the skin is dry, scaly, cold, and pale, and the hair is dry. The skin may itch, and the nails can be more brittle.

If hypothyroidism goes on for years unattended, the skin may become yellow and thick throughout the body. The lips and tongue may become thickened, and people often lose hair in the outer portions of their eyebrows. The yellow skin results from an inability to get rid of the carotene pigment (this is found in our daily diet in such foods as carrots). Once the proper diagnosis has been made, thyroid replacement hormones can be prescribed and the skin changes will soon disappear.

If the thyroid gland is overproducing thyroid hormone, a condition called hyperthyroidism occurs. This is much less common than hypothyroidism. When the thyroid gland overproduces, the skin becomes moist, warm, smooth, and red. The skin may still be itchy, and the nails can separate from the nail bed.

▪ HORMONES AND THE SKIN

Hormones made by various organs, such as the thyroid gland or pancreas, can affect the appearance of the skin. These hormones might interact directly with cells in the skin, or an excess of hormones can cause a condition within the body that leads to specific skin conditions.

Male-type hormones known as androgens have a great effect on both the oil glands and hair. Women also produce androgens in low quantities in their ovaries and the adrenal glands. Excess androgens in women may cause a severe form of acne, as well as increased facial hair and balding of the scalp. These women may also develop an increased brown coloration of the skin around the genitals and nipples. Any woman experiencing such symptoms should see her physician to check for a possible hormone imbalance. Remember, however, that most severe acne or facial hair in women is hereditary and not related to this hormonal problem.

ADDISON'S DISEASE

For a variety of reasons, the adrenal glands may slow production of their hormones. The key body chemicals produced by these small glands that sit atop the kidneys are cortisol and aldosterone, which is necessary for the absorption and retention of salt in the body.

People who do not produce enough of these hormones release an increased amount of a stimulating hormone called ACTH from the pituitary gland at the base of the brain. ACTH itself comes from a more plentiful hormone, whose breakdown products affect the pigment of the skin. This is the telltale skin sign for the condition known as Addison's disease. People with Addison's disease maintain a summer tan far into the winter months and develop darkening in areas of pressure and friction, such as the elbows, knees, skin folds, and creases of the palms, as well as the nipples, armpits, and groin. They also crave salt.

▪ RHEUMATIC CONDITIONS AND THE SKIN

The group of diseases now known as the collagen-vascular diseases (*rheumatic disease* is the old-fashioned term) have in common antibodies that attack normal cells in the skin and internal organs. These antinuclear antibodies often attack different molecules in the nucleus of cells. Diseases in this group include the various types of lupus erythematosus, dermatomyositis, scleroderma, and rheumatoid arthritis. In these diseases, there is also involvement of the blood vessels in which telangiectasias (broken blood vessels), purplish discolorations of the skin, and inflammation may be seen.

LUPUS

Lupus comes from the Latin word for wolf; this name was applied because the skin of patients often looked as if their skin had been gnawed by a wolf. There are three main types of lupus: lupus of the skin only (discoid lupus erythematosus, referred to also as DLE), lupus mainly of the skin with mild involvement of internal organs (subacute lupus erythematosus), and lupus involving internal organs to a great extent, with or without skin symptoms (systemic lupus erythematosus).

People with lupus are typically very sensitive to the sun. The acute rash seen in people who have lupus involving their internal organs is often called a butterfly rash. The cheek rash represents the wings while the small involvement on the nose simulates the body of the butterfly.

People with lupus may also develop what is called a subacute rash. This can take on a number of forms on sun-exposed areas of the body, but it predominantly occurs on the face and backs of the forearms. This rash can look scaly (like psoriasis) or it can have a number of smooth, round red areas without scaling. The rash may include small, raised red dots in sun-exposed areas.

DLE, a chronic type of rash, is also seen in sun-exposed areas. It may appear in people who have subacute or systemic lupus. In DLE, firm, rough dark patches may be seen with raised rough bumps around hair follicles.

Sores inside the mouth, not unlike canker sores, can also occur in people with lupus. Involvement of the kidneys, joints, linings of the heart and lungs, brain, and blood cells can develop in the internal form of lupus and may occur without any skin symptoms. Just because you experience a sunburn on your face that looks like the butterfly rash does not mean that you have lupus or are at high risk for contracting it.

SCLERODERMA AND DERMATOMYOSITIS

Scleroderma is a rare connective tissue disease in which the skin becomes tense and tight over the entire body, eventually resulting in limited motion.

Dermatomyositis is also an uncommon condition. In this disease, there is weakness of some of the large muscles associated with certain skin findings over the knuckles and eye areas.

RHEUMATOID ARTHRITIS

Rheumatoid arthritis is probably the best-known collagen-vascular disease. The skin of people with chronic rheumatoid arthritis is often pale, translucent, shiny, and thin. This is seen most commonly over the hands and fingers.

Rheumatoid nodules develop in 20 to 30 percent of those with rheumatoid arthritis. These nodules are non-tender firm, fixed, or mobile nodules in the subcutaneous fat, typically found next to bone or cartilage. They occur at the elbow, but they also may be found on the backs of the fingers, the palms, the Achilles tendons, or on the hips. Patients with rheumatoid arthritis may develop red palms as well.

In general, skin signs of internal disease often show up after the internal problem is otherwise easily diagnosed. On the other hand, your dermatologist is always on the lookout for signs of internal problems that should be brought to the attention of your internist or gynecologist. There are many, many other skin clues, such as rare tumors, that can be a sign of internal problems. Ask your doctor if you have any concerns.

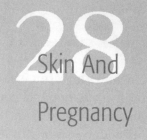

28 Skin And Pregnancy

Enormous changes occur in a woman's body during pregnancy, and the skin is not exempt. These changes range from the hardly noticeable right through to the uncomfortable and even the serious. But every new mother who holds her healthy baby would probably say all the physical travails are worth it; in addition, most skin changes return to normal by the time the new baby is learning to crawl.

▪ CHANGES IN COLOR

HYPERPIGMENTATION

The darkening of the skin known as hyperpigmentation is one of the most common skin changes that occurs during pregnancy. It usually affects only areas of skin that already have a great deal of pigment, such as the nipples and the areola that surrounds the nipples, the armpits, and the genital area.

Fully 90 percent of all pregnant women experience some pigment changes in these areas. This applies to women of all races and skin types. In rare instances, skin may darken all over the body. Such widespread hyperpigmentation may be the result of a specific hormonal problem, so check with your doctor if you notice this happening.

It is thought that hyperpigmentation is common in pregnancy because estrogen and maybe even progesterone stimulate pigment production by the melanocytes. Since birth control pills contain some of these hormones, women taking oral contraceptives may also experience some degree of hyperpigmentation.

THE LINEA NIGRA

The linea nigra is a dark line of skin that develops from the pubic area to the lower chest area, bisecting the abdomen externally, as the backbone might be said to bisect the back internally. From the Latin meaning "dark line," the linea nigra in almost all cases vanishes soon after the baby has been delivered.

MELASMA

Three out of four pregnant women develop a skin condition called melasma. Known also as chloasma or the "mask of pregnancy," melasma affects the cheeks primarily but can occur on the forehead, upper lips, and chin. The skin in these areas darkens and takes on a masklike quality. While the actual cause of melasma has yet to be determined, it's clear that its occurrence has a great deal to do with hormonal fluctuations. Women who are not pregnant but who are taking birth control pills may also have to cope with melasma, which is additional proof that levels of estrogen and progesterone in the blood have a great effect on the skin.

If you have an olive-toned complexion, you are more likely to develop melasma during a pregnancy. If your melasma is very noticeable, you may want to try a bleaching cream to minimize it. Although it is considered safe to use during pregnancy, my rule of thumb is don't try to rock the boat in the middle of the storm. After pregnancy, the stimulating causes of melasma will subside and any therapy you start will be easier. This rule certainly applies to Retin-A, which might be helpful in the management of melasma but in my opinion should not be used during pregnancy.

Most pregnant women are perfectly happy to forgo anything that might endanger their pregnancy or their baby when it comes to the appearance of their skin.

MINIMIZING MELASMA

- Use sunscreen. Ultraviolet radiation will make the pigmentation worse.
- Start with hydrocortisone cream 1% applied twice a day. It is safe to use on the face.
- Discuss with your doctor a regimen that includes Retin-A and/or hydroquinone 4%. Several brands are available, including some that have sunscreen. (Note: some people are sensitive to hydroquinone bleaching cream. Do a test spot on your inner arm for three or four days to make sure you don't develop a rash.)

Follow your regimen for at least two months before expecting to see results.

It's afterward that the concern begins. Once your baby is born, and you're living through those exhausting first months and years, you can begin to worry about what to do about your hard-earned mask of pregnancy. If you're nursing, you may or may not want to apply Retin-A, even though this is probably a low-risk choice in terms of how the topical application will affect your breast milk.

The bad news is that melasma can linger for months or years after it first develops. While no specific treatment can cure melasma, topical regimens can be helpful. A few patients do respond to the ruby laser. The success rate is generally low, however, and many treatments are needed. Moreover, the people in whom melasma is the biggest problem—that is, those with darker skin—run additional risks of side effects with the ruby laser because it can lead to the loss of underlying normal skin pigment making the previously dark area appear blotchy and irregular.

▪ STRETCH MARKS

Stretch marks, known officially as *striae gravidarum*, occur during pregnancy due to the slow but steady stretching of the skin's elastin fibers. Usually they become noticeable only during the third trimester, though some pregnant women notice them almost right away. Stretch marks occur most frequently on the breasts, abdomen, hips, and buttocks. It's estimated that almost 90 percent of pregnant women will have stretch marks.

Darkly pigmented women will notice the stretch mark gradually fade to a lighter and lighter shade, while white women of various ethnicities will notice a pinkish line indicating the beginning of a stretch mark. After childbirth, the skin where a stretch mark has formed will never fully recover to its original appearance; instead, it will always remain somewhat thinned out and noticeable—almost like a scar.

Retin-A may be helpful in minimizing stretch marks after the baby is born. Some of my patients also report that topical application of vitamin E helps, and I don't discourage its use. You will also hear, on prepackaged local-television news spots, that lasers cure stretch marks. Lasers can remove the redness, but the redness will often fade on its own. As far as narrowing the width of the stretch marks or thickening the thinned skin, the verdict isn't in yet. Remember, not all medical "breakthroughs" reported in the media have been confirmed scientifically. In general, when it comes to medicine, what applies in the rest of life holds as well: If it sounds too good to be true, it probably isn't true.

Whatever you decide to do, I advise waiting until after your healthy baby is born and you've stopped breast-feeding.

▪ BLOOD VESSELS

Pregnancy can wreak as much havoc on your outer skin as it can on your blood vessels. This is inevitable because as your circulatory system adapts to meet the needs of two instead of one, your blood vessels have to expand rapidly. (It's a bit like expanding the household overnight.) Major side effects of this great blood vessel expansion are varicose veins and spider nevi.

VARICOSE VEINS

Many women who have never had varicose veins develop them during pregnancy, due to the rapid and necessary growth of blood vessels and the increased fluid volume their bodies are carrying. Women who have suffered varicose veins already may find them worsening with each pregnancy. Varicose or dilated veins usually appear in the legs and can be superficial or deep.

Varicose veins may look like slightly raised blue lines or wavy red lines. Sometimes they are closely grouped in what is called a star-burst pattern. While these are superficial veins, they will likely persist after pregnancy.

The treatment of choice for superficial varicose veins is called sclerotherapy (see chapter 17, "Veins or Vanity") though laser is an option that is pursued more frequently. Results to date are not as predictable as with sclerotherapy.

SPIDER VEINS

Spider veins can appear anywhere on the body, but they are most common on the arms, neck, and face. Most vanish within two months after delivery, but about 25 percent persist. For those that don't resolve after pregnancy (give it some time), laser treatment is now an excellent option. A fair number of patients come for treatment and tell me that the particular red spot they are concerned about came up during pregnancy three years earlier and has not resolved. Women are usually satisfied with this treatment, even though it often takes two or more laser sessions to completely eliminate the growth.

HEMANGIOMAS

Hemangiomas are tightly packed balls of tiny blood vessels that form bright red bumps, usually dome-shaped and no bigger than the tip of a lead pencil. Although they are quite red, they do not bleed. A pregnant women may develop anywhere from a few to a hundred hemangiomas, and these may grow bigger during the pregnancy. Most of them vanish after birth of the baby, but if they persist they can be removed by laser therapy or can be cauterized.

RED PALMS

The red palms of pregnancy (palmar erythema) affect more than 60 percent of white pregnant women. Only 35 percent of black women experience the condition. Palms may be pinkish or bright red, sometimes accompanied by a blue tinge. By the third trimester, the color of the palms is more pronounced. This condition is not related to pigmentation changes, as commonly thought, but rather is caused by changes in blood flow through the blood vessels. Palms return to normal once the baby is born.

▪ SKIN GLANDS

The stimulation of both sweat and oil glands goes way up when you're pregnant. You can guess what happens. You sweat more, and if you are prone to acne, you may break out more. The only treatment that is considered safe for acne flares during pregnancy is topical erythromycin.

Eccrine, or sweat glands, are needed to regulate the body's temperature. Particularly in the last trimester of pregnancy, eccrine activity increases dramatically. This may be why women who give birth in the winter can walk around comfortably in only a sweater, and why we pity the expectant mother who's due in August as she sweats and sweats. Sweating a lot may be uncomfortable in summer months, but it is not dangerous. One side effect of this increase in sweat production is that a pregnant women may develop *miliaria*, which are minute whiteheads on the skin triggered by the plugging of sweat glands.

Sebaceous glands, or oil glands, also increase their activity during pregnancy, once again particularly in the last trimester. In addition, a specific group of glands on the skin of the breasts enlarge during the first few months of pregnancy and almost always form small bumps in the nipple area.

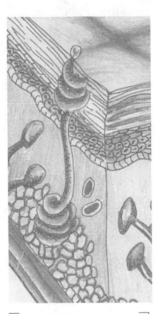

• CHANGES IN HAIR AND NAILS

Not only does pregnancy affect every layer of the skin, it also affects your hair and nails.

HAIR

Hair goes through many changes when you're pregnant—some good, some not so good.

Sweat glands
embedded in skin

Women who say their hair feels thicker during pregnancy are not exactly right, but they're close. The number of hairs that are actually growing at any given time increases during pregnancy, due to hormonal changes. In addition, the hair sheds less. So, it's not true that the hair becomes thicker, there is simply more of it, giving it a thicker, more luxurious texture. This phase of hair growth is called anagen and continues throughout pregnancy. Then the next phase in the hair growth cycle, telogen, begins, and the reverse situation occurs, as the postpartum woman begins to shed more than she ever has before. In this phase of the hair growth cycle, hairs are in a resting pattern. Thus, as the anagen hairs fall out, they are not replaced. The thinning of hair after pregnancy is called *telogen effluvium*. It usually lasts for a couple of months as the natural growing and resting cycle of hair growth re-regulates itself.

In a small number of women, thinner hair may be a permanent effect of pregnancy. Until recently, there was not a lot to be done for such hair loss. Now, however, Rogaine, the brand name for minoxidil, is available over-the-counter and has been proven to stimulate modest hair growth. Wait until you are finished breast-feeding before using any elective medication.

Hirsutism, also known as excess body hair, can develop when a woman isn't pregnant, but the increase in and fluctuation of estrogen and other hormonal levels during pregnancy can contribute to it. Usually, the increase in hair growth is mild.

NAILS

The increase in hormone production during pregnancy stimulates nail growth, and during the last months of pregnancy, nails grow particularly quickly. In addition to an increased growth rate, pregnancy may affect your nails in a number of other ways.

The irregular production of keratin during pregnancy (sometimes there's more and other times less) causes nail ridges. *Transverse grooving* refers to the new horizontal lines or furrows you may notice running across the width of your nails. *Distal onycholysis* is the splitting that may occur at the tips of your nails, resulting in V-shaped nicks. Dead skin may also develop underneath your nails during pregnancy in a condition called *subungual hyperkeratosis*.

Nail problems are difficult for dermatologists to treat at any time. Unless problems with your nails during pregnancy are particularly bothersome, they're best left alone until after the baby is born.

OF MOLES, WARTS, SKIN TAGS, COLD SORES, ET AL.

Many preexisting skin conditions may worsen during pregnancy. *Cold sores or fever blisters* are caused by the herpes virus, which most often breaks out on the lips. During pregnancy, however, herpes virus infection may occur in other areas of the body if it was previously contracted there.

A prime example is genital herpes, which can extend to the anal area. If you experience an outbreak of genital herpes near the time of your due date, your doctor will likely schedule you for a Cesarean-section delivery.

Moles, or nevi, tend to increase in size during pregnancy and can darken in color. New moles may also appear. In most cases, these changes are natural and benign, and the moles will return to their original size and color after childbirth. If you notice, however, that other changes accompany the growth of an existing mole or the appearance of a new mole, such as redness around the area or a raised appearance, consult your physician. (See chapter 22, "Melanoma.")

Freckles and age spots (liver spots) also tend to grow and change color during pregnancy. Once again, these changes are normal and present no danger.

Skin tags can multiply during pregnancy. These occur most frequently on the neck, under the arms, and in the groin area. The theory is that they are spawned by excess friction. My guess is that they are also affected by the increase in a whole host of hormones that have a growth-stimulating effect. People who are overweight tend to have more skin tags than those of normal weight.

While skin tags may be annoying, they are harmless. If they remain after you give birth, they can be easily removed by your dermatologist by lifting them with a forceps and snipping the small stalk that attaches them to the skin. This procedure is so quick that local anesthetic isn't even required in most cases.

Preexisting warts can also grow larger during pregnancy. Whether pregnancy encourages new warts to appear is still not clear. If you have genital warts and they increase significantly in size, a Cesarean delivery will be indicated. Plantar warts—those that appear on the soles—can increase in size and become painful. In this case, there are topical treatments that are safe and effective to use during pregnancy.

▪ SKIN CONDITIONS UNIQUE TO PREGNANCY

DERMATITIS

Certain rashes occur only during pregnancy. Most look like common dermatitis. Many of them mimic acne. Some mimic herpes conditions. Many forms of dermatitis are common only to pregnancy, and most appear as small, itchy, red bumps that are easily treated with topical cortico-steroids. The most common eruption of pregnancy is PUPPP, which is short for Pruritic Urticarial Papules and Plaques of Pregnancy. These bumps, which usually develop in the third trimester, subside within weeks of delivery, but during pregnancy they typically respond well to topical steroids.

Another variety, *autoimmune progesterone dermatitis*, is caused by higher than normal levels of progesterone in the system. It is characterized by acnelike blemishes on the extremities and buttocks.

ITCHING

Itching, or *pruritus gravidarum*, makes you feel itchy everywhere. For pregnant women who experience this mild condition it is usually at its worst during the last trimester. The one plus to pruritus gravidarum is that it is invisible—there is no obvious rash. The itching is thought to be caused by the backup of bile in the bile ducts which can occur during pregnancy.

AN IMMUNIZATION WARNING

If you are thinking of becoming pregnant and know that you have never had rubella, or German measles, your doctor will recommend a rubella vaccination. It's important to be vaccinated, since rubella can cause severe birth defects or miscarriage.

APPENDIXES

Dermatology is a field that lends itself well to intervention, usually in the office. Aside from rashes and
other conditions that are easy to diagnose by looking no
further than the surface of the skin or the history that you
provide, there are many situations in the care and health
of your skin where different procedures may be helpful or
required.

I am a firm believer that *an informed person makes
the best patient.* I routinely see people relax, their blood
pressure drop, and their mood change once they have a
better understanding of the procedure they are having or
are about to have. So in the interest of preparing you for
what to expect, here are some brief descriptions of how
we do things in the dermatology field.

▪ BIOPSIES

SHAVE BIOPSY

The most commonly performed type of biopsy for
skin lesions is called a shave biopsy. This method is used
to diagnose growths that lie in the top surface of skin
(the epidermis) and are usually sticking up above the
surrounding skin surface. For this procedure, a local

anesthetic, typically lidocaine, is used to numb the area.

As the tip of the needle is introduced you'll likely feel a sting. After that, the doctor or nurse will slowly put in enough medication to numb the skin. The effect is usually quite rapid, and people are often surprised at how quickly it works. Some people may require a little more waiting or a higher percent of anesthesia than others.

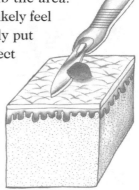

Some patients are sensitive to the epinephrine that is added to the lidocaine to control bleeding and keep the anesthetic in the biopsy site longer. If you get palpitations or otherwise know you have trouble with local anesthetics, be sure to tell your doctor directly.

New topical anesthetic creams (EMLA, ELA-Max, and Topicaine) may help to reduce the pain of injection or avoid the need for a needle if the growth is superficial.

> **Shave Biopsy**
>
> All types of skin growths can be sampled in this easy method, which is performed with local anesthesia.

A shave biopsy may be performed by the deft use of a scalpel. However, it is also common to use one side of a sterilized double-edge razor. The razor, honed to approximately one-millionth of an inch at the edge, is of great aid in the hands of an experienced dermatologist.

There will be a small amount of oozing after the biopsy, and the doctor will usually apply a liquid that will stop the bleeding. This usually contains aluminum chloride, the active ingredient in a styptic pen. For approximately one week following biopsy, you need to keep the area moist with a topical antibiotic ointment or petroleum jelly. The area typically heals quite well. Don't let a scab form, since that may delay final healing and result in a worse cosmetic result. Remember that after any biopsy the skin may stay red for some time, even after healing of the surface has finished. This will resolve itself with time, but it may take many months.

PUNCH BIOPSY

When a dermatologic condition appears deeper in the skin than just the accessible top layer, such as a rash, the cells that we need to see under the microscope are typically in the dermis, or middle layer of the skin. In this case, a punch biopsy is performed.

A punch is simply a small, round, cookie cutter–like instrument that can core out a small piece of skin. This piece is typically smaller in diameter than a pencil eraser. The area is anesthetized with lidocaine. The skin is stretched around the area so that after inserting the circular punch and removing a small piece of skin, the skin will relax into an oval instead of a circle. This oval is then typically closed with one or two stitches; these are removed one to two weeks later or, if reasonable, allowed to heal on its own. A wound the size of a pencil eraser will heal up into a small white or flesh colored scar about 2 millimeters in diameter.

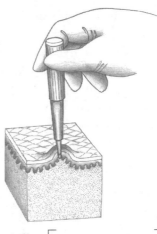

Punch biopsy method

SNIP BIOPSY

A snip biopsy is often performed on growths that have narrow bases and wide tops. This is commonly seen with skin tags, which hang in the armpits or around the eyes, or some warts. In this instance, it is often possible to take a pair of sharp scissors and snip off the lesion without the need for anesthetic. Do not try this yourself!

EXCISIONAL BIOPSY

In an excisional biopsy, a scalpel is used to cut out a full-thickness piece of skin for examination. This is a specimen that extends from the epidermis down to the fat and is shaped like a small football. This procedure is commonly done when the disease process is presumed to extend or be situated in the deep fat. It may also be done when a growth is highly suspected of being a melanoma.

This biopsy method is performed in the same way as any excision. The area is numbed, the design marked, and the area draped with sterile towels after cleansing. After the specimen is removed and set aside to be sent to pathology, preparation begins to close the wound. In order to make sure no puckers of skin result at either edge of the wound, the excess cone of skin at either end is removed. Very often, people are surprised at how long a suture line is after a small growth is removed. The extra wound length results from removal of these puckers. In general, a scar will be about three times the diameter of the specimen that was removed.

Once the excision is made, the wound is stitched either with a combination of dissolving deep sutures and superficial sutures, or dissolving sutures alone. If used, the superficial stitches are usually removed five to seven days later.

After that the skin is well on its way to healing. Infection of facial skin is rare, as is bleeding, but if the site should become hot, red, or painful after surgery call your doctor.

▪ SCRAPING AND BURNING

This is an indelicate way to refer to the common procedure of electrodessication and curettage, employed to remove superficial benign and malignant tumors of the skin. This effective method is often used for benign lesions, such as warts and seborrheic keratoses, or for certain types of basal cell and squamous cell cancers. In this technique, the skin is anesthetized as for a shave or punch biopsy. Then a sharp, round-ended instrument known as a curette is used to scrape the surface of the lesion. The cells within these benign and malignant tumors do not attach effectively to the normal skin surrounding them; therefore the curette will easily remove the abnormal cells while leaving the normal skin intact. The treated area usually oozes a small amount of blood, and the bleeding is stopped with cauterization by a small electric needle.

After an electric needle is passed over the skin and stops the bleeding, a second or third round of curetting may be done to treat small basal and squamous cell cancers. There are, however, many cases of basal cell and squamous cell cancer for which electrodessication and curettage is not appropriate; your dermatologist will know when this procedure should or should not be done. Depending on the depth of curettage, healing will take anywhere from one to four or more weeks. The area is kept moist with an ointment and washed daily in the shower. The resulting appearance will range from near normal skin (if the curettage was superficial) to a smooth white scar (if the curettage went relatively deep into the dermis).

▪ CRYOSURGERY

Cryosurgery refers to the application of cold to destroy certain lesions on the skin. The most common agent used in dermatology is liquid nitrogen, which forms at −196.8 degrees Celsius (−320 degrees Fahrenheit). The application of this incredibly cold liquid is very useful in the practice of dermatology. We most commonly use it to eliminate superficial scaly lesions such as warts, seborrheic keratoses, and the precancerous actinic keratoses. Cryosurgery also helps to remove age spots that form as a result of years of exposure to the sun.

The liquid nitrogen may be applied through a spray apparatus under pressure or on the end of a cotton-tipped applicator. No anesthesia is required for this procedure. For example, a small actinic keratosis on the face would merely be sprayed with liquid nitrogen for several seconds. A small "iceball" would form, the area turning bright white. This fades within a matter of seconds, and the area becomes red and slightly swollen. The scaly keratosis typically peels off within one to two weeks, and the underlying area heals smoothly. Possible side effects of liquid nitrogen therapy include scarring, if the physician sprays an area too hard, and a lighter color of pigmentation. The latter is especially notable in patients with very dark skin, because the pigment-producing melanocytes are the cells most sensitive to damage by cold.

In the past, physicians used to perform what were called "cryopeels" in which dry ice (solid carbon dioxide) was dipped into acetone and spread over the face to cause a superficial chemical peel. This was once used for the treatment of acne but is very uncommon today.

▪ ACNE SURGERY

To extract the common lesions of acne in a physician's office, a special instrument known as a comedone extractor (*comedone* is the medical term for blackheads) is used. One at a time, the contents of the blackheads and whiteheads—a combination of dead skin, skin oils, and bacteria—are extracted. For the whiteheads, we sometimes have to make a small prick in the top of the whitehead, but this should cause no discomfort.

The same procedure is also used to remove *milia*, which are merely very tiny cysts that look like smooth white pearls. They commonly occur under the eyes or in areas where a scar has occurred, as after laser resurfacing. It is a safe procedure and can be done by virtually any dermatologist. Facialists, also called aestheticians, also remove whiteheads and blackheads in some states.

▪ INJECTION OF MEDICATION INTO THE SKIN

It is often helpful to inject corticosteroid medication directly into a skin lesion. The most common form of the medication injected is triamcinolone acetonide. The triamcinolone has many anti-inflammatory properties that are of great benefit in certain skin conditions. It is used to treat keloids (tumors of scar tissue), prurigo nodularis (nodules that can occur in some people from repeated scratching), alopecia areata (a form of hair loss due to immune system overactivity), and other slightly raised scars that are not yet flat.

Intralesional steroid injection is also helpful for some of those acutely inflamed tender cysts that may appear on the face during an acne flare. In this case, I prefer a very low concentration. This low concentration is still enough to get rid of the nodule or cyst, but will help prevent the risk of skin thinning or indentation of the skin that could be permanent.

▪ QUICK TESTS FOR FAST ANSWERS

Occasionally we want to determine whether or not there is blood present in a certain skin lesion. In a procedure called diascopy, we press a glass slide against the growth. If the redness in the area goes away, it means all the redness was within blood vessels. If the redness remains, it means that a small amount of blood has leaked into the skin.

The dermatologist may perform certain microscopic procedures in the office. If a fungal infection is suspected, a KOH preparation can be done. To perform this, a scaly area on the skin is moistened with an alcohol pad, then a scalpel blade or microscope slide is scraped across the skin sideways and the scaly skin is scraped onto a microscope slide. While you wait, the slide is treated with a certain liquid that highlights the fungus under the microscope to confirm the diagnosis.

Viral infections, such as those that cause cold sores or the kind that cause chicken pox or shingles, may be confirmed by poking open one of the blisters and taking some of the skin cells from the base of the blister to study under the microscope. This is called a Tzanck smear.

ablation The process by which tissue is surgically destroyed, as in removing a wart or other benign skin growth.

abrasion The loss of surface skin tissue (epidermis) due mainly to scrapes.

acne An inflammatory disease involving the hair follicles and sebaceous glands and causing a variety of skin eruptions or pimples, usually on the face, neck, shoulders, and/or upper back; the most common variety is called acne vulgaris.

actinic Related to the sun.

actinic keratosis Pink or red raised and rough papules that arise in groups or alone on sun-damaged skin; precancerous.

acupuncture A traditional form of Chinese medicine or medical therapy and anesthesia, using fine needles to puncture the skin at specific acupressure points along the meridians of the body.

adrenal glands Glands that secrete hormones such as cortisal. There are two adrenal glands. One sits above each kidney.

albinism   An inherited genetic condition in which an individual is unable to form melanin, the pigment that gives skin its color, resulting in unpigmented skin, hair, and eyes.

allergic reaction   A hypersensitive reaction in which histamine is released from mast cells, causing inflammation, redness, hives, and in severe cases, breathing problems.

alopecia areata   A disease characterized by the appearance of well-defined, round, or oval bald patches on the head and on other parts of the body. The condition usually reverses itself but may require treatment.

alopecia totalis   A condition that involves the loss of all scalp hair.

anagen   The growth phase of the hair growth cycle.

androgenetic or male pattern alopecia   A common form of baldness in men, beginning in the forehead area and spreading gradually until a fringe of hair remains at the temples and around the back of the head. A similar hair loss pattern may develop in women after menopause.

arrector pili   The muscle attached to the hair follicle, which allows the hair to respond to fluctuations in temperature and other stimuli via contraction or expansion; causes goose bumps.

arteriovenous anastomosis   A connection between an artery and a vein, either because of a congenital anomaly or because of a surgically produced link between vessels that allows blood to bypass a capillary bed.

autograft   The surgical transplantation of tissue from one part of the body to another part of the body on the same individual, as in hair transplantation.

axillary   Of or relating to the armpit, or axilla, the pyramid-shaped space forming the underside of the shoulder where the upper arm joins the chest.

bacillus   Any spore-producing, rod-shaped strain of bacteria in the family Bacillaceae.

basal cell cancer   A malignant growth of cancerous cells that may erode, crust, or bleed and that can penetrate the deeper layers of the skin (a.k.a. basal cell carcinoma); destructive locally but does not metastasize or travel in the bloodstream.

basal   When pertaining to the skin, the deepest layer of the epidermis (a.k.a. the stratum basale).

benzoyl peroxide   An agent found in common acne medications.

biopsy   A surgical procedure that involves the removal of a small amount of body tissue, which is then examined to determine or establish a medical diagnosis and/or estimate a prognosis.

blanche   To make pale by applying pressure.

bubo   The origin of the name bubonic plague. A bubo (buboes, plural) is an inflamed and enlarged lymph node that appears in the axilla (armpit) or groin region. In addition to bubonic plague, it may also indicate such diseases as chancroid or syphilis.

bulla   A blister filled with fluid. A bulla is a large vesicle.

carcinogen   Any substance that causes cancer.

clindamycin hydrochloride   An antibiotic frequently used as a topical gel for the treatment of acne.

collagen   A vital protein consisting of tiny interwoven fibers. In skin, collagen constitutes most of the dermis and gives this second layer of the skin its strength. Other types of collagen make up tendons, ligaments, and skin.

comedone   A hair follicle that has been clogged with dried sebaceous and keratinous material.

condylomata acuminata   An infectious wart caused by the human papilloma virus and found in genital areas.

connective tissue   The connective tissue supports and binds other body tissue and body parts together. It is composed largely of collagen.

contact dermatitis   A skin rash resulting from an allergic compound to which an individual has been exposed. Poison ivy or poison sumac are classic examples of contact dermatitis.

corpuscle   Usually refers to a red or white blood cell.

cortex   The term is used to refer to the outer layer of any body organ or any other structure. We usually associate it with the brain, but in matters of skin and hair, it refers to the middle layer of the hair shaft, which is housed between the medulla and the cuticle, the inner and outer layers of the hair shaft.

corticosteroid   Any of the natural or synthetic hormones produced in the adrenal cortex, which can be used to control inflammation. Used very commonly as a medication in dermatology.

corynebacterium acnes   Bacterium of the skin found in acne lesions.

cosmetics   Any product applied to the skin for purposes of beautification.

cosmetic surgery   The alteration of skin or underlying tissue for purposes of beautification.

cutaneous   Of or pertaining to the skin.

cuticle   The thin edge of tissue at the base of a nail; also the sheath of a hair follicle.

cutis   The skin.

cystic acne   A severe form of acne distinguished by large cysts and eventual scarring.

demodex folliculorum   A mite that lives in the hair follicles of the face and nose.

dermabrasion   A treatment to remove scars or wrinkles with diamond fraize, revolving wire brushes, or sandpaper; largely supplanted by newer technology such as laser.

dermal   Pertaining to the second layer of the skin.

dermatitis   An inflammatory skin condition that is manifested by redness, irritation, and even blisters. Dermatitis may result from an allergen, disease, or infection.

dermatoglyphics   The ridge patterns on the fingers, palms of the hands, toes, and soles of the feet. The patterns are used for purposes of identification and have some diagnostic value because certain patterns are associated with chromosomal disorders.

dermatologist   A medical doctor who specializes in skin disorders.

dermatology   The study of the anatomy, physiology, and pathology of the skin, as well as the diagnosis and treatment of skin disorders.

dermis   The second layer of the skin, found right beneath the epidermis. It contains blood and lymphatic vessels, hair follicles, nerves, and glands.

eccrine glands   Sweat glands that help regulate body temperature by secreting water to the skin's surface which then evaporates.

eschar   Crusted dead skin produced at the site of injury to the skin.

eczema   A skin inflammation that causes itching, scales, and redness.

epidermis   The outer or surface layer of the skin.

erythroderma   Abnormal redness of the skin.

erythromycin   An antibiotic used frequently when a person is allergic to penicillin.

eumelanin   A form of melanin that produces a brown or black color in the skin, hair, and eyes.

fibroblast   A flat, elongated cell within the dermis that produces collagen fibers and contributes to the formation of the dermis and scar tissue.

fibroma   A benign tumor made of fibrous connective tissue.

flat warts   Multiple warts (occurring in groups of up to 100) found on the face, neck, backs of the hands, forearms, and knees. They are flat and flesh colored and are more common in children.

flexural psoriasis   Psoriasis occurring over the joints.

frostbite   Frozen skin and underlying tissues due to extremely low temperatures. In severe cases, tissue damage can be permanent.

granulomatous   A term used to describe inflamed skin tissue (usually red and grainy in appearance) that often accompanies certain infection.

guttate psoriasis   A form of psoriasis characterized by small, distinct "teardrop" patches of red, scaly skin.

hair follicle   The structure that produces a hair.

herpes simplex infection   A skin infection caused by the herpes simplex virus. The type I herpes virus is usually associated with outbreaks of cold sores on the lips and around the mouth area. The type II virus is associated with genital herpes. All outbreaks are characterized by small clusters of blisters.

hyperpigmentation   Pigmentation producing darker than usual skin.

hypertrichosis   Excessive hair growth.

hypertrophic scarring   Scarring caused by the excessive formation of new tissue during wound healing. Hypertrophic scars are hard and raised; different from keloids, which are actual tumors of scar tissue.

impetigo   A contagious skin infection caused by staphylococcal bacteria, exhibiting small pustules that can cluster quickly into large blisters.

integument   The skin.

keloid   A tumor of scar tissue at the site of a wound or a surgical incision.

keratin   A protein that is the prominent constituent of the skin, hair, and nails.

Langerhans cell   A cell in the epidermis that mediates immune function in the skin, helping to direct the removal or destruction of germs and other foreign substances that penetrate the surface of the skin.

lentigo   Flat, tan, or brown spot on the skin that results from stimulation of pigmentation by the sun.

lesion   Used in dermatology to refer to a wound, sore, blister, or other form of tissue damage caused by injury or disease.

lunula   The small, pale crescent at the root of the nail.

macule   A flat spot on the skin; may range from white to dark brown or even black.

medulla   When used in dermatology, the central core of a strand of hair.

Meissner's corpuscles   The egg-shaped nerve receptors located between the dermis and epidermis that inform the brain precisely where the skin is being touched.

melanin   The dark pigment of the hair, skin, and eyes.

melanocyte   A cell that synthesizes melanin.

minoxidil   A vasodilating drug that was originally developed to treat high blood pressure but also causes hair growth in cases of male pattern baldness. The brand name is Rogaine.

mites   Tiny, eight-legged members (including ticks) of the Acarina family that suck blood from animals and humans.

nevus   Same as mole; a pigmented lesion that may be smooth or rough, raised or flat, regularly shaped or irregularly shaped, colored or absent of color. Normal moles do not require attention; see your dermatologist promptly if you notice a change in a mole.

PABA   Abbreviation for para-aminobenzoic acid, a compound in some sunscreen products which absorbs ultraviolet radiation, preventing damage to the skin. Notable because many people are allergic to this chemical and should avoid it.

pacinian corpuscles   Quick-acting, onion-shaped nerve receptors in the dermis that provide instantaneous information about movement.

papillary layer   The upper layer of the dermis, where the dermis meets the epidermis and exhibits papillae, the microscopic protrusions that reach into the epidermis.

phaeomelanin   A form of melanin responsible for red hair.

pigment   A natural or fabricated substance that gives color to the skin.

pilar   Having to do with the hair.

pityriasis   A common skin condition usually found on the face and characterized by small, flat lesions resembling scaly dandruff.

pityrosporum ovale   A yeastlike fungus that normally lives in the skin of the face and scalp.

plantar wart   A wart located on the sole of the foot. It is caused by the common wart virus.

prurigo   General term for itching skin conditions.

psoriasis   A chronic, inheritable skin disorder characterized by red patches covered by thick, dry, silvery scales. These patches usually appear on the scalp, elbows, and knees. Ears and genitalia may also be affected.

purpura   Bruising; results from any hemorrhage of skin.

Raynaud's syndrome   Intermittent episodes of vasoconstriction in the extremities causing blanching in the fingertips or toes, sometimes followed by blue or red discoloration.

ringworm   A skin infection caused by fungi and resulting in circular, itchy, and scaling patches on the skin (a.k.a. tinea).

rubella   A short-lived, highly contagious viral infection that causes a skin rash similar to that of measles. It is most dangerous to pregnant women (a.k.a. German measles).

rubeola   The medical term for measles, a viral condition causing red eruptions all over the skin. The rash is often accompanied by fever and swelling of the mucous membranes.

scabies   A contagious disease caused by *Sarcoptes scabiei*, the itch mite. It is characterized by an itchy, irritating rash caused when the female mites burrow into the outer layers of the skin to lay their eggs. Secondary bacterial infections may also occur after the first infection.

scleroderma   Autoimmune disease affecting the connective tissue and the blood vessels that causes the thickening and hardening of the connective tissue of the skin and other organs.

sclerosis   Hardening (of the skin).

sebaceous glands   Located in the dermis throughout the body, these glands are especially abundant in the scalp, face, mouth, internal ear, and anus. There is a single duct in each gland that opens onto the surface of the skin through which sebum is secreted in the oils of the gland. Sebum can be responsible for clogging pores and resultant outbreaks of acne.

seborrhea   Excess sebum (oil) production by the skin.

subcutis   The fatty layer of skin beneath the dermis.

systemic   Refers to medications taken orally or through injection so that they affect the entire body. The term also applies to illnesses that affect the entire body.

terminal hair   Visible pigmented hair, such as the hair that grows from the scalp; also called mature hair.

telangiectasia   Small, dilated blood vessels usually seen on the face; also known as broken blood vessels.

topical medication   Drugs applied to the skin's surface.

urticaria   Hives or raised white or red patches of skin.

varicella   A contagious disease of childhood (a.k.a. chicken pox) caused by the varicella-zoster virus resulting in red, itchy, pimple-like eruptions on the skin accompanied by fever. The same virus also causes shingles. Many pediatricians now recommend children receive the chicken pox immunization.

vellus   The lightly pigmented, almost invisible hair that covers the fetus (a.k.a. lanugo).

verruca   A wart.

vesicle   A blister less than 1 centimeter in diameter.

vitiligo   White patches on the skin caused by the absence of melanocytes.

xerosis   Dry skin.

Yersinia pestis   The species of bacteria responsible for bubonic plague.

Zostrix   An ointment used to ease the pain of shingles. All blisters must have disappeared before the ointment can be used. The active ingredient in Zostrix is capsaicin, which is derived from the same red peppers used to make chili powder.

Zyderm   The brand name for injectable bovine collagen used to improve the appearance of fine lines, wrinkles, lips.

With all that the environment sends to bombard our skin, it's amazing we aren't bothered more frequently by injuries of one kind or another. With just a little information, you'll be able to determine what is a real emergency and which problem will get better on its own. No one wants to sit in an emergency room for hours on end unless absolutely necessary.

▪ BRUISES AND ABRASIONS

Bruises (or contusions) are caused by blows that do not break the skin. The blow breaks the blood vessels in and beneath the skin, however, which causes the bruising. Most bruises require no medical treatment and disappear within a day or two of the injury, though severe bruises can cause pain and might warrant medical attention.

Frequent or prolonged bruising should alert you to see your doctor. Problems with your blood such as abnormal platelets or clotting factors can be responsible. Many older patients take blood thinners such as Coumadin to prevent stroke or heart attack, and increased bruising can happen in this situation because of the decreased blood clotting.

To alleviate pain and reduce swelling, an ice pack wrapped in a thin, soft cloth may be applied to the area. Ice and ice packs should never be applied directly to the skin. Alternatively, a package of frozen vegetables, such as peas, which is soft and can mold to the bruised site is helpful.

If a blow or blows and the resultant bruise(s) seem particularly severe, internal bleeding may have occurred. If you think there is a possibility of internal bleeding, especially when the bruise is over your flank or abdomen and the trauma is substantial, seek medical attention immediately. If numbness or lack of function result, check it out quickly, because a severe blow may cause a broken bone as well.

Spontaneous bruising with no apparent cause may be indicative of a serious illness. If you notice bruises on your skin and can't remember a bump, bang, or blow causing them, you should contact your doctor. (See chapter 27, "Your Skin is a Window to Your Health.")

Abrasions occur when the skin has been scraped. They may or may not bleed. Often a welt may appear where the skin was scraped, or a burning sensation may accompany the abrasion.

Abrasions should be washed with tepid tap water and gentle soap. Sand, dirt, or any small particles should be removed from the scrape. You should then apply an antibiotic ointment. In general the skin defends itself well against invaders. The advantage of using topical antibiotics is that the ointment base helps stimulate regrowth of the epidermis, which has been sheared off. Finally, bandage the area with a nonstick dressing. This is preferable to a piece of gauze since the fibers may stick to the wound.

If heavy bleeding accompanies a severe scrape, it should be treated as a puncture wound. (See "Cuts and Wounds," p. 379).

▪ BURNS

Regardless of the emotional implications of an old cliché, it's certainly true that no one gets through life without getting literally burned. From that hot pot on the stove to scalding water out of the tap or the chemical we used without remembering to don protective gloves, potential burn sources lurk everywhere in our environment. And of course the sun, which nourishes life, can be a burn danger to our skin.

There are three levels of burns: first degree (confined to the epidermis), second degree (involving the dermis), and third degree, in which the complete skin layers have been damaged. The latter situation is actually painless because the nerves in the skin have been destroyed. The first two degrees can be quite painful since the nerve endings reside just where the thermal injury has occurred.

Symptoms of burns include swelling, redness, pain, and peeling skin. In the case of second-degree burns, blistering may occur. If third-degree burning has occurred, the skin may turn white. It may also become blackened and charred.

MINOR BURNS

If the skin on a minor burn has not been broken, let cool water run over the area or immerse it in cool water for about five minutes. While doing so remain calm. Next apply a bland emollient cream such as Eucerin or an ointment such as Aquaphor. Aloe vera gel may be soothing but it's best to use a thicker ointment. If the skin is broken, consult your doctor regarding how to avoid infection.

A sterile dressing, one that does not apply pressure, should be applied to the burn. This dressing should be changed frequently, checking the burn for swelling and infection as you do so. An over-the-counter analgesic may be used for pain.

Although you could probably manage small second-degree burns at home, I recommend seeing a doctor if you think you have a burn that is more than first degree.

MAJOR BURNS

If you believe a burn is major (second or third degree), covering a large surface area, check the person's airway and call EMS immediately. Keep the patient as calm as possible while waiting and check breathing and circulation frequently. Remove restrictive clothing and jewelry. If any fabric is stuck to the burned area, cut it away with a scissors to avoid tearing away burned skin. Watch for signs of shock. These include cold, clammy, or bluish skin, dizziness, rapid heartbeat, and a dazed expression. Cover the person with a blanket to avoid chills.

All third-degree burns should be treated by a doctor on an emergency basis.

CHEMICAL BURNS

Chemical burns can be caused by either acidic or alkaline chemicals. Symptoms of chemical burns are similar to those for heat burns and include swelling, redness, and sometimes blistering and peeling.

Thorough washing with clean tap water is the immediate treatment recommended for acidic chemical burns. Alkaline burns should be kept dry initially, as moisture can cause further burning. Instead, brush the area with a cloth (not your hand). Remove all clothing that may contain traces of the chemical. Once the chemical has been brushed away from the area, water may be applied in the same manner as for acidic burns.

In either case the area should be washed with cool tap water for about a half an hour. If a burning sensation still remains in the area, continue to flood the burn with water. EMS should be called if the burn is extensive or if the patient is in shock. If the person has inhaled the chemical, EMS should be called immediately.

ELECTRICAL BURNS

Since the body is mainly water and water conducts electricity, even the smallest amounts of electrical current can cause electric burns. Most of the damage caused by an electrical burn affects tissues beneath the surface of the skin. Don't let an electrical burn that looks insignificant fool you. It could be serious. Electrical burns should be treated in the same way heat burns are treated, but in all cases, consult a doctor since internal injury is always a possibility with an electrical burn. The most severe electrical burn causes electrocution, which can cause cardiac and respiratory arrest. If you suspect someone has been electrocuted and think he or she may still be in contact with the electrical current, *do not touch the person*—call EMS immediately.

▪ CUTS AND WOUNDS

As great a defender as our skin is, there are those sharp objects for which it is no match—from the prick of a thorn to a knife wound, the skin can be punctured. A puncture wound may be either penetrating or perforating.

A puncture wound perforates the skin. These are small perforating wounds from common household objects that barely penetrate the surface

STAUNCHING THE FLOW

Bleeding is an impressive phenomenon. There always appears to be more blood at a skin injury than there is. Fortunately, the healthy body is designed to stop bleeding with a range of strategies: blood vessels constrict, platelets plug up holes, and the clotting cascade just rolls on.

In some cases it helps to slow or stop bleeding until help can be obtained. Because so many people are on aspirin now for its cardiac benefits, we all ooze a little more. Aspirin's effect lasts for ten days while that of non-aspirin painkillers like Advil last only about three hours.

There is little superficial bleeding that cannot be stopped with firm pressure. Follow these steps:

1. After identifying the *exact* source of bleeding, apply pressure to the bleeding area firmly but not so pain is caused.
2. Hold pressure for *ten minutes by the clock.* Most people vastly underestimate what ten minutes is, especially when they are eager to look and see if they've stopped the bleeding. Distract yourself by counting the seconds along with the clock but don't take pressure off before it's time.

of the skin. Then there are bigger puncture wounds, such as those that result from bullets. Those perforating wounds bleed internally as well as externally. Items that cause perforating wounds of the skin include knives, bullets, nails, shattered glass, wood splinters, staples, and straight pins.

When dealing with a puncture wound, first stop the bleeding. You can do this by using a clean pad to apply pressure to the wound. Then secure a bandage with a dressing that's fixed with a strong knot. Do not apply a tourniquet unless you can't control the bleeding by other means. Use tourniquets very cautiously in diabetics.

When the object that caused a penetrating puncture wound remains in the wound, leave it there. In other words, if someone steps on a nail, your efforts to remove the nail may make the situation worse. Instead, take the person to an emergency room and have a medical professional do the job right. In addition, it may be advisable to have a tetanus shot after a penetrating puncture wound. Your doctor will advise you as to whether this precaution is necessary.

Because of our interest in skin health and looking younger, there are thousands of products on the market worldwide devoted to helping us maintain our skin in the best condition possible. Some of these products are medications that are available only by prescription; others are creams, lotions, cleansers, and oils that assist us in our daily skin care. This list is not a comprehensive review of these products. It is not possible to list here all the products that are of excellent quality which help maintain your skin in good health.

For details about medications mentioned in this book but not listed here, see the *Physicians Desk Reference*. The products listed represent some of the products my colleagues and I use in practice. This does not mean that many other excellent products are not available, only that most dermatologists settle on one or two in each class and become comfortable using them. Note that when it comes to cosmetics, any of the brand-name products are of the highest quality and undergo rigorous testing.

Class	Examples	Comments
Acne	Topical: Neutrogena Oil-Absorbing Acne Mask	Good for maintenance, not for acute acne flare.
	Clearasil Adult Care Cream	Active ingredient is sulfur, resorcinol.
	Adapalene*	Retinoid-type compound.
	Benzoyl peroxide*	Alone as 5% gel or in combination with topical erythromycin, this is an effective anti-acne medication.
	Tretinoin*(Retin-A, Renova, Retin-A Micro)	Available in range of concentrations; effective as topical gel or cream for acne and decreasing facial lines and wrinkles due to sun damage.
Bleaching agents	Lustra* Solaquin Forte*	Hydroquinone 4%; compound can be irritating—do a skin test on your forearm before using on face
Cleansers	Basis Facial Cleanser Eucerin Bar Neutrogena Cleansing Bar	Wash your face once a day.
	Nonsoap cleansers: Liquid Neutrogena Facial Cleansing Formula Aquanil Lotion Cetaphil	Excellent for daily facial cleansing.
Corticosteroids* (These differ in strength as topical medications. One example from each group is given.)	**Super-potent:** Temovate cream Diprolene ointment Psorcon ointment	Do not use on face; for limited use only.
	Potent: Topicort cream	
	Medium-potent: Cutivate	As directed by your physician.

*denotes prescription item

Class	Examples	Comments
	Mild: Aclovate cream	May be used for prolonged periods and on the face
	Mild, over-the-counter: Hydrocortisone cream 1%	Excellent to have handy for mild irritations of the skin; if no response after a few days of use, call your dermatologist.
Cosmetics	**Foundations:** *Oily skin:* Oil-control makeup (Almay) *Normal skin:* Extra Protection Liquid Makeup (Almay) Active Protection Makeup (Max Factor) *Dry skin:* All-In-One Makeup (Coty)	Avoid these ingredients that can cause pimples (comedogenic): linseed oil, oleic acid, butyl stearate, isopropyl myristate, cocoa butter, olive oil, sesame oil, peanut oil. Where possible select makeup that has sunscreen in it.
	Foundation for Skin Irregularities: Soft Finish Compact Makeup (Estee Lauder) Workout Makeup (Clinique)	
	Opaque Cover Cosmetics: Dermablend (Dermablend) Covermark (Lydia O'Leary)	To cover irregularities in pigmentation.
Herpes	**Topical:** Denavir*	Topical must be applied at first sign of cold sore outbreak.
	Oral: Famvir* Valtrex*	Oral medication may be used for prevention in severe, chronic situations.
Moisturizers and Emollients	Neutrogena Rainbath Moisture Rich Shower and Bath Gel Nivea Moisturizing Bath and Body Oil	It is best to moisturize the skin while it is still moist from a shower or bath; this helps lock in the moisture your skin needs that might otherwise evaporate off.

*denotes prescription item

Class	Examples	Comments
Moisturizers and Emollients	Products containing 20% urea or alpha-hydroxy acid—too numerous to list	Many brands available; excellent compounds.
	Acid Mantle Skin Acidifier (Doak)	For slightly irritated skin.
	AmLactin 12% LacHydrin 12%*	Contains lactic acid, a very effective moisturizer; may sting at first.
	Complex 15 Eucerin Cream	Excellent routine moisturizers; as with all creams, do not apply in excess.
Self-Tanning	Clarins products Clinique products Estee Lauder products Melasyn	All of these are patient recommendations.
Sun protection	Choose between sunSCREEN and sunBLOCK	Look for SPF greater than 15; broad spectrum rating—protects against UVA and UVB rays; waterproof. Apply every two hours
	Sunscreen See page 99	Avoid products with para-aminobenzoic acid (PABA)
	Sunblock Neutrogena Chemical Free See also page 99	Usually contains micronized titanium dioxide or similar compounds that reflect the sun's rays off the skin.
	Protective clothing: Sun Precautions 1-800-882-7860 www.sunprecautions.com http://www.sunprotective clothing.com/ http://www.solareclipse.com/	 1-800-353-8778 1-800-878-9600

*denotes prescription item

T his list provides the names, addresses, and contact information for some organizations devoted to common and more specific skin problems. Some organizations are committed to research in particular areas, others represent patient advocacy groups. Still others are, or include, patient and family support groups.

Condition or Disease	Organization	Comments
General information about skin disease; dermatologist referral	American Academy of Dermatology 980 North Meacham Road Schaumburg, IL 60173-4965 847-330-0230; Fax 847-330-0050 www.aad.org	National organization to which most board-certified dermatologists in the country, and many in the world, belong
AIDS	American Foundation—AIDS 120 Wall Street, 13th Floor New York, NY 10005-3902 212-806-1600	Premier private sponsors of AIDS research and support
AIDS in children	Pediatric AIDS Foundation 1311 Colorado Avenue Santa Monica, CA 90404 310-395-9051; Fax 310-314-1469	

Condition or Disease	Organization	Comments
Albinism and Hypopigmentation	National Organization for Albinism and Hypopigmentation 1530 Locust Street, # 29 Philadelphia, PA 19102-4415 215-545-2322 or 800-473-2310 e-mail: noah@albinism.org www.albinism.org	Information and patient support
Alopecia areata	National Alopecia Areata Foundation P.O. Box 150760 San Rafael, CA 94915-0760 415-456-4644 Fax 415-456-4274 e-mail: naaf@compuserve.com www.naaf.org	Excellent literature
Behçet's syndrome	American Behçet's Foundation, Inc. P.O. Box 54063 Minneapolis, MN 55454-0063 800-723-4238 or 800-7BEHCETS	Provides information about this painful chronic condition
Cancer, skin; melanoma	Skin Cancer Foundation 245 Fifth Avenue, Suite 2402 New York, NY 10016 212-725-5176; Fax 212-725-5751	Active patient education program; excellent brochures and newsletters; supports research
	American Skin Association Incorporated 150 East 58th Street, Floor # 33 New York, NY 10155-0002 212-753-8260	Patient education
Cancer	American Cancer Society 1599 Clifton Road, NE Atlanta, GA 30329 800-227-2345 or 404-320-3333;	Committed to public education and funding research on all types of cancer.

Condition or Disease	Organization	Comments
Cancer, skin; Mohs micrographic surgery	American College of Mohs Micrographic Surgery and Cutaneous Oncology 930 North Meacham Road Schaumburg, IL 60173 847-330-9830; Fax 847-330-1135 www.mohscollege.org	Official organization for Mohs micrographic surgeons who have completed thorough training in the specialty
Cancer	National Cancer Institute Office of Communication National Institute for Health 9000 Rockville Pike, #2a 33 Bethesda, MD 20892 301-496-0549 or 800-4-CANCER; Fax 301-402-0043	National resource for information about all forms of cancer
Cosmetic surgery, skin surgery, skin cancer	American Society for Dermatologic Surgery 930 North Meacham Road Schaumburg, IL 60173 847 330-9830; Fax 847-330-1135	Information about facial rejuvenation and a variety of other dermatologic procedures
Cosmetic surgery	Plastic Surgery Association 4150 Regents Park Row # 260 La Jolla, CA 92037-1417 619-550-9697	Supports research projects that advance all areas of plastic surgery.
Dermatitis herpetiformis	Gluten Intolerance Group of North America (Dermatitis Herpetiformis) 15110 10th Avenue Seattle, WA 98166 206-246-6652 Fax 206-246-6531	This skin condition is affected by diet. In part, this organization provides up-to-date information on dietary and other resources for patients.
Eczema	National Eczema Association 1221 SW Yamhill, Suite 303 Portland, OR 97205-2110 503-228-4430	Resources for patients and families with eczema.

Condition or Disease	Organization	Comments
Epidermolysis bullosa	National Epidermolysis Bullosa Registry Clinical Coordinating Center University of North Carolina Dept. of Dermatology, Room 137–NCMH Chapel Hill, NC 27514 919-966-3321	Registry of patients with this disease; database helps understand genetics of the disease
Hair loss	International Society of Hair Restoration Surgery 930 North Meacham Road Schaumburg, IL 60173-6016 847-330-9830; Fax 847-330-1135	Information and referrals about hair transplantation
Herpes	National Herpes Hotline 919-361-8488 National Herpes Resource Center American Social Health Association P.O. Box 13827 Research Triangle Park, NC 27709 919-361-8400; Fax 919-361-8425	Information about current treatment for cold sores and genital herpes
Ichthyosis	National Registry for Ichthyosis and Related Disorders Dept. of Dermatology, Box 356524 University of Washington Seattle, WA 98195-6524 e-mail: geoff@u.washington.edu; 800-595-1265	Registry of patients for this genetic disease in which epidermis is affected
Lupus	Lupus Foundation of America, Inc. 1300 Picard Drive, Suite 200 Rockville, MD 20850-4303 301-670-9292 or 800-558-0121; www.lupus.org	Information about lupus, including the skin type

Condition or Disease	Organization	Comments
Neurofibromatosis	National Neurofibromatosis Foundation 95 Pine Street, 16th Floor New York, NY 10005 800-323-7983 or 212-344-6633 www.nf.org	Information about neurofibromatosis, a genetic skin disorder
Nevus; congenital moles	Congenital Nevus Support Group 2585 Treehouse Drive Lake Ridge, VA 22192 405-377-3403	Devoted to support of patients, parents, and families
Papilloma virus	Human Papillomavirus Support Program American Social Health Association P.O. Box 13827 Research Triangle Park, NC 27709 800-227-8922	Addresses concerns about genital warts
Pediculosis (lice)	National Pediculosis Association P.O. Box 610189 Newton, MA 02461 781-449-6487; Fax 781-449-8129 www.headlice.org	Information
Pemphigus vulgaris	National Pemphigus Vulgaris Foundation 1098 Euclid Avenue Berkeley, CA 94709 510-527-4970	Research and patient information.
Psoriasis	National Psoriasis Foundation 6600 SW 92nd, Suite 300 Portland, OR 97223 503-244-7404 or 800-723-9166; Fax 503-245-0626 e-mail: getinfo@npfusa.org www.psoriasis.org	Supports research and patient and family education

Condition or Disease	Organization	Comments
Psoriasis	Psoriasis Society of Canada P.O. Box 25015 Halifax, NS B3M 4H4 Canada 1-800-656-4494 902-443-8680; Fax 902-457-1664 e-mail: info@psoriasissociety.org www.psoriasissociety.org	Supports research and patient and family education
Rosacea	National Rosacea Society 800 South Northwest Highway, Suite 200 Barrington, IL 60010 800-NO-BLUSH e-mail: rosacea@aol.com www.rosacea.org	Provides patient information and resource materials
Sarcoidosis	Sarcoidosis Family Aid and Medical Research Foundation 460 Central Avenue East Orange, NJ 07018 201-399-3644 or 800-203-6429	Research and support for this condition, which occurs in the skin and internally.
Scleroderma	Scleroderma Federation 89 Newbury Street, Suite 201 Danvers, MA 01923 800-722-HOPE 978-750-4499; Fax 978-750-9902 www.scleroderma.org	Information, research funding, and patient and family support
	United Scleroderma Foundation 734 East Lake Avenue Watsonville, CA 95076-3566 831-728-2202; Fax 831-426-1083	
Shingles; varicella zoster	VZV Research Foundation 40 East 72nd Street New York, NY 10021 800-472-8478; Fax 212-861-7033	Research support

Condition or Disease	Organization	Comments
Sturge-Weber syndrome	The Sturge-Weber Foundation P.O. Box 418 Mt. Freedom, NJ 07970-0418 973-895-4445; Fax 973-895-4846 www.sturge-weber.com	Patient and family information for this condition which includes facial port wine stain, visual problems, and other symptoms
Vitiligo and pigment disorders	National Vitiligo Foundation 611 South Fleishel Avenue Tyler, TX 75701 903-531-0074; Fax 903-525-1234 e-mail: vitiligo@trimofran.org www.nvfi.org	Research support and patient information

The information explosion requires us to be more selective about the information we read and the sources of information we rely on when it comes to our health. Technical articles on skin problems can now be accessed through the Internet or at any medical school, health center, hospital library, or public library.

Reliable sources of internet-based information include the following websites:

American Academy of Dermatology
www.aad.org

This national organization represents more than eight thousand practicing dermatologists. Educational materials and physician referrals are available.

American Society for Dermatologic Surgery
www.asds-net.org

This organization includes members with a special interest in dermatologic surgery, laser surgery, and cosmetic dermatologic surgery.

American Academy of Cosmetic Surgery
www.cosmeticsurgery.org

This organization includes a range of specialists who

have a common interest and proficiency in different aspects of cosmetic surgery. Information about board-certified general plastic surgeons can be found at the website of the American Society of Plastic and Reconstructive Surgeons (see below).

American Society of Plastic and Reconstructive Surgeons
www.asprs.org

While plastic surgery is a technique practiced by a wide range of specialists with different medical training backgrounds, this organization represents physicians who have completed at least a two-year residency in general plastic surgery.

CenterWatch
www.centerwatch.com

This site provides information about clinical trials. Clinical research into new medications, procedures, and devices is an active aspect of dermatology. You can find information here about studies in which you might be eligible to participate.

DermGuide
www.dermguide.com

This search engine devoted to dermatology will quickly help you find out about a topic of concern.

Dr. David J. Leffell is Professor of Dermatology, Plastic Surgery, and Otolaryngology at the Yale School of Medicine and Chief of Dermatologic and Laser Surgery at Yale-New Haven Hospital. He was educated at Yale, McGill, Cornell, and the University of Michigan and is board certified in internal medicine and dermatology. He conducts a broad range of clinical research, publishing extensively in the areas of aging skin, skin cancer, and new biotechnologies in skin health. He is on the editorial boards of several dermatology journals and on the board of directors of national dermatology organizations. Dr. Leffell is also Associate Dean for Clinical Affairs at the Yale School of Medicine. He lives in New Haven with his wife and two children, where he practices dermatology.